W9-ABJ-332

DATE DUE

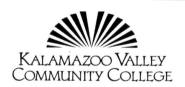

HEINERMAN'S
ENCYCLOPEDIA OF

NATURE'S
VITAMINS
— and —
MINERALS

JOHN HEINERMAN, PH.D

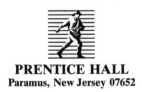

PRENTICE HALL
Paramus, New Jersey 07652

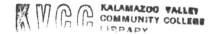

Library of Congress Cataloging-in-Publication Data

Heinerman, John
  [Encyclopedia of nature's vitamins and minerals]
  Dr. Heinerman's encyclopedia of nature's vitamins and minerals /
John Heinerman
    p. cm.
  Includes index.
  ISBN 0-13-258500-6 (PPC). —ISBN 0-13-258492-1 (Cloth)
  1. Vitamins in human nutrition—Encyclopedias. 2. Minerals in
human nutrition—Encyclopedias. 3. Dietary supplements—Encyclopedias. I. Title.
QP771.H362 1997
613.2'86—dc21   97-25868
                                            CIP

Printed in the United States of America

10 9 8 7 6 5 4 3 2 1   10 9 8 7 6 5 4 3 2

ISBN 0-13-258500-6 (PPC)   ISBN 0-13-258492-1 (Cloth)

ATTENTION: CORPORATIONS AND SCHOOLS

Prentice Hall books are available at quantity discounts with bulk purchase for educational, business, or sales promotional use. For information, please write to: Prentice Hall Special Sales, 240 Frisch Court, Paramus, New Jersey 07652. Please supply: title of book, ISBN, quantity, how the book will be used, date needed.

PRENTICE HALL
Paramus, NJ 07652

A Simon & Schuster Company

On the World Wide Web at http://www.phdirect.com

Prentice Hall International (UK) Limited, *London*
Prentice Hall of Australia Pty. Limited, *Sydney*
Prentice Hall Canada, Inc., *Toronto*
Prentice Hall Hispanoamericana, S.A., *Mexico*
Prentice Hall of India Private Limited, *New Delhi*
Prentice Hall of Japan, Inc., *Tokyo*
Simon & Schuster Asia Pte. Ltd., *Singapore*
Editora Prentice Hall do Brasil, Ltda., *Rio de Janeiro*

Author's Foreword

The world we live in is quite imperfect. Everybody knows and pretty much agrees with that fact. Because it's imperfect, things go wrong much of the time. When this happens stressful situations are created that have a severe negative impact on the health of individuals. We constantly interact with each other from positions of strength and weakness. But being the mere mortals that we are, the weaker features show through more often than the strengths do. (Why do you think that noble aspect in each of us is always referred to as "the strong *silent* type"?)

When a large number of individuals from varying backgrounds intermingle for very long, their faults tend to show. When this happens, tension is created. As a consequence, the human body itself becomes irritated. The "ripple effect of stress," as I like to call it, originates in mortal frailties and slowly gathers speed and size as it rolls through social exchanges between people. By the time it reaches our own shores, it has enough momentum to even make a subconscious impact at a cellular level.

As that particular wave of mental or emotional discontent effortlessly glides back out into that ocean of humanity's mistakes, another type of reaction is instantly triggered within our cell nuclei. A molecular disturbance is evident (though we can't feel it on the physical plane right away) that seriously disrupts the finely synchronized "ebb and flow" of energy that constantly circulates within our beings. Outside stress, regardless of its source, produces electrical interferences within the body's delicate and intricate workings.

The necessary restoration of harmony comes about in several ways. The first and most obvious, of course, is to remove self from the source of stress. The next most logical thing would be some simple spiritual exercise such as meditation, prayer, or imaging in order to bring calmness back to the soul again. After this come dietary measures in which *nutritious* foods and beverages are consumed so that the organic system may be properly nourished.

This is the stage where my book comes into play. The nutrients contained within the substances ingested are what help to rebuild the temporal parts of our "stressed out" beings. It is those life-giving vitamins and energizing minerals that reanimate our bodies and make them feel well and whole again. Disease is nothing more or less than a prolonged state of molecular disturbance and electrical interference within the human biological system. And wellness, when it finally is achieved, is the removal of that atomized static that chemically irritates everything within, from tiny cells to major organs.

The many different vitamins and minerals mentioned within these pages work in specific ways to help restore biological tranquillity to the body. These nutrients assist the body in reconnecting itself so that the natural rhythmic patterns of energy return to their normal "ebb and flow."

This book plows new ground in several directions, both for my own titles as well as for more conventional works by other authors. So as not to be too wordy, I've synthesized some of the major advantages below for you to check (✓) out.

✓ It's the largest and most thorough health encyclopedia I've ever written.

✓ The "easy-to-find" layout style is patterned after my juice book.

✓ About *twice* the nutrients are covered here as in similar references.

✓ It contains the *most complete* section on Vitamin B Complex found anywhere.

✓ Little-known features about Vitamin C are mentioned.

✓ Vitamin E is approached in a way you *never* expected.

✓ It includes the *only* data you'll ever find on Vitamins F, K, L, P, and U.

✓ Like some clever and witty writing? Then check out Vitamin T.

✓ 26 trace elements are covered—the *most* ever included in a book of this type.

✓ Microminerals you never knew about are here: Cobalt and Tin.

✓ It covers Hydrogen, Oxygen, and Nitrogen—trace elements that *no one* else covers.

✓ The benefits of Chlorine are discussed here.

✓ Learn a lot about the mountain men, fur trappers, and frontier scouts under Iron.

✓ Iodine is for more than just thyroid; read about it in the mineral section.

✓ "Get the Lead out" safely and efficiently with my recommendations.

✓ You need *twice* the Magnesium over Calcium and this book explains *why*.

✓ Improve your mental health and emotions with Manganese-rich foods suggested by me.

✓ A wonderful nutritional discovery is made in China and discussed under Molybdenum.

✓ I show you how to acquire that *competitive edge* in all you do under Phosphorus.

✓ Reduce stroke risk when you read what I have to say in the Potassium entry.

✓ Find out from my book how drug-resistant bacteria can be conquered with Selenium.

✓ Feeling stiff? Then loosen up with my Silicon suggestions.

✓ Let me show you some tricks on controlling your *prehistoric* Sodium gene.

✓ Discover within my pages the many nutritional purposes for Sulphur.

✓ Become better informed on the role Vanadium plays in hypoglycemia and diabetes.

✓ Enter the intriguing world of Zinc and be prepared for some amazing things.

This book is all about *you helping yourself.* I'll tell you which foods are good sources for every vitamin and mineral mentioned by me. I also cite reliable nutritional products made by honest manufacturers that can be trusted for their wholesome goodness, and inform you how much should be taken of each. Plus, I back up what I say with ample scientific references.

But the best part is that I do all of this in a way that both educates and entertains. This is a book that will hold your interest, even fascinate you many times, and certainly will make for a lot of compelling reading. In a word, it informs with a writing style that is personable and very enlightening. I hope this volume will remain among your most prized possessions for many years to come!

Your Friend, John Heinerman (Summer 1997)

Dedication

To John A. and Leah D. Widtsoe,
pioneers in good health and nutrition.

Contents

Section One: Vitamins

Section Two: Minerals

Health Situations and Their Nutritional Solutions

ACNE (SEE ALSO SKIN PROBLEMS)
Vitamin F 175, Silver 331, Sulphur 346, Zinc 355

AIDS (SEE ALSO IMMUNE SYSTEM DYSFUNCTIONS)
Fluorine 256, Selenium 317, Zinc 550

ALCOHOLISM
Vitamin B-1 19, Vitamin B-3 25, Vitamin B-5 30, Vitamin C 100, Vitamin D 154, Calcium 223, Chromium 246, Magnesium 296

ALLERGIES
Vitamin B-5, 30, Vitamin C 100, Vitamin F 175, Molybdenum 307

ALZHEIMER'S DISEASE
Choline/Lecithin 11, Vitamin B_T 93, Vitamin P 191, Fluorine 256

ANEMIA
Vitamin B-2 23, Vitamin B-6 37, Vitamin B-12 67, Chromium 246, Cobalt 249

ANGINA
Vitamin B_T 93, Vitamin E 159, Magnesium 296, Silicon 326

ANGIOMA
Vitamin C 100

ANGULAR STOMATITIS
Vitamin B-6 37

ANKYLOSING SPONDYLITIS
Vitamin C 100

ANOREXIA (SEE ALSO EATING DISORDERS)

Biotin 54

ANTISOCIAL BEHAVIOR (SEE ALSO DELINQUENCY, MENTAL DISORDERS)

Vitamin C 100

ARRHYTHMIAS

Vitamin B-1 19, Vitamin B-Complex 9, Vitamin B$_T$ 93, Copper 250, Selenium 317, Silicon 326

ARTERIOSCLEROSIS

Vitamin B-6 37, Vitamin B-9 56, Chromium 246, Lead 280, Sulphur 346

ARTHRITIS (SEE ALSO RHEUMATOID ARTHRITIS)

Vitamin D 154, Copper 250, Fluorine 256, Sulphur 346

ASTHMA

Vitamin B-6 37, Vitamin C 100, Vitamin F 175, Calcium 223, Fluorine 256, Magnesium 296, Molybdenum 307

ATHEROSCLEROSIS

Vitamin A 1, Vitamin B-3 25, Vitamin C 100, Vitamin E 159, Magnesium 296

ATHLETE WEAKNESS (SEE ALSO CHRONIC FATIGUE SYNDROME, FATIGUE)

Vitamin B-5 30, Vitamin B-15 79, Iron 269, Phosphorus 311, Potassium 314

ATTENTION DEFICIT DISORDER

Vitamin B-1 19, Vitamin B-5 30, Vitamin B-6 37

AUTISM

Vitamin B-6 37, Magnesium 296

BACK PAIN

Sulphur 346

BACTERIAL OVERGROWTH

Vitamin E 159, Selenium 317

BALDNESS

Vitamin F 175, Sulphur 346

B-COMPLEX DEFICIENCY SYNDROME

Vitamin B-5 30

BERIBERI

Vitamin B-Complex 9

BIRTH DEFECTS (SEE ALSO GENETIC DEFECTS)

Inositol 14, Vitamin B-9 56, Vitamin B-2 23, Vitamin C 100, Lead 280

BLEEDING GUMS

Vitamin P 191

BLINDNESS

Zinc 355

BLOOD CARAMELIZATION

Sulphur 346

BLOOD CLOTS

Vitamin B-6 37, Vitamin F 175, Vitamin K 184, Vitamin P 191, Calcium 223, Oxygen 366, Selenium 317

BONE FRACTURES/BONE LOSS

Biotin 54, Vitamin D 154, Vitamin K 184, Boron 217, Cobalt 249, Calcium 223, Copper 250, Fluorine 256, Lead 280, Magnesium 296, Phosphorus 311, Potassium 314, Silicon 326, Zinc 355

BRAIN DYSFUNCTION (SEE ALSO MENTAL DISORDERS)

Choline 11, Vitamin B-6 37, Copper 250, Lead 280, Magnesium 296, Manganese 303, Oxygen 366

BREAST-FEEDING DIFFICULTIES

Vitamin B-6 37

BRITTLE NAILS (SEE ALSO SPOTTED NAILS/STRETCH MARKS)
Biotin 54, Sulphur 346

BROKEN BONES (SEE ALSO BONE FRACTURES/BONE LOSS)
Vitamin D 154, Calcium 223, Fluorine 256, Zinc 355

BRUISING
Vitamin P 191

BURNS
Vitamin A 1, Vitamin C 100, Vitamin E 159, Selenium 317, Oxygen 366, Zinc 355, Silver 331

BURSITIS (SEE ALSO ARTHRITIS)
Sulphur 346

CAFFEINE ADDICTION
Vitamin B-12 67

CANCER
Vitamin A 1, Vitamin B-3 25, Vitamin B-9 56, Vitamin C 100, Vitamin E 159, Niacin 25, Vitamin B-12 67, Vitamin B-17 83, Vitamin K 184, Vitamin P 191, Boron 217, Calcium 223, Chlorine 243, Copper 250, Selenium 317, Fluorine 256, Germanium 261, Iodine 264, Magnesium 296, Molybdenum 307, Nitrogen 366, Potassium 314, Selenium 317, Sulphur 346, Tin 352, Zinc 355

CARAMELIZATION (SEE BLOOD CARAMELIZATION)

CARDIAC FAILURE (SEE ALSO MYOCARDIAL INFARCTION, CARDIOVASCULAR DISEASE, HEART DISEASE)
Vitamin B-1 19

CARDIOVASCULAR DISEASE (SEE ALSO HEART DISEASE)
Vitamin A 1, Vitamin B-5 30, Copper 250, Zinc 355, Magnesium 296, Selenium 317

DETOXIFICATION

Vitamin B-3 25, Vitamin C 100, Hydrogen 361, Molybdenum 307, Silicon 326

DIABETES

Vitamin A 1, Inositol 14, Vitamin D 154, Vitamin E 159, Vitamin P 191, Chromium 246, Magnesium 296, Oxygen 366, Sulphur 346, Tin 352, Vanadium 354

DIARRHEA

Vitamin A 1, Vitamin C 100, Vitamin F 175, Magnesium 296, Silver 331, Sulphur 346

DIGESTIVE DISORDERS

Chlorine 243, Magnesium 296

DIZZINESS

Vitamin B-2 23

DRUG ADDICTION

Vitamin A 1, Vitamin B-6 37, Vitamin C 100, Vitamin D 154, Vitamin E 159

DRUG RESISTANT BACTERIA

Zinc 355

DYSLEXIA

Vitamin F 175

EATING DISORDERS

Zinc 355

ECZEMA

Vitamin B-6 37, Vitamin F 175, Silicon 326, Sulphur 346

EDEMA

Vitamin B-1 19, Vitamin B-6 37

FATIGUE (SEE ALSO CHRONIC FATIGUE SYNDROME)

Vitamin C 100, Vitamin B-12 67, Vitamin E 159, Calcium 223, Chromium 246, Iodine 264, Iron 269, Magnesium 296, Manganese 303, Biotin 54, Nitrogen 366, Phosphorus 311, Sulphur 346, Zinc 355

FEVER

Nitrogen 366

FIBROCYSTIC BREAST

Iodine 264

FREE RADICAL CELL DESTRUCTION

Vitamin A 1, Vitamin C 100, Vitamin E 159, Vitamin P 191, Copper 250, Manganese 303, Selenium 317, Zinc 355

FEVER BLISTERS (SEE COLD SORES)

FUNGAL INFECTION

Vitamin B-5 30, Iodine 264

GALACTOSEMIA

Vitamin P 191

GALL STONES

Vitamin F 175

GANGRENE

Vitamin C 100, Oxygen 366

GENETIC DEFECTS

Zinc 355

GIARDIASIS

Sulphur 346

GLANDULAR PROBLEMS

Vitamin B-2 23, Biotin 54, Vitamin F 175, Vitamin P 191, Iodine 264, Nitrogen 366, Selenium 317

GLOSSITIS

Vitamin B-6 37, Biotin 54

GLUTEN ENTEROPATHY

Vitamin E 159

GOITER

Iodine 264

GUM DISEASE

Sulphur 346

HEART DISEASE

Vitamin B-3 25, Vitamin B-6 37, Vitamin B-15 79, Vitamin B$_T$ 93, Vitamin C 100, Vitamin D 154, Vitamin E 159, Vitamin F 175, Vitamin P 191, Calcium 223, Hydrogen 361, Magnesium 296, Potassium 314

HEAT STROKE/HEAT EXHAUSTION

PABA 18, Vitamin C 100

HEAVY MENSTRUATION

Vitamin P 191

HEMORRHAGING

Vitamin C 100, Vitamin K 184, Calcium 223

HEMORRHOIDS

Vitamin P 191

HEPATITIS

Vitamin C 100, Vitamin K 184

HERNIA

Vitamin E 159

HERPES SIMPLEX/HERPES ZOSTER

Vitamin D 154, Vitamin P 191, Silver 331

INFERTILITY (SEE ALSO CRIPPLED SEXUALITY)

Vitamin B$_T$ 93, Vitamin C 100, Boron 217, Lead 280, Selenium 317, Zinc 355

INFLAMMATION

Vitamin E 159, Vitamin F 175, Vitamin P 191, Calcium 223, Copper 250, Magnesium 296, Selenium 317, Silver 331

INFLAMMATORY BOWEL DISEASE

Vitamin D 154, Magnesium 296

INFLUENZA (SEE ALSO COMMON COLD)

Vitamin A 1, Vitamin P 191, Zinc 355

INSECT BITES/STINGS

Vitamin B-12 67, Silver 331, Sulphur 346

INSOMNIA

Vitamin B-3 25, Vitamin B-Complex 9, Vitamin B-12 67

INTESTINAL MALABSORPTION SYNDROME

Vitamin D 154

INTESTINAL PARASITES

Sulphur 346

INTOXICATION

Calcium 223

JOINT/TENDON INFLAMMATION/WEAKNESS

Chlorine 243, Copper 250, Fluorine 256, Silicon 326, Sulphur 346

KIDNEY DISEASE

Vitamin B-6 37, Vitamin B$_T$ 93, Lead 280, Magnesium 296

KIDNEY FAILURE

Vitamin B-1 19, Vitamin B-6 37, Fluorine 256, Hydrogen 361

Premenstrual Syndrome (PMS)

Vitamin B-6 37, Vitamin E·159, Calcium 223, Magnesium 296, Zinc 355

Prickly Heat

Vitamin C 100

Pruritis

Sulphur 346

Psoriasis (see also Skin Problems)

Vitamin D 154, Vitamin F 175, Vitamin P 191, Sulphur 346

Psychosis (see Mental Disorders)

Radiation Poisoning

Calcium 223, Magnesium 296

Rash (see also Skin Problems)

Chlorine 243

Respiratory Distress Syndrome (see also Infection, Viral Infection)

Vitamin C 100, Vitamin E 159, Selenium 317, Oxygen 366, Nitrogen 366, Zinc 355

Restless Legs Syndrome

Vitamin F 175, Magnesium 296

Reye's Syndrome

Vitamin B_T 93

Rheumatoid Arthritis (see also Arthritis, Joint/Tendon Inflammation/Weakness)

Vitamin B-3 25, Vitamin C 100, Vitamin F 175, Vitamin P 191, Selenium 317, Sulphur 346

Rickets

Vitamin D 154, Calcium 223

SCHIZOPHRENIA (SEE ALSO MENTAL DISORDERS)

Vitamin B-1 19, Vitamin B-6 37, Vitamin B-9 56, Vitamin B-12 67, Vitamin C 100, Manganese 303, Magnesium 396

SCLERODERMAL BOWEL DISEASE (SEE ALSO INFLAMMATORY DOWEL DISEASE)

Vitamin E 159

SCURVY

Vitamin C 100

SEBORRHEIC DERMATITIS (DANDRUFF)

Vitamin B-6 37

SECONDHAND SMOKE INHALATION (SEE ALSO SMOKING)

Vitamin B-5 30, Vitamin B-6 37, Vitamin B-9 56

SEIZURES

Vitamin B-6 37, Manganese 303

SENILITY (SEE ALSO MEMORY FAILURE)

Vitamin B-1 19, Vitamin B-3 25, Vitamin B-12 67, Vitamin B_T 93, Vitamin P 191

SENSORY DYSFUNCTIONS

Zinc 355

SEPSIS (SEE ALSO INFECTION)

Vitamin C 100, Selenium 317

SEXUAL NON-PERFORMANCE (SEE ALSO CRIPPLED SEXUALITY)

Vitamin C 100, Vitamin E 159, Vitamin B_T 93, Vitamin A 1, Zinc 355, Calcium 223, Iron 269, Potassium 314, Phosphorus 311, Choline (lecithin) 11, Vitamin B-6 37

SHINGLES

Vitamin C 100

SHORT BOWEL SYNDROME

Vitamin E 159

SICKLE CELL ANEMIA

Vitamin B-9 56

SKELETAL MUSCLE WEAKNESS (SEE ALSO MUSCLE TISSUE WEAKNESS)

Vitamin B_T, 93

SKIN PROBLEMS

Vitamin A 1, PABA 18, Vitamin B-2 23, Vitamin B-5 30, Biotin 54, Vitamin D 154, Vitamin F 175, Vitamin P 191, Calcium 223, Fluorine 256, Silicon 326, Silver 331, Sulphur 346

SMOKING (SEE ALSO SECONDHAND SMOKE INHALATION)

Vitamin B-5 30, Vitamin B-6 37, Vitamin B-9 56

SNAKEBITE

Sulphur 346, Zinc 355

SPOTTED NAILS/STRETCH MARKS

Vitamin C 100, Zinc 355

SPRUE

Vitamin E 159

STOMACH UPSET

Vitamin A 1

STRESS

Vitamin P 191, Chromium 246, Magnesium 296

STROKES

Vitamin B-6 37, Vitamin C 100, Vitamin E 159, Vitamin F 175, Vitamin P 191, Oxygen 366, Potassium 314

STUNTED GROWTH

Vitamin B-6 37, Vitamin F 175, Calcium 223, Cobalt 249, Nitrogen 366

SUN DAMAGE

Silver 331, Sulphur 346, Zinc 355

TARDIVE DYSKINESIA

Choline (lecithin) 11, Vitamin B-6 37, Vitamin E 159

TENDONITIS (SEE ALSO JOINT/TENDON INFLAMMATION/WEAKNESS)

TOOTH DECAY

Vitamin A 1, Vitamin D 154, Calcium 223, Chlorine 243, Fluorine 256, Tin 352

TETANUS (SEE ALSO INFECTION)

Vitamin C 100

THERMOREGULATION DYSFUNCTION (SEE ALSO OVERWEIGHT)

Vitamin C 100

TOOTHACHE

Sulphur 346

THROAT CANCER (SEE ALSO CANCER)

Vitamin B-6 37

THROMBOSIS (SEE ALSO BLOOD CLOTS)

Vitamin C 100, Vitamin K 184

TUBERCULOSIS (SEE ALSO VIRAL INFECTION)

Vitamin D 154

UNCONTROLLABLE CRYING

Zinc 355

UNDERWEIGHT

Vitamin A 1, Vitamin F 175

VARICOSE VEINS

Vitamin F 175, Vitamin P 191

VASCULAR PROBLEMS (SEE ALSO CIRCULATORY PROBLEMS)
Vitamin C 100, Vitamin F 175, Vitamin P 191

VIRAL INFECTIONS (SEE ALSO INFECTIONS)
Selenium 317, Vitamin E 159, Silver 331

VISION PROBLEMS (SEE ALSO BLINDNESS, CATARACTS, MACULAR DEGENERATION, NIGHT BLINDNESS)
Vitamin A 1, Vitamin B-2 23

VITAMIN B-12 DEFICIENCY
Vitamin B-9 56, Vitamin B-12 67

VITILIGO
Vitamin B-3 25

VOMITING (SEE ALSO STOMACH UPSET)
Biotin 54

WATER RETENTION
Vitamin B-6 37, Sodium 337

WOUNDS
Vitamin B-5 30, Nitrogen 366, Silver 331, Sulphur 346

WRINKLES (SEE ALSO SKIN PROBLEMS)
PABA 18, Biotin 54, Sulphur 346

YEAST INFECTION
Vitamin C 100, Vitamin P 191

ZINC INSUFFICIENCY
Zinc 355

ZINC OVERSUFFICIENCY
Zinc 355

Nature's Healing Vitamins

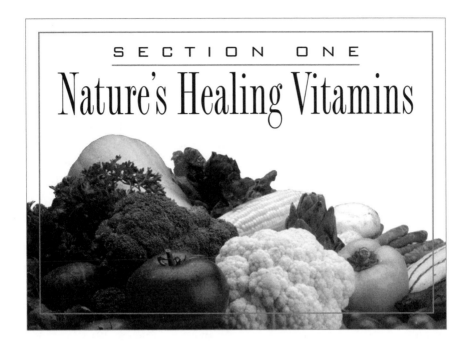

Vitamin A

AN ANTIOXIDANT THAT OFFERS THE BODY BALANCE AND PROTECTION

Vitamin A Precursors

Carotenoids are responsible for the red, yellow, and orange colors given different fruits and vegetables. These plant-synthesized pigments also capture energy from the sun that fuels photosynthesis or plant metabolism. There are well over 600 carotenoids, but only a very small number (probably fewer than 15) have been determined by scientists to be vital in human biology.

Foods rich in beneficial carotenoids include tomatoes, carrots, corn, and orange juice. Tomatoes have a substance called lycopene that makes them red. This is known to combat prostate cancer, according to research published in the *Journal of Nutrition & Cancer*

1

Inst. (87:1767-76, 1995). Carrots contain a great deal of alpha- and beta-carotenes. Both are powerful antioxidants, meaning they help to control the activity of free radicals within the body. Without such carotenes present, these scavenger molecules (lacking an electron) run amok within the body, creating biochemical havoc wherever they venture. Corn and orange juice share two yellow pigments between them known as lutein and zeaxanthin. Both of these are especially helpful in strengthening failing vision. Green plants in general are wonderful sources of carotenoids, although the red, yellow, and orange pigments are masked by chlorophyll.

Special enzymes within the gastrointestinal tract help to catalyze the conversion of some carotenoids to actual vitamin A. About four dozen such carotenoids possess varying degrees of vitamin A or retinol activity. But the one showing the most promise is beta-carotene, of course. In theory, 2 micograms of beta-carotene can supply 1 micogram of retinol. But, in actuality, it's more like 6 micrograms of beta-carotene needed for every 1 microgram of retinol. This is due to incomplete conversion.

Retinol is necessary for the normal functions of the eyes, lungs, and intestines. Low vitamin A intake is known to lead to decreased immune function. But too much of a good thing can be harmful. The liver is capable of storing excess retinol up to a certain point, but beyond that it becomes toxic to the system. I recall during the late 80s and early 90s having considerable discussions on this very issue with Kurt Donsbach, when we both were celebrated speakers for the National Health Federation. Kurt thought nothing of gulping down 200,000 or 300,000 I.U. daily of vitamin A and recommending the same for others. I was much more conservative in my approach and suggested *short-term* intake of 100,000 I.U. during a cold, flu, or bout with infection, and maintenance doses of a mere 25,000 I.U. every *other* day.

The fact remains, though, that excessive intake of vitamin A can cause genetic birth defects, according to a study published in *The New England Journal of Medicine* (333:1369-73, 1995).

Prevents Cancer and Cardiovascular Disease

For many years, scientists believed that beta-carotene was the Number One carotenoid antioxidant. More recently, research has demonstrated that the lycopene found in tomatoes and the alpha-carotene in carrots manifest a great deal more free radical inhibition than beta-carotene does. An intriguing article published in the *Archives of Biochemistry and Biophysiology* some time ago (274:532-38, 1989) demonstrated this in a simulated cellular system, or what is commonly known as the *in vitro* process. Lycopene extracted from ripe tomatoes was found to have *double* the antioxidant capabilities that beta-carotene has.

Carotenoids work at a molecular level to prevent the formation of carcinogens, those nasty chemical compounds that are responsible for tumor growth. Lycopene, alpha-carotene, and beta-carotene sort of "handcuff" those renegade chemicals that like to link up with each other to induce cell mutations. Safely separated from those chemicals, healthy cells continue to behave in the normal fashion of multiplying and dividing. Oxidative cellular damage is eliminated, and with that the prospect of developing cancer.

Cardiovascular disease is the most common type of heart ailment among adults 40 and older. Atherosclerosis, or the progressive hardening and narrowing of heart blood vessels, is the chief cause of this. The process usually begins with injury to the arterial wall. The immune system immediately kicks in and extra white blood cells are produced.

This, in turn, unleashes the production of free radicals. These scavenger molecules damage "bad" cholesterol-rich molecules known as LDLs (low-density lipoproteins). The oxidized LDLs next enter the vessel walls and discharge their fatty contents. Over many years, fatty streaks develop, creating plaque that shuts down much or all of the blood vessel. When this happens, the regular supply of oxygen to the heart and other vital body organs is cut in half or more.

What fruit-and-vegetable-based carotenoids do is to prevent such LDL oxidation from occurring in the first place. With their full presence in the body, atherosclerosis is prevented and the risk of heart attacks, which are common to cardiovascular disease, is substantially reduced.

One glass of tomato or carrot juice every other day is certainly going to help the body resist the development of cancer or heart disease. Eating such vegetables raw or in salads or lightly cooked is good for you, too. *Periodic* supplementation, say 25,000 I.U. of vitamin A every day for two weeks of every month, may also be necessary.

Stomach Acid Necessary for Vitamin A Absorption

Millions of people in this country pop antacids into their mouths almost on a daily basis. They suffer stress-induced stomach acid and seek quick relief. But, according to a fascinating report recently published in the *American Journal of Clinical Nutrition* (64:622-26, 1996), such stomach-acid-blocking OTC (over-the-counter) drugs can dramatically reduce the absorption of carotenoids like beta-carotene. People who suffer from atrophic gastritis, in which there is virtually no stomach acid produced, are also unable to properly absorb vitamin A.

Therefore, it behooves a person to switch to herbal antacids such as *cool* chamomile or peppermint teas in lieu of the others. Or, if *more* stomach acid is needed, take internally 2 to 3 tablespoons of apple cider vinegar or sauerkraut juice just before taking beta-carotene.

If You Exercise, You Need Vitamin A

A lot of health-minded folks these days are exercising for different reasons. For some it is to keep trim, while others may do it to lose weight. While exercise is good for the body, it also has a "down side" to it: Overexercise can generate huge amounts of free radicals within the system.

According to Kenneth H. Cooper, M.D., the man who coined the term "aerobics" back in 1968, antioxidant nutrients are the solution to this vexing problem. He prefers vitamins A (25,000 I.U.), C (1,000 mg.), and E (400 I.U.) for this on a daily basis. He once told an interviewer that whenever he was scheduled to participate in heavy exercise of some kind or be in some other situation that would produce high oxidative stress on his body cells, he invariably increased these nutrient amounts accordingly.

The Antioxidant Drink That's Good for You

One of the nice things about working with different foods is that they can be fun as well as flavorful and healthy. I'm a strong proponent of carotenoids for the following health reasons:

- Improved eyesight
- Prevention of night blindness
- Strong bone growth and thickness
- Resistance to infection and disease
- Assistance with diabetes
- Prevention of acne, boils, and open skin sores
- Maintenance of healthy hair, skin, and mucous membranes
- Strong tooth enamel
- Reduction of diarrhea and weight loss

Years ago I started making a very simple drink for myself every other day that was extremely high in those carotenoids valuable for the body. The recipe is very simple and takes less than two minutes to make. I call it my Super Antioxidant Drink Tonic.

Super Antioxidant Drink Tonic

1/2 cup tomato juice (canned or fresh)

1/2 cup carrot juice (canned or fresh)

1 tsp. Pines' beetroot juice powder

1 tbsp. Pines' Mighty Greens drink powder

Mix together and stir thoroughly. Drink one glass alone or with a meal every other day. (See Product Appendix.)

Leg Ulcer Healed

Roy Arliss is a retired auto mechanic residing in Miami, Florida. When we met and Roy learned what I did for a living—writing books on natural remedies—he volunteered a story of his own about alternative healing.

Roy is diabetic and has been for some years. Awhile back (he never specified exactly when it was) he developed an open skin ulcer on his lower right leg, midway between the knee and ankle on the inside of the calf. His doctor readjusted his daily insulin intake and wrote out a prescription for an antibiotic ointment, informing Roy that the runny sore was due to an infection. But after faithfully applying the ointment several times every day for a week or more, Roy could see no improvement in his condition.

It was then that he decided to take a different course of action. He went to a local health food store in Miami and spoke with a clerk about his problem. He pulled up his pant leg and showed her just how bad this ulcer had become. She suggested that he take some cayenne pepper and ginger capsules (2 of each every day) with meals to help improve his blood circulation. She also advised him to get some vitamin A to take with them.

He took one 25,000 I.U. softgel capsule in the morning with breakfast and another one in the evening with dinner. He also did something else quite unusual: He pricked the end of several of these capsules with a needle and squeezed out their liquid onto the surface of his skin ulcer. He very gently rubbed this vitamin A, derived from fish liver oil, over the sore morning and evening. He claimed that in just a few days, "the danged thing started clearing up and got me all excited." Within ten days the ulcer was totally healed and new skin growth in place.

An aside to Roy 's story concerns the *reason* why he picked this particular brand of vitamins from Arizona. (See Product Appendix, p. 381.) "As I looked at all those bottles on the shelves," he told me, "I couldn't find *any* of them except this one that came in a *glass* container. The rest of them were all made of plastic. I figured to myself that if glass is more natural than plastic, then these vitamins probably had to be better than those in plastic bottles." I laughed at his rather unscientific but apparently very logical way of choosing his supplements.

The Best Time to Take Antioxidant Vitamins

Something that has received very little attention in medical science and virtually *no* coverage that I know of in the many self-treatment books in print these days is the little-known subject of chronobiology. This has to do with *when* is the ideal or optimal time to take a drug, herb, or nutrient of any kind. It involves a lot more than personal biorhythms, for it suggests a specific time frame within which a particular substance is apt to be at its *peak* performance. The progress of a disease at certain hours of the day or night, conditions of light or dark, and periods during which the body's own "master glands" are at maximum activity are just some of the factors that go into determining the *best time* to take something such as vitamin A.

More work on this theme has been done in cancer research than in research on other health problems. While various tumors are obviously going to have different hours for their *peak* growth throughout the day, it seems from a careful scanning of the medical literature in this area that the majority of cancers progress more rapidly in the *morning* than at any other time. Therefore, antioxidant vitamins such as A, C, and E, which have historically been used together to fight cancer, work better from 6 to 10 a.m. than later in the day. Also, they appear to be more efficient in early or late stages of tumor expansion than in middle periods of development.

The suggested intake will, of course, vary considerably when the type and length of cancer progression is taken into account. But a good rule of thumb that many doctors who treat cancer with natural means have suggested to me in the past, goes something like this:

Vitamin A-	50,000 I.U. morning*
Vitamin C-	10,000 mg. morning/afternoon
Vitamin E-	800 I.U. morning

Some Food Sources for Beta-Carotene

The following list has been compiled from several different U.S. Department of Agriculture publications of past years: *Composition of Foods* (No. 8, 1975); *Composition of Foods: Vegetables and Vegetable*

---

*I prefer the fish-oil-derived vitamin A and beta-carotene in the form of chlorophyll powder.

Products (Nos. 8-11, 1984); *Nutritive Value of American Foods in Common Units* (No. 456, 1975); and *Composition of Foods: Fruits and Fruit Juices* (Nos. 8-9, 1982).

Because of some of the inherent problems connected with the overconsumption of beta-carotene supplements that had been making headlines in the last couple of years, it is highly advisable to obtain your daily intake of this form of vitamin A from food sources *only*. Rely on a quality brand of vitamin products for your sea-algae-derived form of this important nutrient (See Product Appendix, p. 381).

Food Source	Amount	Vitamin A Content I.U.
Apricots	3	2,769
Avocado	1	1,230
Broccoli (cooked)	1 spear	2,537
Cantaloupe	1/4	4,304
Carrot (raw)	1	20,253
Carrot (cooked, sliced)	1/2 cup	19,150
Kale (cooked)	1/2 cup	4,810
Nectarine	1	1,007
Papaya	1	6,197
Spinach (cooked)	1/2 cup	7,363
Squash, winter, butternut (cooked)	1/2 cup	7,124
Sweet potato (baked)	1	24,867
Tomato (raw)	1	1,528
Turnip greens (cooked)	1/2 cup	3,943
Watermelon	1/16 slice	1,758

Vitamin B Complex
INTERACTING WITH THE B VITAMINS: WATER-SOLUBLE NUTRIENTS FOR ADULTS

Introducing the Vitamin B Group

Of all the vitamins cited in this first section, none are as extensive in size and scope as the B group. Think of them as a family. There are 16 members; this number, however, widely fluctuates depending on which nutritional authorities you're talking to at the time. They may be arranged in the following three subcategories for easier comprehending:

A. There are generally nine recognized B-complex vitamins: B-1 or thiamine; B-2 or riboflavin; B-3 or niacin; B-6 or pyridoxine; B-12 or cobalamin; folic acid; pantothenic acid; biotin; and choline. In some nutritional circles, the total number is given as eleven, due to the fact that two of the recognized B vitamins have twins: B-3a (nicotinic acid or niacinamide or nicotinamide) and B-5a (pantethine).

B. Four others may be considered to belong to this group because they have achieved limited acceptance by the medical and scientific communities. They are comparable to adopted children becoming part of a biological family of children. These are inositol, PABA or paraaminobenzoic acid, B-15 or pangamic acid, and L-carnitine (B_T). The last one enjoys the greatest respect from doctors.

C. The lone B vitamin considered a questionable member of the family by most nutritional experts is B-17 or amygdalin (but better known by its more popular name of laetrile). Although nutritional science virtually ignores it and scoffs at the idea of its even being considered a B vitamin, a reference work no less prestigious than *The Merck Index* (9th Ed.) regards it as a recognized nutrient of some therapeutic worth (see entries #630 and #5197.)

Vitamin B Behavior.

Members of the B-complex family dissolve in water, are rapidly absorbed, circulate freely, are rapidly excreted, and must be regularly replenished since they are poorly stored in body tissue. Concentrations exceeding levels of cell or tissue saturation are quickly expelled in urine and perspiration, and ingestion of these vitamins in extremely large quantities, for the most part, is relatively safe for healthy individuals.

Most of the B vitamins function in the human body as coenzymes. That is, they enable regular enzymes to chemically react with many other compounds in order to initiate a wide number of different bodily functions. Since the B group all seem to work together synergistically, it is usually a good idea to take them together in a *single* high-potency supplement. The amount needed, of course, will vary from person to person, depending upon individual physical builds, weights, and diets. Sometimes, certain health conditions demand that some of this B group be taken separately. But as a general rule, it is better to focus on eating foods or taking a supplement in which the majority of them are always included.

Signs of Deficiencies.

Usually, when there is one B-vitamin deficiency, there are likely deficiencies in others of the same family. Fatigue, mental lethargy, depression, nervousness and irritability, skin problems, insomnia, lack of appetite, elevated cholesterol, and disturbances in heart functions are the most prominent symptoms. It is amazing how the short-term supplementation of high-potency B-complex vitamins can eliminate most, if not all, of these symptoms rather quickly.

Numerical Arrangement within the Text.

To better assist the reader in identifying with each of these vitamins, I've taken the unusual liberty of listing them numerically. A couple of the numbers may seem a bit foreign to the reader, but I can assure you that they are not my creations. I'm referring specifically to B-5 (pantothenic acid) and B-9 (folic acid), which appear in *The*

Complete Guide to Vitamins, Minerals & Supplements by H. Winter Griffith, M.D. (Tucson: Fisher Books, 1988; pp. 63, 51). Those having no official numbers connected with them appear in the very beginning. Their positions in this list correspond with how they appear in the rest of the text belonging to the B vitamins.

The B-Vitamin Group

B	CHOLINE
B	INOSITOL
B	PABA / PARAAMINOBENZOIC ACID
B-1	THIAMINE
B-2	RIBOFLAVIN
B-3 / B-3$_a$	NIACIN / NIACINAMIDE / NICOTINAMIDE / NICOTINIC ACID
B-5 / B-5$_a$	PANTOTHENIC ACID / PANTETHINE
B-6	PYRIDOXINE
B-8	BIOTIN
B-9	FOLIC ACID / FOLATE / FOLACIN
B-12	COBALAMIN / CYANOCOBALAMIN
B-15	PANGAMIC ACID
B-17	AMYGDALIN / LAETRILE
B$_T$	L-CARNITINE

B (CHOLINE): Protect Your Brain, Nerve, and Muscle from Damage by Oxidation

Choline is one of those water-soluble B vitamins you don't hear too much about, except when it's associated with lecithin. This is because choline is the key, base ingredient in the formation of lecithin. Lecithin is one of the most widely used food additives, appearing in everything from ice cream and ready-made whipping cream to margarine and mayonnaise. Lecithin is the bridge that connects water to the fats in these products and, thereby, helps maintain their consistency.

Choline is very beneficial to human health. It sometimes appears as an extra ingredient in vitamin formulas. But more often than not, its use internally is primarily confined to liquid or granulated lecithin.

Rhoda P. of Shreveport, Louisiana shared her own experience with me a few years ago concerning how lecithin *delayed* the onset of Alzheimer's disease in her aged mother.

"My mother," she wrote in a letter dated August 17, 1992, "started getting memory lapses when she turned 71. I took her to a physician, who said she was in the very early stages of Alzheimer's disease. Well, someone in our church where we worship weekly told me about lecithin. I got some in the liquid [form] from a health food store and had her start taking one teaspoonful of this every morning and evening. This seemed to stop the progress of her memory loss. She lived with us for another 13 years before succumbing to a stroke. But her mind was just as good as ever because of the lecithin."

A psychiatrist in the eastern U.S. who treats his patients with natural means once related the following true case study to me, which I found totally amazing! Patient M.F., a white female, age 37, weight 143 lbs., came to see him. She was suffering from a combination of manic-depression (a mental illness) and tardive dyskinesia (a neurologic disorder). Psychiatric counseling over an extended period of time helped to improve her mental and emotional outlook on life. He prescribed for her 1 tablespoon of lecithin granules and 20 grams of 90% phosphatidylcholine every day. He also put her on lithium (standard therapy for manic-depressive illness). In one week her facial muscle twitching and jerking ceased, and within a month her manic-depression was in a turnaround phase.

Food Sources

Besides supplements, there are some valuable food sources for obtaining pure choline. These would include *fresh* egg yolks from organically-raised chickens; mix two medium-sized egg yolks in 6 oz. of carrot or orange juice and drink every other morning for breakfast.

Fish and organ meats are rich in choline, too. Sardines and mackerel, in particular, are exceptionally high in choline, as are beef brain and liver, sweetbread (calf thymus), kidney (beef and lamb), and chicken livers. All of these may be better for you, but don't sound quite as appetizing as sirloin, veal, roast, or chops might.

The fish can be eaten right out of a can, or else put on flavorful breads such as rye, pumpernickel, or sourdough. Some of the organ meats go well with eggs in a soufflé or quiche, while others of them may be baked or slowly roasted in the oven; *none* of them should be fried or deep-fried, however, as that may destroy some of their choline content.

Legumes and soybeans are also fairly good sources of choline. Chickpeas do especially well in this regard. For those unable to handle soybeans directly, alternative forms may do just as well—sprouts, tofu, etc.

Finally, wheat germ and brewer's yeast carry in them more than enough choline to meet the body's daily nutritional requirements. One teaspoonful of wheat germ sprinkled on cooked or dried cereal in the morning is a nifty way to take it. The real problem, though, comes with the latter. The truth is, no matter what you mix brewer's yeast with, it's still going to have a somewhat nauseating smell and taste about it. There's just no getting around this dilemma completely. But there are a few tricks to *masking* some of its odor and taste. Try mixing 1/2 teaspoonful of brewer's yeast in a breakfast protein shake of some kind. Egg nog is another flavorful way to take what's good for you without gagging. Taking brewer's yeast in capsules is convenient, but it's better to swallow it with a little milk or something thick and flavorful in the way of a beverage so as to prevent any vitamin after-burp from occurring later on. (Brewer's yeast after-burps are enough to make you shudder!)

CHOLINE-RICH NOG

2 cups regular or Jersey milk

2 medium egg yolks

2 teaspoons almond butter

1 tablespoon honey

1/2 teaspoon brewer's yeast

Pinches of cinnamon and nutmeg

Combine everything in a food processor and blend for 1 1/2 minutes or until thoroughly combined. Sip slowly to enjoy the full flavor.

Recommended Daily Intake

The average daily intake of choline is somewhere between 100 and 200 mg. for adult men and women. It would be slightly higher (275 mg.) for phosphatidylcholine. In the form of lecithin, about two capsules or one level teaspoon of granules or one teaspoon of the liquid is proposed.

B (INOSITOL): Treating Depression and Panic-Anxiety as Well as Diabetes and Obesity the Natural Way

Nearly two decades ago, medical researchers discovered that the level of inositol (which is a close cousin of glucose) in the spinal fluid of people who suffered from bouts of mild to severe depression was usually lower than among people who were upbeat and cheerful. This led to the hypothesis that this water-soluble B vitamin could be used to treat depression.

In 1995, a psychiatric team at Israel's Ben Gurion University of the Negev published several double-blind studies in which inositol was used to treat mental illness successfully. Their conclusion: Inositol could very well serve as an ideal treatment for depression and for that type of anxiety known as panic disorder. Depressed patients who benefited from high doses of inositol included those with both monopolar and bipolar depression or manic-depressive disease. (The bipolar type is marked by interchangeable periods of depression and euphoria.)

The Israeli psychiatric team also focused its research on people with panic disorder, a form of anxiety in which people get sudden attacks of extreme agitation, as if they were in the throes of death or the end of the world were at hand. These attacks are far worse than the grouchiness or nervousness most of us are more familiar with.

Panic-anxiety patients who took inositol regularly experienced fewer incidents of such attacks per week (a decrease from 9.7 to a mere 3.7 instead). The intensity of the panic attacks also significantly decreased in patients who took this important B vitamin.

This important research appeared in several very respected medical journals: *American Journal of Psychiatry* (152:792-94; 152:1084-86, both in 1995); *Psychopharmacology Bulletin* (31:167-75, 1995); and the *Israel Journal of Psychiatry and Related Sciences* (32:14-21, 1995). All of this shows just how helpful inositol is in treating these kinds of mental disorders.

This member of the B group also plays a significant role in the treatment of diabetes and obesity. Type I insulin-dependent diabetes afflicts about 4 percent of the total U.S. population. Quite often it is an outgrowth of obesity. One of the most frequent and crippling complications of diabetes is diabetic peripheral neuropathy. The nerves of the lower limbs are generally affected first. There can also be interrupted digestion, nighttime diarrhea, low blood pressure, and muscle numbness and pain. Retention of urine and impotence can also be problems.

Different medical investigations into the reason for this wide-spread complication (diabetic peripheral neuropathy) has turned up a greatly reduced level of myo-inositol, which is the nutritionally active form of the water-soluble B vitamin inositol. But when doctors administered 500 mg. of myo-inositol to their diabetic patients twice a day for two weeks, many of these nerve-related symptoms completely disappeared. Some physicians increased this intake to 1,500 mg. daily and saw even quicker results.

So it is fair to say that myo-inositol will certainly decrease or prevent one of the *symptoms* of diabetes. But it needs to be taken in conjunction with other things, like garlic (2 capsules daily) and barley grass juice powder (1 level tablespoon in 8 ounces of water), to effectively reduce the risks of ever developing this disease. Fine supplements such as these are only part of the solution, though. A comprehensive program of healthy eating habits and exercise is in order, too.

Watching your daily intake of white sugar and the more dangerous "hidden" sugars, is, by far, one of the most important things to do. Early in 1997, I took a short flight on during which the flight

attendants distributed fat free apple cereal bars to each of the pas-
sengers. As always, I checked out the fine print on the label before
quietly blessing and then eating it. I was astonished at just how
many "hidden" sugars there were. They were a clever combination
of either straight or secondary sugars: sugar, dehydrated apples, corn
syrup, dextrose, ground raisins, apple juice concentrate, high fructose corn syrup, and molasses. Out of a total of 28 ingredients, fully
one-third were sugars in some form!

Americans do much too much sitting; we need to get up and
move about more every day. Even something as simple as walking
a lot, but in many small trips throughout a day, will do amazing
things for the body in helping to keep the pancreas active and
healthy. In my own research center, I've deliberately located my fil-
ing cabinets in a room far from my office, so that I am forced to take
many steps back and forth every day to retrieve materials I need in
my writing. Add to that a four-block walk to the parking garage, and
it is fair to say that I probably walk about 1 1/2 miles every day as
part of my normal daily routine, without considering any kind of
regular exercise program.

The point of all this is quite simple: Watch out for "hidden" sugars in the things you eat by being a more careful label reader; and
exercise often by *unconscious* walking that isn't planned or regi-
mented (that way it won't seem such a physical chore, psychologically). Of course, by all means don't forget the myo-inositol! Use
one-half teaspoon daily in cooked cereal, milk, juices, or healthy
shakes. (See Product Appendix, p. 381.)

Food Sources

There are, of course, some nice food sources of myo-inositol. Most
of us get close to or above one gram every day principally in the
phospholipid form or as phytic acid in plant sources. Hard-shelled
foods that require shelling, considerable chewing, or cooking, such
as nuts, seeds, grains, and beans, are loaded with myo-inositol. So,
too, are some fruits: 1/2 cantaloupe contains about 675 mg.; a sweet,
navel orange has approximately 310 mg.; 1/2 ruby-red grapefruit has
207 mg.; 1/2 cup of frozen concentrate of grape juice contains 461

mg.; 1/2 cup of frozen concentrate of orange juice has 243 mg.; and one slice of whole wheat toast contains 297 mg. (I'm grateful to the Sunkist Corp. and the Florida Citrus Board for the foregoing figures concerning myo-inositol contents in certain citrus fruits.)

Recommended Daily Intake

There is always lecithin, of course, which will supply the body with a small amount of inositol (in the form of phosphatidylinositol). The lecithin can be taken in granules (1/2 teaspoon daily) or else in liquid form (one level teaspoon every morning with juice or water). Inositol, like its other B cousin, choline, should help keep blood sugar levels in balance and hold body weight in check, when other factors (label reading and exercise) come into play.

The amounts of inositol that were given in the previously cited studies involving patients suffering from depression and panic-anxiety were unusually high—6 grams (6,000 mg.) twice a day. But these very high doses were administered under strict medical supervision and for short periods running into weeks, not months or years. Also, no one has yet looked into the matter of inositol possibly interacting with prescription or over-the-counter medications that so many people take today.

In another, more recent study published in the *American Journal of Psychiatry* (153:1219-21, 1996) Israeli psychiatrists administered even greater doses of inositol (18 grams per day for 1 1/2 months) to 13 patients afflicted with obsessive-compulsive disorder. The doctors discovered that all of their patients responded well to this vitamin therapy and displayed "significantly less" of this abnormal mental behavior.

Still, in spite of the extremely large doses that some doctors have given to their patients suffering from various mental disorders, it is a good idea to confer with your doctor before attempting to take doses of inositol beyond the prudent and safe amounts of 150 to 250 mg. per day for very long.

Inositol also works quite well in company with vitamin B-9 (folic acid) for reducing genetic birth defects in newborn babies. British medical researchers discovered that when expectant mothers took 300 micrograms of folic acid and 150 mg. of inositol every day, beginning at the time of conception, they experienced dramatically fewer birth defects. Both B vitamins can be used with relative safety during the entire pregnancy.

B (PABA): Wonderful Skin and Hair Protection

Another water-soluble B vitamin, paraaminobenzoic acid (PABA) is actually a component of B-9 (folic acid) and acts as a coenzyme within the body. It teams up with folic acid to assist in the metabolism of proteins and in the manufacture of blood cells; it works alongside B-5 and B-5$_a$ to make the body feel and look younger and helps internal systems such as the cardiovascular and immune systems to function more dynamically.

Starting with the top of the head, PABA's influence may be seen in helping to minimize hair loss and eradicate grayness. On the skin, it is simply wonderful for a variety of disorders: dermatitis, herpes, lupus erythematosus, lymphoblastoma cutis, and scleroderma.

PABA also affords the skin protection from intense sunlight. I remember something that a woman by the name of Kathy Roth from Clarks Summit, Pennsylvania, wrote to me years ago, describing how PABA worked for her. "Every summer I'd break out all over with nasty red bumps that itched like crazy. So, I started slathering PABA lotion all over the exposed parts of my body. I also decided to take PABA internally—400 mg. every day without fail. From that time on, these bumps disappeared, never to come back again. And, my pale skin didn't even so much as peel and burn under such hot conditions. For me, that was highly unusual, but pleasantly received. Now I'm never without PABA when exposed to the brutal heat of the summer sun!"

However, some dermatologists with whom I've previously consulted on this matter have told me that PABA's main value is largely in its external applications. They recommend that their patients combine PABA externally with B-6 *internally* to minimize heat stroke and sunburn.

A few medical studies, particularly those coming out of Scandinavian countries in past years, have shown that a combination of PABA and B-5/B-5$_a$ expedites wound healing. Surgical incisions healed much more quickly in animal models and patients when PABA and pantothenic acid/pantethine were routinely prescribed together. Oral consumption and external application were the two ways in which these B vitamins were administered.

Another thing that may come as a surprise to some people is that PABA helps prevent wrinkling of the skin. Look for lotions high in PABA content. When this B vitamin and aloe vera are applied together over the surface of the skin, there will be far less wrinkling from the harsh elements of wind, sun, air, and water. A facial mask made at night of equal parts of PABA, aloe vera, and honey and left on the face while sleeping will tighten up loose skin to help some wrinkles disappear. It can be removed the next morning with cotton balls saturated in rubbing alcohol followed by warm water.

Food Sources

Certain foods contain varying amounts of PABA. These include, but are not limited to, the following: blackstrap molasses, wheat and oat bran, rye, millet, eggs, liver, kidney, brown rice, and wheat germ.

Recommended Daily Intake

When the body needs to be supplemented with PABA, it should be for short-term periods of no more than a couple of weeks at a time. The daily intake should not exceed 100 mg., unless a doctor advises higher amounts. Caution: If your doctor has you on any of the so-called "sulfa drugs" (sulfonamide antibiotics) for serious infections, stay away from PABA. Externally, though, PABA can be used as much as is necessary, without regard to safety.

B-1 (THIAMINE): Keeps You Mentally Alert and Emotionally Stable

While lecturing in Florida in 1979 for an international direct-marketing herbal company, I had the good fortune of meeting the late W. Henry Sebrell. He was then a very young 73 years of age, and his quick mind showed no signs of fading memory at all. He had just then retired from the post of medical director for Weight Watchers International. We spent several pleasant hours in Tampa together and I learned much from him about the B vitamins in general.

Sebrell became identified as an expert on the entire B-complex group in the 1930s. He spent more than 30 years with the United States Public Health Service and the Institutes of Health. In these trusted positions, he was able to promote the enrichment of flour and bread with thiamine, riboflavin, and niacin, which went far in helping to wipe out pellagra, beriberi, and other B-deficient ailments.

I asked Dr. Sebrell what made him so mentally alert at an age when many other seniors were in the throes of faulty memory recall, senile dementia, or even Alzheimer's disease. He attributed his own razor-sharp memory to a *daily* supplementation of 150 mg. of B-1 for almost 29 years. He claimed that "I can outthink many of those young upstarts around me, half my age, who have this attitude that because they're younger they have some sort of monopoly on energy and brain power."

Dr. Sebrell also called my attention to the fact that many of the mentally ill and institutionalized elderly have always shown subclinical thiamine deficiencies. In fact, he noted, "It is quite common for 50 percent or better of patients under psychiatric care to regularly show low levels of B-1." He explained to me that this can affect the levels of other brain nutrients, such as the neurotransmitters glutamate and aspartate. Reduced thiamine content can also spell trouble for another B vitamin, choline, which is required for acetylcholine that plays a major role in the transmission of nerve impules at the synapses.

Dr. Sebrell was of the definite opinion that "most of the current cases we hear or read about in the news concerning emotionally or mentally unstable individuals can be directly linked to severely depleted levels of B vitamins" such as thiamine, choline, and pyridoxine. "But if they could just be supplemented with adequate amounts of the B's, then just about all of their instabilities would vanish."

Lead poisoning is still fairly common in America, especially among lower-income households. Dr. Sebrell explained how important thiamine is in helping to excrete excess lead from the body. The thiamine binds itself to lead molecules, thereby preventing lead poisoning. These thiamine-lead complexes are later discharged from the system with other waste materials. Sebrell estimated that a minimum daily intake of 100 mg. of thiamine would afford protection against lead poisoning.

This pioneer in vitamin research loved to hold forth in long discussions about the B vitamins, which he spent so much of his scientific life studying. Vitamin B-1 "can help turn around disturbed heart rhythms, elevate low blood pressure, stabilize shortness of breath, reduce swelling of the legs and feet, and protect against kidney and cardiac failures." Chronic alcoholics, who often suffer from many of these clinical manifestations, "benefit from B-1 in a big way."

(Dr. Sebrell died in late September, 1992 at his home in Pompano Beach, Florida at the age of 91. Had he been asked by someone shortly before his demise what he attributed his long life and good health to, I'm almost sure he would have said thiamine and the rest of the B vitamins. For more of my interview with this brilliant man, see the section on B-3, or niacin.

Food Sources

Processing procedures such as milling flour or grains, curing meats, irradiating, canning, freezing, adding sulfites, and pasteurizing and evaporating milk all destroy many of the B vitamins, says Lauri M. Aesoph, N.D., a natural health practitioner, educator, and writer residing in Sioux Falls, South Dakota. The peeling of a fruit or vegetable, cooking foods in water, and long-term storage cause loss of B vitamins. Also, exposing foods to light results in loss of B vitamins, "especially B-6 and B-2."

Some cholesterol-lowering drugs can decrease folic acid absorption, she insists. Anti-ulcer medications can interfere with B-12 absorption; so, too, does sodium bicarbonate, because it neutralizes stomach acid, which some B vitamins need for proper distribution throughout the body. Anyone on medication should be taking B vitamins, she notes.

Another thing that greatly reduces blood levels of B-1 is the consumption of beverages high in tannic acid. These include black tea (both hot and iced) and coffee. Colas and soft drinks are, likewise, believed to be culprits in thiamine depletions.

Excellent food sources for deriving your daily intake of thiamine include: blackstrap molasses, brewer's yeast, brown rice, millet, rye, oatmeal, dried beans (especially soybeans), poultry, liver, fish, lobster, sunflower seeds, some nuts (cashews and pecans especially), other seafood and seaweed (dulse, kelp), and enriched bread.

Bear in mind though that thiamine is heat-sensitive, with a fair amount being destroyed when food is cooked. So, the trick here is to eat what foods you can in a raw form or else lightly cooked.

Recommended Daily Intake

Young children really don't need B-1 supplementation, since the enriched bread many of them gobble down already has plenty of thiamine in it. Adult men and women, however, should take at least 100 mg. every day for a couple of weeks, and then discontinue doing so for a few weeks more. This on-again, off-again routine will prevent excess thiamine buildup, which could result in an offsetting deficiency of other members of the B group.

Food should, of course, always be the main source for B vitamins. But when supplementation becomes necessary, look for high-quality supplement suppliers. I recommend a B-1 100 mg. tablet as well as three B-complex products (see Product Appendix, p. 381).

In my conversation with Dr. Sebrell many years ago, I was struck by one statement he made that has remained with me ever since. He observed in a very matter-of-fact way, emphasizing with right-hand chops in midair: "People spend incredible sums of money for psychiatric counseling. And several hundred thousand of the elderly languish in rest homes and institutions in states of semi-senility. Parents and teachers are frustrated with hyperactive kids, who don't know how to behave and who have attention spans shorter than my thumb. And yet, all it would take to solve these different but interrelated problems is an inexpensive bottle of B-1 and another bottle of high-potency B-complex."

So simple and within reach, but denied to them because of public ignorance in this matter.

B-2 (RIBOFLAVIN): Making Glands Work Right for You

To a chemist looking at riboflavin under a microscope in the laboratory, vitamin B-2 would appear as a yellow crystalline substance. While found throughout the human body, the liver and kidneys have greater stores of this important nutrient than other body tissues; but even in these two organs reserves are minimal. This B vitamin assists in body growth, tissue repair, and cell respiration. It is also essential for the proper digestion of food, the health of the nervous system, the assimilation of iron, and, in conjunction with vitamin A, for good vision.

But where B-2 does most of its good is with those body glands responsible for the production of energy and vitality. These include the various glands that comprise what are collectively referred to as the endocrine glands: adrenals, parathyroid, pituitary, and thyroid. The hypothalamus (located within the forebrain) also benefits from riboflavin, since it is prominently involved in the functions of the different endocrine glands and plays a role, through the nervous system, in underlying moods and motivational states. Another large gland of a dark-red color situated in the upper portion of the abdomen on the right side requires adequate amounts of B-2 as well. This is the liver, where food sugars (carbohydrates) are converted into glycogen and then stored; riboflavin assists in the release of glycogen for energy production. B-2 also helps release energy from consumed fats and proteins.

Ruth L. is a secretary in her mid-forties, working for the state government in Phoenix, Arizona. Her indiscriminate eating habits formerly consisted of a diet such as a jelly doughnut and coffee for breakfast, a burger and fries for lunch, lots of soft drinks throughout the day, and a TV dinner or pizza at night. She soon developed chronic fatigue, oily skin, and a lot of intestinal gas. In spite of the fact that she has near-perfect or 20/20 vision, she also developed eye problems: sensitivity to light, visual strain, and an itching, burning sensation. She also experienced mild dizziness occasionally.

Ruth consulted several local doctors, who didn't do her much good. One told her it was all in her head and, for that quick assessment, charged her $55 for her office visit, which she thought was outrageous to say the least. Another doctor prescribed some "little yellow and black pills, which cost me $72 for 10 of them." A third physician recommended that she "not work so hard, but take more time to play and have fun."

Feeling thoroughly discouraged with all of this medical incompetence, she related her woes to her hairdresser one day, who told her of an alternative medical doctor who worked with nutrition. She consulted with him and had some blood tests and a hair analysis done. Both doctor and patient learned that she was extremely deficient in vitamin B-2. He put her on a program of riboflavin-rich foods (see Food Sources in this section) and had her take 75 mg. twice daily of B-2 along with 15 mg. of supplemental iron. This regimen was kept up for one month, at the end of which time she was told to decrease her B-2 intake to only 50 mg. daily and her iron consumption to just 5 mg. every other day.

"I couldn't believe how good I felt after the first couple of days," she claimed. "It was almost as if I had taken some kind of 'wonder drug' or 'miracle pill.' I couldn't believe the energy I had. By the end of the first week I felt like a brand new woman. Isn't it funny, how a couple of nutritional supplements put me back into shape again, when no drugs could? And by just making a few changes in my eating patterns, I am now able to work long hours *and* play just as hard (racquet ball and tennis) as one of my former doctors told me I should."

This B vitamin is also useful for those who exercise a lot. Dedicated exercise is obviously good for the heart and for keeping your weight down, but it also increases free radicals within the body. Riboflavin exerts antioxidant properties to protect against any potential damage that these scavenger molecules could otherwise inflict on muscle tissues and joints.

Riboflavin deficiencies have been linked with increases in throat cancers in some parts of the world. Supplementation with B-2 seems to reduce the number of precancerous cells, especially in the esophagus. As mentioned before, riboflavin and iron work in harmony to protect against anemia.

Food Sources

Dairy products are, undoubtedly, some of the very best sources for B-2. Just one quart of milk contains 1.7 mg. of riboflavin. Those dairy products that have been fermented actually contain a lot more B-2—different cheeses, yogurt, and buttermilk.

There are a number of other food sources for B-2 that might be more suitable for those who don't like dairy products. Blackstrap molasses, brewer's yeast, eggs, fruit, green leafy vegetables, legumes, nuts, organ meat, poultry, tongue, and whole grain breads and cereals are some of them.

Recommended Daily Intake

There is a big difference between the thinking of U.S. government scientists and alternative nutrition experts about B-2 intake for adults. The government's RDA suggests a mere 1.6 mg. for men and a bit less for women, 1.2 mg. But the *real* levels necessary for optimum health are much higher than this—anywhere from 50 to 300 mg. for both genders. There is no evidence that suggests such high doses might be toxic.

B-3 (NIACIN): Big Surprises from a Little B Vitamin

Niacin or nicotinic acid may be used interchangeably with each other since they are one and the same. If taken in large amounts (100 mg.), a flushing action is noticed; The skin begins to tingle and turn red, as if you had an instant sunburn. This is due to the enlargement of blood vessels and the prompt release of histamine and heparin into the bloodstream by niacin. Niacinamide is another form of niacin that doesn't produce this untoward reaction. However, it's virtually worthless in reducing fat levels in the blood.

I shall now pick up where I left off in the section on B-1 with the rest of my interview with the late Dr. W. Henry Sebrell. My interview with this great genius occurred in 1979 while I was in Tampa for a number of speaking engagements.

In the 1930s this man became one of the recognized experts on vitamin B-complex. He helped to discover the prevention and cure for pellagra. His mentor in this work was Dr. Joseph Goldberger, a bacteriologist who devoted his entire career to the study of pellagra. This was once a pervasive clinical deficiency syndrome throughout the world due to a lack of niacin (or the body's inability to convert the amino acid tryptophan to niacin). People with pellagra suffered from dermatitis, inflammation of the mucous membranes, diarrhea, and psychic disturbances. The dermatitis occurred on those portions of people's bodies that were exposed to light or trauma. Their mental symptoms included depression, irritability, anxiety, confusion, disorientation, migraine headaches, delusions, and hallucinations. Alcoholics, drug addicts, and consumers of junk food most often suffered from such symptoms. In. former times they would often be diagnosed as being schizophrenic or even psychotic and some were locked away in mental institutions. There, some of them were subjected to electroshock therapy, massive doses of powerful sedative drugs, and even prefrontal lobotomy (mild brain surgery), in hopes of making them passive and fairly "normal" again.

Goldberger died in 1929 and his unfinished research was carried on by Dr. Sebrell and others. Among other areas, Dr. Sebrell studied B-5 (pantothenic acid) deficiency and its impact on the adrenal glands; he also focused on blood abnormality from B-9 (folic acid) deficiency, liver necrosis, and cirrhosis.

As a nutrition expert, he advised the League of Nations and United Nations. In World War II he made strategic recommendations for the diets of civilian workers and rationing for civilian survivors in Western Europe. It was largely through his efforts as a public health official that white flour and bread became enriched with niacin, thiamine, and riboflavin. This almost single-handedly helped to wipe out pellagra and beriberi (another vitamin B deficiency problem).

In the postwar prosperity that followed, Sebrell shifted from the receding problem of malnutrition to the dangers of eating too much. In 1952 he proclaimed that obesity had replaced dietary deficiencies "as the No. 1 nutrition problem" in the nation, with a fourth of the population being overweight. That is what eventually led him to join Weight Watchers International, where he became its first medical director after leaving a tenured professorship at Columbia University.

Dr. Sebrell served for a time as president of both the American Institute of Nutrition and the Society for Clinical Nutrition. He published over 300 scientific papers in his lifetime and was coeditor of a five-volume reference work on vitamins that became a mainstay for nutritionists and doctors for many years.

Next to thiamine, Dr. Sebrell felt that niacin was the "second most important of the B vitamins for all-around good health." I've arranged the rest of my interview material with him according to the different conditions for which he felt niacin would be particularly useful.

Ménière's Disease. This syndrome is characterized clinically by vertigo, nausea, vomiting, ringing in the ears, and progressive deafness. Dr. Sebrell related several experiences he knew of personally when physician colleagues of his had prescribed niacin to some of their patients suffering with this disorder, with very good results.

Rheumatoid Arthritis. He mentioned that several rheumatologists had prescribed "high doses" ranging from 150 to 300 mg. to some of their arthritic patients. Improved joint function, lessening of joint discomfort, and improved mood were the happy results of this unique therapy.

Heart Disease. Dr. Sebrell showed me some of the published work of a friend of his, Edwin Boyle, M.D., a past clinical professor at the Medical University of South Carolina in Charleston. "Before Boyle was treating heart disease with niacin," he said with obvious pride in his voice, "I had been recommending it myself for many years to any doctor who would listen to me. Those who took me seriously found out for themselves that their patients with heart disease improved remarkably when placed on niacin."

I asked him, on that occasion long ago, how they resolved the flushing problem. "Oh, that's an easy one," he replied. "They would have their patients take the niacin with meals, or else place them on smaller doses spread over the day (100 mg. morning, noon, and night), and eventually increasing the amount gradually (300 mg. daily). In a number of cases they would have their patients take an aspirin beforehand. All of these things eliminated the burning sensation to the skin."

About eight years later, a major piece of published research that reported the same effect appeared in the *Journal of The American Medical Association* (257:3233-40, June 19, 1987). Entitled "Beneficial Effects of Combined Colestipol-Niacin Therapy on Coronary Atherosclerosis and Coronary Venous Bypass Grafts," it told of "significant regression" of plaque buildup in the hearts of 162 nonsmoking men aged 40 to 50 years with previous coronary bypass surgery, after taking both vitamin supplements for two years. The combined therapy of an antihyperlipidemic agent and a powerful B vitamin resulted in "a 26% reduction in total plasma cholesterol, a 43% reduction in low-density lipoprotein [bad cholesterol]" and "a simultaneous 37% elevation of high-density lipoprotein cholesterol [the good kind]."

As I read this report through, I thought of my friend in Florida and wondered if his own work with niacin many years before may not have served as some kind of inspiration for the California doctors who conducted this particular cholesterol-lowering atherosclerosis study.

Senility. During my several hours' visit with Dr. Sebrell, he brought up the advantages of niacin for treating senility. He walked across the room to a bookcase and withdrew a volume by Abram Hoffer, Ph.D. entitled *Niacin Therapy in Psychiatry* (Springfield, IL: Charles C. Thomas, 1962). Handing it to me, he remarked, "This psychiatrist put a number of middle-aged and elderly people on large amounts of niacin [12 tablets daily] with the result that most of them recovered from their senility and their minds became as sharp as ever."

Insomnia. "I used to suffer from it occasionally myself," he stated. "But when I started taking 100 mg. of niacin every evening an hour before bed, I fell fast asleep and slept like a baby. Never was bothered with it anymore after that."

Vitiligo. This is a blemish that appears on otherwise normal skin in nonpigmented white patches of varied sizes that are usually symmetrically distributed and bordered by hyperpigmented areas. Sebrell

said he knew of a certain dermatologist "over Miami way, who treated his patients with large doses of niacin" for this condition. He met
this doctor at a nutritional science convention, where the other made
passing reference to it in casual conversation between the two. Dr.
Sebrell was sorry that he couldn't remember the doctor's name, nor
exactly how much niacin was administered or for how long. I insert
this here because of its highly unusual nature. Regrettably, I can't verify its success.

Cancer. Dr. Sebrell was of the definite belief that niacinamide
could be used to prevent certain forms of cancer. *Cancer Research*
(45:809-14; 3609-14, 1985) and *Journal of the National Cancer
Institute* (73:767-70, 1984) reported that niacinamide is useful in preventing and decreasing cancers of the kidneys, mammary glands,
and pancreas.

Food Sources

There are several ways of obtaining adequate amounts of niacin from
foods. Obviously, one is to eat those foods that are already high in
niacin content. The other is to consume those foods that are high in
tryptophan, which is soon converted into niacin within the body.

Foods already rich in niacin include: shelled, roasted peanuts
(one cup gives you 24 mg.); tuna fish sandwich on enriched white
bread (the two together should yield about 23 mg.); liver (5 1/2
slices have 75 mg.); mackerel (a 15 oz. can contains nearly 40 mg.);
and spaghetti with meatballs in tomato sauce (one serving has 52
mg.). Other foods with lower niacin content are eggs, lean meats,
organ meats, milk products, poultry, seafood, whole grain breads
and cereals, and brewer's yeast.

Tryptophan is the least abundant essential amino acid to be
found in foods. It has a most unusual distribution in foods, some of
which may not be deemed too healthy by pure food enthusiasts.
Ham, meat and beef extract, salted anchovies, certain cheeses (parme-
san and Swiss, in particular), turkey, sausage, and almonds are all high
in this amino acid. Within a short time after any of these staples are
eaten, the trytophan will become converted into useful niacin. Stay
away from sugar, though, which can severely deplete niacin!

Recommended Daily Intake

Adult men and women over the age of 50 require a daily niacin intake of between 30 and 50 mg. The equivalent amounts of dietary tryptophan would range from 1,800 to 3,000 mg. Keep in mind, though, that excess amounts of *supplemental* (as opposed to food-derived) tryptophan can do the body harm. So be sure to check with your doctor before self-dosing with niacin or tryptophan!

B-5 (PANTOTHENIC ACID): Is Your Body Suffering from B-Complex Deficiency Syndrome?

The root name of this particular B vitamin may interest readers: "panthos" comes from the Greek, which means "everywhere." Quite literally, B-5 is found in a wide range of foods, suggesting its availability is just about "everywhere" in the diet. But because it is water-soluble, it can easily be removed from the body. Hence, those who are constant drinkers of beer, wine, coffee, and black tea or iced tea will always be short of this vitamin. The same goes for smokers and those inhaling secondhand smoke.

Vitamin B-5 works primarily in the adrenal glands to produce energy, in the digestive tract to help in the absorption of other nutrients, in the immune system to protect the body from infection, in the nerves to keep things calm, and in the skin to keep the complexion beautiful.

But some medical doctors with extensive practices honestly believe that there is a critical shortage of *all* the B vitamins (including pantothenic acid) in the diets of *most* of their patients. Dr. Bruce West has a thriving clinical and telephone practice out of Carmel, California. He publishes a monthly *Health Alert* newsletter that reaches tens of thousands of readers around the country. Every day, for an hour in the morning (California time, of course), subscribers can call in with their health problems and receive diagnoses and appropriate therapies *by telephone.*

Some time ago, Dr. West reported that this "B-complex deficiency syndrome" is a common "scenario played out every day in doctors' offices around the country." The typical patient comes in "with symptoms ranging from a chronic headache to insomnia to bouts of depression."

Usually a number of expensive and difficult tests are run, "all of which come back negative." The doctor is then left with the baffling question of what to do when nothing shows up in the way of an actual illness. Soothing words may be spoken, some hand-holding done, a prescription written for a powerful sedative or some other "knock-out" drug, and the patient sent on his or her way with a nod of the head and a patronizing smile. Once rid of such a presumed hypochondriac, the doctor can then turn his or her attention back to those who are truly ill.

But those suffering from B-complex deficiency syndrome aren't imagining any of their symptoms—they indeed *are* sick! The problem is that their serious malady "mimics a wide range of other ailments," which makes it virtually impossible for the average physician to correctly diagnose.

Typical symptoms commonly associated with B-complex deficiency syndrome are as follows:

- recurring hunger or excessive appetite
- heart palpitations or skipped beats
- periodic bouts of depression
- chronic headaches
- hypoglycemia
- a continual craving for sweets
- difficulty sleeping
- frequent exhaustion or chronic fatigue
- overwhelmed and unable to cope with life
- panic attacks or fear of the unknown

Ted Benjamin, M.D. is another practicing physician who works along natural lines in much the same way that Dr. West does. Dr. Benjamin had a woman of 43, whom he referred to as Jill, come to him with many of these symptoms. After running a number of tests on her, he determined that she was suffering from "gross B vitamin deficiencies." He placed her on foods rich in the B vitamins. He also recommended that she take pantothenic acid tablets (1,000 mg.) (see Product Appendix, p.381). He had her take one tablet in the morning with breakfast and one again in the evening. She did this for three weeks, and then he switched her to 100 mg. pantothenic acid tablet instead; she took two of these twice a day with food, thereafter.

At the end of one month's nutritional therapy, Jill reported back to him that she was feeling "100 percent better, sleeping like a log, feeling happy and good" about herself, and had "no more headaches or fears." Dr. Benjamin attributed much of this success to her daily intake of pantothenic acid and the B-rich foods she regularly consumed.

Pantothenic acid can rightfully be called "the vitamin for hard times." Of all the B vitamins, it seems to target the important areas of stress with a finesse that none of the others seem capable of doing. Consider these different stressful situations and see for yourself if B-5 doesn't address them in a much better way than the rest of the B group does.

Environmental Stress. In the 1930s, medical researchers divided a bunch of laboratory rats into three separate groups. Group I got a diet deliberately deficient in pantothenic acid. Group II got a diet with moderate pantothenic acid. And Group III received a diet very high in this important vitamin.

Then all the rats were put in cold water and made to swim until they were exhausted. Group I rats didn't last very long—only 16 minutes on the average. Group II managed to survive for about 29 minutes. But Group III did the best of all—they stayed afloat for over an hour on average!

This rat study eventually inspired another study, this time involving humans. In 1952, a group of normal men were immersed in cold water that was precisely 48° F for no more than eight minutes. Unlike the rats, they didn't have to swim around. Precise chemical measurements of their blood and urine were taken before and after the stress test.

Then, for the next 1 1/2 months, the men received 10 grams of pantothenic acid every day. After this time they were again immersed in the cold water and the same measurements were taken over again.

Now, under ordinary circumstances, such stress induces an immediate decrease in some of the white blood cells that protect the body against viral and bacterial invasions. But after taking the B-5, the men had much less of a drop in these important white blood cells. Also, levels of vitamin C—a nutrient normally burned up by stress—were noticeably higher. The men also excreted less uric acid, a sign that their bodies had not undergone as much wear and tear the second time around. Additionally, they had lower levels of "bad" (LDL) cholesterol.

Medical Stress. For 21 days before and 30 days after surgery, rabbits were fed a pantothenic-acid-deficient diet or a control diet (20 mg. B-5 added per kilogram of deficient diet). A third group was fed the control diet and given daily injections of B-5, 20 mg. per kg. of body weight. Under anesthesia, a midline incision was made in the abdomen and immediately sutured. The breaking strength of scars was measured every five days postoperatively. From the 15th to the 30th day, the breaking strength of the aponeurosis was consistently lower in the pantothenic-acid-deficient rabbits and higher in the B-vitamin-supplemented rabbits than in controls. Fibroblast count in the aponeurosis tended to be higher with B-5 supplementation and lower with the B-5 deficiency than with the control diet. Pantothenic acid supplements given both before and after surgery appeared to have a beneficial effect on wound healing, according to the *American Journal of Clinical Nutrition* (41:578-89, 1985). (Note: The aponeurosis can be either a fibrous sheet or an expanded tendon, giving attachment to muscle fibers and serving as the means of origin or insertion of a flat muscle. The fibroblast count is the correct medical terminology for an increase in cellular multiplication observed in the aponeurosis during the first postoperative period.)

Infection Stress. In July 1979, Jessie Forystek of Ocqueoc, Michigan, wrote the following letter to me:

Dear John:

I heard you on the local talk station in this area last week. You had asked listeners to write in with their favorite remedies, which you were collecting for some book. [The book was Science of Herbal Medicine, *which is now out of print.]*

Well, sir, I'd like to share with you this little cure I come up with for a fungal infection that settled sometime ago in my finger and toe nails. I tried the medications of different doctors I visited, but just got sick from all of their drugs.

So I decided to start taking 500 mg. of pantothenic acid every day for one month. I also crushed some of the tablets (about 15 at a time) into a powder, mixed a quart of water with it, set the solution in a pan and then soaked first my toes and then afterwards my fingers in it for 30 minutes every day.

Healing set in almost at once. Within 11 days most of the pain, swelling and fissures were gone.

/s/ Jess Forystek

Electromagnetic Radiation. Due to our advanced technology, we are constantly being bombarded with many invisible waves of electromagnetic radiation emitted from a wide variety of electrical objects. These can range from high-tension power lines and cellular telephones to computer screens, color TV sets, and microwave ovens. Think of such radioactive waves, coming from these and other things like electric shavers and handheld hair dryers, as tiny bullets shooting into your body and smashing cells into minute pieces.

In an experiment conducted in the early 1960s, a Hungarian scientist by the name of Dr. I. Szorady of the Department of Pediatrics at the University Medical School in Szeged, Hungary exposed 200 lab mice to total body irradiation with x-rays.

The rodents were equally divided into four groups. One group received healthy doses of pantothenic acid for a week before massive irradiation. Half were still alive following heavy exposure to x-rays. But among 50 other mice *not* afforded such nutritional protection, over half were dead within just eight days of being irradiated.

"It follows that, as compared to controls, survival was pro-longed by 200%," Dr. Szorady concluded in his report, which appeared in the East European medical journal, *Acta Paediatrica Hungaricae* (vol. 4, no. 1, 1963). "Due to its metabolic key position, pantothenic acid thus seems to induce slow biochemical processes which ensure enhanced protection against radiation injury."

In the early 1990s, a metabolite of B-5 called pantethine was discovered. The scientific literature shows that it has definite use in lowering "bad" (LDL) cholesterol and protecting the body against cardiovascular disease. Some doctors have even used it with great success in many of their recovering alcoholic patients, since it is a good detoxifier after such substance abuse. Other doctors who care for AIDS patients and those already infected with HIV but not yet manifesting any symptoms have found fairly good success with pantethine as an immune booster of killer T cells and lymphocytes.

Vitamin B-5 and its metabolite have also shown considerable promise as nutrients for athletic strength and stamina. In one study performed some years ago, highly conditioned long-distance runners were given 1,000 mg. of B-5 and 200 mg. of pantethine every day for 14 days. Their performance on a treadmill was then compared with equally well-conditioned distance runners who received only placebos during the study period. A slight but discernible difference in performance was observed. But when the same well-trained runners had their dosages doubled to 2,000 mg. every day for the same time period, more impressive results were noticed. Those getting B-5 out-performed other, equally well-trained distance runners who received placebos for comparison purposes. The B-5 athletes also used 8 percent less oxygen to perform equivalent work and had close to 17 percent less lactic acid buildup. Such evidence indicates that both pantothenic acid and pantethine deserve a prominent place in sports nutrition.

Food Sources

Milk has always been a good source for pantothenic acid. Unfortunately, many adult Americans can't tolerate very much milk in their systems, in spite of the pervasive "milk mustache" print ads put·out by the National Fluid Milk Processor Promotion Board throughout 1996 and 1997. They are unable to digest the lactose (a prominent sugar) occurring naturally in milk. Numerous allergies develop as a result of drinking cow's milk. Dairy products have also been directly linked to a number of behavioral disorders, including attention deficit disorder and hyperactivity. Worse still, cow's milk can promote a great deal of mucus that clogs the lungs, nose, sinuses, throat, and ear canals. Finally, the homogenization process that milk must pass through has been shown to be one of the major contributing factors in hardening of the arteries and heart disease.

But now there is a milk substitute available made entirely from whey (the watery part of milk left over from cheese-making). Called Fresh Country White, it looks, smells, and tastes like the real thing, but it isn't. Its ingredients are all natural, which makes it safe to use. Fresh Country White contains 25 percent of the pantothenic acid cited in the U.S. Government 's own RDAs (Recommended Dietary Allowances). (See the Product Appendix under Total Life Concepts International for more information on this remarkable milk substitute.)

Other good sources for pantothenic acid and pantethine are as follows:

Food Item	mg per 100 grams
Beef liver	7.7
Brewer's yeast	12.0
(1 tbsp. = 8 grams)	
Broccoli	1.2
Brown rice	1.1
Cashews	1.3
Eggs	1.6
Mushrooms	2.2
Oats (rolled)	1.5
Peanuts (roasted)	2.1
Pecans	1.7
Trout	1.9
Wheat germ (toasted)	1.2

Recommended Daily Intake

The nutritional guidelines set forth by the federal government some years ago indicated that somewhere between 4 and 7 mg. of pantothenic acid was adequate for most adults on a daily basis. Vitamin B-5 is converted in the body to coenzyme A, which helps metabolize fats, carbohydrates, and protein..It also helps produce fats, cholesterol, bile, vitamin D, red blood cells, neurotransmitters, and steroid hormones.

Doses of from 50 to 100 mg. of pantothenic acid combined with some royal jelly and injected intramuscularly every day in patients suffering from severe rheumatoid. arthritis resulted in greater improvement than when B-5 was used alone. However, when these injections were discontinued after awhile, the symptoms of swelling and pain soon returned. This suggests that the therapy's result was short-term relief, rather than actually doing something about the problem itself.

B-6 (PYRIDOXINE): Many Metabolic Processes Are Dependent upon This Particular Nutrient

Pyridoxine is probably one of the most important of the B vitamins. It is a cofactor for some 80 different biochemical reactions within the human body. Among these are the conversion of the amino acid tryptophan into the powerful neurotransmitter serotonin. When there is a drop in serotonin levels, migraine headaches set in. Other serotonin-related disorders include some cases of depression and attention deficit disorder (ADD) in children and teenagers.

Muscle contains between 70 and 80 percent of vitamin B-6 in the body. Most of it is in the form of pyridoxal phosphate associated with glycogen phosphorylase. While B-6 in other parts of the body is easily depleted, pools of this vitamin in skeletal muscles remain fairly stable and aren't subject to as much depletion. According to the *American Journal of Clinical Nutrition* (53:1436-42, 1991), periodic supplementation of B-6 didn't result in increased levels in muscle, although levels of it rose elsewhere in the body.

Pyridoxine plays a vital role in protein, lipid, and carbohdyrate metabolism. Therefore, depletion of B-6 in people is followed by a broad spectrum of abnormalities, including deranged amino acid metabolism, decreased enzyme activities, and a variety of other discernible manifestations. I've put together a short list of some of the

most frequent clinical symptoms associated with a deficiency of vitamin B-6. I've placed the correct medical terminology first and then
beside each one a description in lay terms of what each disorder
really is about. What this list shows is the extent to which B-6 is
needed in the system for a wide variety of functions.

Abnormal Electroencephalograms (EEGs): Recording of electrical activity within the brain that isn't the norm.

Anemia: (Hypochromic) Average corpuscular hemoglobin concentration that's less than normal. (Microcytic) Average size of circulating erythrocytes is smaller than normal.

Angular Stomatitis: Inflammation of the mucous membrane of
the mouth.

Cheilosis: Dry scaling and fissuring of the lips.

Convulsive Seizures: Violent attacks of sudden muscle spasms
during an epileptic episode.

Eczema: Acute or chronic inflammatory conditions of the skin.

Glossitis: Inflammation of the tongue.

Hyperacusis: Abnormal acuteness of hearing due to an irritability of the sensory neural mechanism.

Hyperirritability: Excessive and excited reaction beyond moderation.

Seborrheic Dermatitis: Scaly eruption of the face, scalp (dandruff), interscapular area, pubic area, and about the anus.

Since excess B-6 may prove toxic in some cases, it is better to
take less (50 mg. daily) than more, just to be on the safe side.

A combination of clinical and anecdotal evidence strongly suggests that *moderate* supplementation of vitamin B-6 (25-50 mg.) may
be helpful in the prevention and treatment of certain types of health
problems. Dosages higher than these should be taken only after con-
ferring with a health practitioner of your choice.

Arteriosclerosis. Homocysteine is a sulphur-containing amino
acid that is known to prevent fatty plaque buildup in the arterial walls
of the heart. Experimental vitamin B-6-deficient diets have resulted in
homocysteine excretion in humans and enhanced risk of arterioscle-

rosis in monkeys. Diets rich in meats and dairy products, which are associated with an increased risk of cardiovascular disease, usually have higher methionine (an essential amino acid) to vitamin B-6 ratios than diets based on vegetables and fruits. And while methionine is important in supplying the system with sulphur and methyl groups for normal metabolism, too much of it from animal flesh, milk, cheese, ice cream, and yogurt can deplete levels of B-6. Also, exposure to the environmental pollutants, carbon monoxide and carbon disulfide, that occur in big-city smog causes pyridoxine deficiency, besides being linked to the development of arteriosclerosis. Therefore, moderate intake of B-6 for several months at a time, with 30-day intervals of no consumption in between, seems a prudent course to follow. (*Medical Hypotheses* 15: 361-67, December 1984.) (See the Product Appendix for more information.)

Asthma. Pyridoxal phosphate (a form of pyridoxine) in the red blood cells of 15 adults with bronchial asthma was measured and then compared with that drawn from 16 healthy controls. The levels were low in all patients but one. Seven asthmatics were supplemented with 50 mg. pyridoxine (in the form of pyridoxine HC1) twice daily for three to ten months. Patients reported a pronounced reduction in frequency, duration, and severity of wheezing and asthmatic attacks. A drastic reduction in the need for emergency room treatment was experienced by one woman. Some patients were even able to reduce their medications. It appears that daily supplementation with vitamin B-6 in 100 mg. doses is a useful nutritional therapy for asthmatics. (*American Journal of Clinical Nutrition,* 41:684-88, April 1985)

Autism. This is a story about deeply-ingrained medical hostility toward something miraculously simple, and favoritism instead for a potent antipsychotic drug like Thorazine (chlorpromazine hydrochloride). In 1981 there were nine studies in the world medical literature showing vitamin B-6 to be helpful to autistic and autistic-type children. According to *Science News* (119:243) for April 18, 1981, "There are no studies which contradict these positive results. In none of the studies have there been any significant side effects. Vitamin B-6 is undoubtedly an extremely safe and inexpensive treatment, as well as a rational one."

The same things could not be said for the more preferred method of drug treatment involving Thorazine. The literature for the same period showed that this antipsychotic agent could induce nervous agitation and facial muscle grimacing in those who took it. In others on the drug, it was observed that tardive dyskinesia was present. This neurological syndrome is characterized by stereotyped involuntary movements consisting in sucking and smacking of the lips, lateral jaw movements, and fly-catching dartings of the tongue. In some instances, there may also be quick movements of the extremities. (See Louis S. Goodman's and Alfred Gilman's, *The Pharmacological Basis of Therapeutics,* 5th ed. New York: Macmillan Publishing Co., Inc., 1975, pp. 169-172.)

No such strange physical manifestations were discerned, however, in kids routinely given daily supplements of B-6. Not only was "highly significant improvement" demonstrated in the children's behavior, but there was also a higher "urinary excretion of abnormal metabolites" and heightened "electrical activity in their brains."

But modern medicine's failure to fully appreciate B-6 and utilize it more often in the treatment of autism stems from a definite bias against nutritional therapy. Many doctors still find it an incredible stretch of their imaginations to be asked to believe that something so simple and inexpensive as a B vitamin could work such wondrous personality miracles in a childhood emotional disturbance of such great severity. Therefore, they favor something more complex in chemical makeup and with uncertain side effects. Drugs, at least, they can understand, but vitamins they can't!

Since 1981, there have been numerous other studies in support of B-6 as rational therapy for autism. One of the best experiments took place at the Explorations Fonctionnelles Psychopathologiques in Cedex, France and was reported in *Biological Psychiatry* (20:467-78, 1985). The effects of pyridoxine and magnesium supplementation on 60 autistic children between the ages of 3 and 4 were examined in a double-blind trial. Autistic behavior was rated on a 10-item scale by two independent observers. Neither vitamin B-6, given as pyridoxine chlorhydrate in daily doses of 30 mg./kg. and even up to one gram per day, nor magnesium, in daily doses of 10 to 15 mg./kg. from magnesium lactate, produced any significant changes.

However, the *combination of the two,* given for two weeks, resulted in very significant improvement in 7 of the 10 items. Eating problems were also substantially improved. Compared to initial values for unsupplemented children, the B-6-magnesium combo reduced urinary homovanillic acid levels and decreased abnormalities in cortical evoked potentials. Dr. J. Martineau and his staff concluded that vitamins B-6 and magnesium could produce clinical improvement in autistic children after all.

Once viewed as being nothing more than "nutritional hocus-pocus," megavitamin therapy is now being used by a growing number of mental health professionals for treating some childhood behavioral afflictions of mysterious origin. This is certainly very encouraging for parents who now have safer and healthier options to pursue for their autistic children than potentially damaging brain medications.

Blood Clots. Seventy-five patients under 50 years of age with occlusive arterial disease were given vitamin B-6 in varying dosages. It helped to reduce their overall incidents of blood clot development, according to a report from the Netherlands that appeared in the *New England Journal of Medicine* (313:709-15, 1985).

Breast-Feeding. Modest supplementation (20 mg. each day) with vitamin B-6 is helpful for women who are breastfeeding their infants, but doesn't necessarily always guarantee that the babies are receiving 100 percent of the daily RDA (under 3 mg.) they're supposed to, according to the *American Journal of Clinical Nutrition* (41:21-31, 1985). This indicates that additional supplementation from food sources is a prerequisite for adequate infant B-6 needs, observed the *Journal of The American Dietetic Association* (84:1339-44, 1984).

Carpal Tunnel Syndrome. Carpal tunnel syndrome (CTS) is a very painful wrist condition typically linked with repetitive motion injuries. It is estimated that roughly two million people in America suffer from CTS, characterized by wrist pain and numbness, tingling, or burning in the fingers or hand. Many doctors are of the opinion that these symptoms could result from compression of the median nerve, which runs from the wrist to the hand through a passageway called the carpal tunnel.

Some doctors have successfully employed B-6 therapy in the treatment of many of their patients who continually suffer from the excruciatingly painful effects of CTS. Researchers at the University of Michigan surveyed 125 workers at two industrial plants about their diet and health history. The men and women then underwent nerve conduction studies and blood tests to identify those with CTS or vitamin B-6 deficiency. Almost 29 percent of the workers displayed signs of CTS. A moderately corresponding deficiency in pyridoxine was also noticed. (This study from the Ann Arbor researchers appeared in the May 1996 issue of the *Journal of Occupational and Environmental Medicine.*)

Clinical and anecdotal accounts exist to show the validity of B-6 therapy in correcting CTS. A 32-year-old man with a 3-year history of CTS was found to have marked deficiencies of the vitamins riboflavin and pyridoxine. He was given B-2 orally, 50 mg. daily for 5 months, and 500 mg. pyridoxine orally every day for the next 3 months thereafter, in addition to his usual riboflavin intake. By then all of his CTS symptoms had completely disappeared. University of Texas researchers were of the opinion that a combination of vitamins B-2 and B-6 appears to be more effective than either vitamin alone in the treatment of CTS, reported the *Proceedings of the National Academy of Sciences* (81:7076-78, 1984).

The second account comes from a friend of mine, Shauna Gee of South Salt Lake City. This full-time mother of seven is also kept busy as a Cub Scout den mother and a volunteer PTA worker. One night while I was at the Gee residence chatting with her and her husband, Merrill (a substitute teacher), Shauna mentioned her own experience with B-6 therapy in relation to CTS.

She developed carpal tunnel syndrome, she thought, some years ago when the diapering, feeding, burping, bathing, and cuddling phases of her lengthy career as a dedicated mom began. She attributed it to the extensive gripping and grabbing she had to do constantly with both of her hands in the fulfillment of all these chores. In time the pain became so great she could barely stand it.

She sought nutritional relief for her problem by going to a local health food store and purchasing some vitamin B-6. She only took one 100 mg. tablet every day, but noticed a definite diminishing of her pain. Her doctor suggested that she take one tablet of ibuprofen every day with it, which she did. The two together worked quite well for her problem. She is still occasionally troubled with CTS, but not at all like before. Her intake of B-6 is rather spotty, though, which may account for some lingering pain and periodic numbness.

Cavities. Pet hamsters were fed a cariogenic diet containing pyridoxine in a concentration of 10 parts per million (ppm). It was observed that they had fewer cavities than a similar group fed the same diet but with a small concentration of just 0.5 ppm of B-6. Other studies have focused on school-age children given a lozenge containing 3 mg. of pyridoxine three times a day after meals. At the end of a year, this group had fewer decayed, missing, or filled teeth than a control group without the benefit of B-6, according to the *Journal of Nutrition* (70:60, 1960).

Epilepsy. Newborn infants sometimes are prone to epileptic seizures in the hospital. At the Hôpital des Enfants Malades in the Paris suburb of Cedex, doctors administered between 100 and 200 mg. of pyridoxine intravenously to infants experiencing intractable epilepsy in the first few weeks of birth and up to four months. Such nutritional measures prevented these emergencies from becoming worse and even terminal. Doctors also recommended that patients with recurrent brief seizures should take oral doses (50 mg.) of B-6 every day.

Excitement. This is one of the darndest stories I've ever run across involving the consistent use of B-6 and how it helped to allay extreme excitement in a near-death situation. It's one of those "read to believe" kind of episodes. It appeared in the February 28, 1997 issue of the *Salt Lake Tribune* (page B-1). I interviewed the gentleman mentioned by phone and got the missing nutritional details from him.

Thern Blackburn is 70 years old. His wife died some years ago. He 's gotten used to being alone, but sometimes likes to take drives in Farmington Canyon (north of Salt Lake City) to help ease the loneliness a bit. On his way up the canyon one Wednesday around 1 a.m., he got lost. His car hit a patch of ice in the road and slid plumb off to the side, where it teetered precariously on the edge of a 200-foot cliff.

The man sat perfectly still for over three hours until a passer-by notified police of his dangerous situation. He had to remain absolutely calm for another three hours, while rescue crews worked very carefully to secure some lines to keep his vehicle from plunging over the edge to certain death and wreckage on the rocks below. What held his car in place was the tailpipe, which had caught on a rock and was the only thing keeping it from going into the abyss. Meanwhile, firefighters climbed into the car to get Blackburn out.

Tow crews managed to save the man's car while he was transported to Lakeview Hospital in Farmington, where he was thoroughly checked over before being released.

"It's the first time that I've done it and the last time, g-u-a-r-a-n-t-e-e-d!" he said, spelling out the last word very methodically for added emphasis. "I won't get in the car and go driving at night like that again."

Thern told me that he is a retired engineer from the Unisys Corporation. I asked how he could have remained so "perfectly calm" in light of his very desperate situation. "I attribute my lack of excitement to my B-6," he responded, "which I take a tablet [50 mg.] of every day. Before I started taking this, I used to be a very anxious fellow, one easily excitable over nothing. But a few years of B-6 have made my nerves as steady as steel."

In fact, he continued, "I've told some of my other friends about this, and have had them take B-6 or else a full B-complex formula to curb their panic attacks, fears, and high anxieties. There's nothing quite like it. If I hadn't been taking my vitamins before this happened, I probably would've panicked and, by now, they'd probably be holding my funeral, for sure."

Heart Disease. There are two kinds of cholesterol. One is bad and is known as low-density lipoprotein (LDL). The other is good and is called high-density lipoprotein (HDL). The former promotes heart disease, while the latter protects against it.

Richard C. Keniston of William Beaumont Army Medical Center in El Paso, Texas thinks he has found a way to boost your good cholesterol. In a recent study he conducted with 600 soldiers aged 35 to 45 with normal cholesterol levels, he had them take 50 mg. of B-6 every day for five months. While pyridoxine didn't lower total cholesterol, it did significantly elevate good HDLs. Also, the vitamin

improved the ratio of beneficial HDL to dangerous LDL-type cholesterol. This ratio is considered one of the best predictors of who
develops heart disease and who doesn't.

Pyridoxine works best, he said, "if your HDL is already low—
less than 35—and you have low levels of B-6 to boot." Doses of B-
6 were also especially beneficial to smokers. Their HDLs went up
just as much as if they had stopped smoking, he noted.

"I'd advise people with low HDLs to take 50 mg. a day of vitamin B-6," Keniston stated. "It's a safe dose." (This news item
appeared in the May 3, 1990 issue of the *Orlando [FL] Sentinel.*

Kidney Failure. Renal failure was diagnosed in a 3-month-old
infant girl who had severe anemia. Renal biopsy revealed fan-
shaped crystals in her kidneys. She was immediately put on 50 mg.
of pyridoxine daily for several days and then 300 mg. daily for an
indefinite period, according to the *New England Journal of Medicine*
(311:798-99, 1984). Within seven months the B-6 therapy had
reversed the course of this tiny girl's renal failure, wrote the Swiss
doctor and his colleagues who treated her in a Lausanne teaching
hospital. It is hypothesized that pyridoxine might also be beneficial
to adults suffering from kidney failure.

Kidney Disease. Eight men with end-stage renal disease underwent hemodialysis three times a week. Five of them were found to
be very low in vitamin B-6. After supplementation with pyridoxine
HC1 (50 mg./day) for 3 to 5 weeks, significant improvement in their
immune functions and overall health was observed. Doctors in the
nephrology unit at Strong Memorial Hospital in Rochester, NY, who
conducted this study, recommended that all patients undergoing
maintenance hemodialysis should be given supplemental B-6 to
reduce potential infection, according to the medical journal *Nephron*
(38:9-16, Sept. 1984).

Another study from the Tygerborg Hospital in Tygerborg, South
Africa, reported that patients suffering from nephritis (inflammation
of the kidneys) did well on pyridoxine supplementation, 25
mg./day. This report appeared in the *International Journal of
Vitamin and Nutrition Research* (54:313-19, Oct.-Dec. 1984)

Melanoma. Vitamin -6 therapy may be useful for melanoma or
skin cancer, according to a study that appeared in *Nutrition Cancer*

(7:43-52, Jan.-Jun. 1985). For two weeks before and three weeks after being injected subcutaneously with B-6 melanoma cells, mice were treated twice weekly with skin injections of pyridoxal, 0.5 grams per kilogram of rodent body weight. The average tumor weight in the pyridoxal-treated group was 62 percent less than in untreated controls. In a second experiment, mice were not given pyridoxal until two weeks after receiving melanoma cells; then pyridoxal, 0.5 g/kg body weight, was injected directly into the tumor mass daily for six days. Tumor growth was inhibited by 39 percent. Preliminary results showed that topical application of B-6 retards growth of locally recurrent malignant melanoma.

Multiple Sclerosis. Doctors writing in the *South African Medical Journal* (66:437-41, 1984) hypothesized that subclinical vitamin B-6 deficiencies could very well be responsible for greater susceptibility to multiple sclerosis in some individuals.

Myocardial Infarction. Plasma levels of pyridoxal-5-phosphate (PLP), the active form of vitamin B-6, were analyzed in blood samples taken from 15 men with myocardial infarction during the preceding 24 hours and from 28 male controls. The average PLP level in the patients was only 47 percent of that in controls, a highly significant difference. Total cholesterol levels were slightly higher, and HDL (good) cholesterol levels slightly lower, in controls than in patients, with the total/HDL cholesterol ratio being 6.4 for controls and 5.4 for patients. The authors of this study, which appeared in *Atherosclerosis* (55:357-61, 1985), postulated that plasma PLP (B-6) levels may be a far more sensitive indicator of risk for myocardial infarction than total or HDL cholesterol values. They argued in favor of B-6 therapy for prevention of myocardial infarction.

Premenstrual Syndrome (PMS). Adult working women who suffer from PMS may benefit from moderate intake of vitamin B-6 daily. Periodic (three weeks on and two weeks off) supplementation with pyridoxine—50 mg. daily—will help to decrease the fatigue, headaches, irritability, and depression that frequently accompany PMS. But anything higher than this amount and for longer periods of time could have just the reverse effect and, in fact, intensify such symptoms, according to a letter in the British medical journal, *Lancet* (1:1168-69, May 18, 1985).

Shortness. A letter submitted by two Italian medical doctors to *The New England Journal of Medicine* (444, 1982) presented clinical evidence to show that pyridoxine can increase the rise in growth hormone, but only when accompanied by physical exercise. For young children having growth problems, B-6 supplementation of around 5 mg. might just be of some positive assistance.

Smoking. Plasma pyridoxal-5-phosphate (PLP, the active form of B-6 in the body) and pyridoxal levels were measured in 106 smokers and 143 nonsmoking men aged 28 to 63 years, who didn't take supplements regularly. Average PLP levels were only 9.20 nanograms per milliliter of blood in smokers, but an astonishing 13.01 ng/mL in nonsmokers. According to South African pathologists, writing in *Atherosclerosis* (59:341-46, 1986), this was "a significant difference." Smoking *or* inhaling secondhand smoke may have a detrimental effect on the status of vitamin B-6 in the system.

Strokes. Following two years of extensive research, scientists at the Massachusetts Institute of Technology in Boston concluded that homocysteine—a by-product of high-protein diets—is really the culprit in hardening of the arteries, which in turn causes heart attacks and strokes. "Cholesterol isn't the cause of heart attacks and strokes—the villain is homocysteine," I recall Dr. Edward R. Gruberg telling me in the summer of 1979.

He and his colleague, Dr. Stephen A. Raymond, believed that "people taking vitamin B-6 will experience a lower rate of heart disease...it should lower their risk of getting a heart attack or a stroke. It's up to physicians to encourage their patients to take more B-6 or, at least, change their diets so that they will have more intake of those foods high in pyridoxine."

Drs. Gruberg and Raymond are both neurophysiologists, researchers who specialize in the study of the central nervous system. Homocysteine can harden and narrow arteries, they asserted. "It does so by somehow stimulating the growth of cells along delicate inner arterial walls," Dr. Raymond pointed out.

But vitamin B-6 easily prevents the accumulation of homocysteine in the blood. This dramatically reduces the risk of hardening of the arteries, the main cause of heart attack and strokes. Both scientists agreed with my own assessment that the FDA 's RDA of just

2 mg. daily of B-6 was "way too low." They thought it should be more in the range of 25 to 50 mg. per day instead. Whole grains, nuts, fruits, and vegetables contain adequate amounts of B-6.

Water Retention. In July, 1979, Phyllis Barrett of Pinckney, Michigan wrote me the following letter to describe her own experience with B-6 in regard to fluid retention.

"Dear Mr. Heinerman:

For over a decade I'd been taking a drug for my edema. When my doctor first prescribed it, he told me that along with losing the fluid I would also lose many nutrients as well. And I was to eat a banana or an orange after taking each small pill. He failed, though, to mention that my skin would become as dry as bark.

"Needless to say, I despised having to take them. But days would come when I would fill up so badly with fluid I actually felt like I was being squashed underfoot like a bug. My breathing became very difficult. And my eyelids would get so puffy it was very hard to keep them open. So, in desperation, I would run for the 'safety'(?) of my water pills, which didn't seem to give any relief unless I took four before going to sleep. I would weigh from 7 to 12 pounds less, and wouldn't feel squashed anymore after that.

"But for years the thought in my mind was "Why is this happening to me?" I figured there must be something in my body that wasn't working quite right. Why not treat the cause instead of the symptom, I reasoned.

"When I brought these questions up in discussion with my doctor, he would start in on how many women retain water before and during their periods. I couldn't make the fool understand that my problem was all the time, not just once a month.

"I figured the sooner I got away from this arrogant, male chauvinist pig, the better off I'd be. I really grew to hate the guy, from his many off-the-wall comments about women and all.

"Then I heard you give a lecture for Nature's Sunshine [a direct-marketing health products company]. In it you referred to vitamin B-6 being used to reduce fluid retention in pregnant women. So, based on your information, I went out and purchased a bottle of 50 mg. tablets and started taking two tablets a day. Nothing happened, though, so I doubled my tablet intake. Again nothing occurred.

"So, I went back to my notes of your lecture and reread what I had jotted down. It was then that I discovered you had mentioned tak-

ing 50 mg. every hour. So, I began taking one tablet every waking hour, just like you said to do.

"Words couldn't even begin to express my feelings when 'Boulder Dam' finally broke and I commenced making numerous trips to the bathroom without even opening the bottle of water pills.

"To cut down on having to take so many pills a day, I finally bought 500 mg. tablets of B-6. At this time I am taking two a day. I have lost ten pounds and haven't taken a water pill in two months."

/s/ P. Barrett

[Caution: My recommendation for such excessive intake of B-6 was *only* for water retention. Even then, it is highly advisable to consult with a health practitioner of your choice before taking excessive amounts of B-6.]

Food Sources

Everything in nature is in balance; it is only when people interfere with the intricate workings of nature that such a delicate balance is thrown out of kilter. Take, for instance, whole wheat bread, which is high in vitamin B-2. During the milling process much of its natural riboflavin is lost. Consequently, a certain amount of synthetic B-2 must be added to replace that which disappeared.

This enrichment of cereal grains and other processed foods with ample amounts of synthetic riboflavin has created a much higher daily intake per capita of this B vitamin than was the case in 1936. In one way this is good, because *riboflavin is absolutely essential for the conversion of another B vitamin, pyridoxine, to its many coenzymes* (which is how B-6 functions within the body).

But, on the other hand, there appears to be a critical shortage of B-6 in the American diet. The B-6 content of meals served in the cafeterias of 50 American colleges and universities from coast to coast was carefully evaluated and discovered to average only 1.43 mg. per person per day. Pyridoxine values ranged from a dismal 0.65 to a positive 2.91 mg. (The suggested RDA intake for adult men and women is 2.2 mg. every day.) But, according to the *Journal of the American Dietetic Association* (66:146, 1975), more than 80 percent of these values were way below the daily RDA figure. The article also mentioned that about one-quarter of these campus cafeterias served meals with just 50 percent of the needed B-6.

Pyridoxine is very sensitive to light and heat. Some of it is destroyed when foods are cooked at extremely high temperatures, which is common in the giant food processing industry but not so common in home meal preparations. Also, the extraordinary consumption of fast foods, junk foods, and colas and soft drinks has had a tendency to further deplete stores of B-6 from the liver, where it appears in the highest concentration within the human body.

So while there is plenty of riboflavin floating around in what is carelessly consumed these days by a nutritionally-ignorant public, there is a nearly equal dearth of vitamin B-6. It is the aim of this section to present some individual food and meal considerations that will provide adequate sources of this important nutrient.

Food Portions	*B-6 Contents*
Amaranth (3 1/2 oz. or 1/2 cup)	0.2 mg.
Barley, pearl (3 1/2 oz. cooked or 1/2 cup)	0.3 mg.
Broccoli (3 1/2 oz. raw, 1 cup chopped)	0.2 mg.
Chestnuts (3 1/2 oz. roasted, 3/4 cup)	0.5 mg.
Ham (cured, extra lean, 3 1/2 oz.)	0.4 mg.
Lentils (3 1/2 oz. cooked, 1/2 cup)	0.2 mg.
Peanuts (3 1/2 oz. dry roasted, 2/3 cup)	0.3 mg.
Pork (top loin, 3 1/2 oz. cooked)	0.4 mg.
Quiñoa (3 1/2 oz. dry, 1/2 cup)	0.2 mg.
Rice, brown (3 1/2 oz. dry, 1/2 cup)	0.5 mg.
Rice, white (3 1/2 oz. dry, 1/2 cup)	0.4 mg.
Sunflower seeds (3 1/2 oz. dry roasted, 3/4 cup)	0.8 mg.
Walnuts, English or Persian (3 1/2 oz. shelled raw)	0.6 mg.

The following three recipes have been carefully put together for their rich B-6 contents due to some key ingredients. Beans, lentils, rice, and duck are all excellent sources of pyridoxine. Consider these meals as typical examples of what can be done with certain foods to insure that you get generous amounts of vitamin B-6.

Vegetarian Lentils

1 1/4 cups wild rice

1 1/4 cups red lentils

3 1/4 cups warm water

1/2 cup olive oil

1 medium-sized onion, peeled and chopped

3/4 tsp. crushed fresh ginger root

3/4 tsp. minced garlic

1-inch piece cinnamon stick

6 cloves

1 bay leaf

1 1/4 tsps. ground coriander

1/2 tsp. turmeric

3/4 tsp. granulated kelp (a seaweed)

Wash the rice and the lentils thoroughly in cold water, then drain well. Put both into a large bowl and cover with the warm water. Soak for 40 minutes, then drain thoroughly, but reserve the water.

Gently heat the olive oil in a large stainless steel saucepan. Stir in the onion and fry slowly on Low heat for about 3 minutes, stirring often to prevent its burning.

Next, add the ginger, garlic, cinnamon stick, cloves, and bay leaf to the onion and continue frying for one minute.

Following this, add the rice and lentils to the fried onion, along with the coriander, turmeric, and kelp. Stir over the heat for about 2 1/2 minutes, or until the rice and lentils are evenly coated with oil.

Pour the reserved water into the rice mixture and bring to a rolling boil. Reduce the heat and cover the pan with a tight-fitting lid. Simmer for 8 to 10 minutes without stirring, or until the water has been totally absorbed.

Stir the rice and lentils together, remove and serve at once. Serves 4.

Oriental Duck with Oranges

3 navel oranges

1 duck

1 tbsp. butter

1 1/4 tbsps. sesame seed oil

1 1/4 cups light chicken stock

2/3 cup Tsingtao or Sapporo (flavorful Chinese or Japanese beers)

2 1/2 tbsps. red currant jelly

salt and freshly ground black pepper to taste

1 1/4 tsps. arrowroot

1 1/4 tbsps. cold water

Using a potato peeler, carefully pare the rind thinly off 2 of the oranges. Cut the rind into very large fine shreds using a sharp paring knife. Put the shredded orange rind into a small bowl and cover with boiling water. Set aside to blanch for 5 minutes, then drain.

Squeeze the juice from the 2 oranges. Set this aside.

Cut away the peel and the pith from the remaining orange and then slice the flesh into thin rounds. Set this aside also.

Next wash the duck inside and out and pat thoroughly dry with paper towels or a clean hand towel.

Put the butter and the oil into a large wok and heat until melted. Add the duck and fry, turning frequently until it is brown all over.

Remove it from the wok and cool down for about 10 minutes. Then using poultry shears, cut away the leg and wing ends. Cut the duck in half lengthwise and then cut each half into 1-inch strips.

Remove the fat from the wok and return the duck to the wok. Add the stock, Chinese or Japanese beer, red currant jelly, squeezed orange juice, and the well-drained strips of rind. Bring to a boil, then season to taste. Reduce the heat, cover the wok and simmer the duck gently for another 20 minutes, or until it is well cooked.

Skim away any surface fat and thicken the sauce by mixing the arrowroot with the water and stirring them into the wok. Bring the mixture back to a boil and simmer for another 7 minutes, or until the sauce is fairly thick.

Arrange the duck on plates and garnish with orange slices and fresh watercress leaves, if desired. Serves 4.

KIDNEY BEAN AND WALNUT CHILI

1 tsp. sesame seed oil

1/2 teaspoon granulated kelp (a seaweed)

1 medium onion, finely chopped

3 cloves garlic, minced

2 bay leaves

1 tbsp. mild chili powder

1 tsp. powdered cumin

1/2 tsp. dried oregano

1/2 cup lightly toasted walnuts, measured, and then coarsely chopped

2 cups cooked, drained kidney beans (from 1 cup dry)

bean cooking juices, soup stock, or combination to cover minced scallions or chives

In a 2-quart stainless steel pot, sauté the onions in oil or water; add the kelp to draw out their moisture. Stir until tender. Add the garlic and spices and stir. Add the nuts, beans, and bean liquid and/or stock to barely cover. Bring to a boil. It might be a good idea to slip a heat deflector beneath the pot. Reduce the heat and simmer for 2 1/2 hours on low. Stir periodically and add more liquid if the chili needs to be moistened. The beans should be thick, soft, and almost as stiff as refried beans. Remove the lid and simmer away excess juice if necessary.

For a vegetarian meal, serve with a grain dish and a green, leafy vegetable. Or, serve this chili with baked fish or chicken, salad or cooked greens, and a grain. All of these side dishes increase the vitamin B-6 content of this meal. Serves 4 to 8.

Recommended Daily Intake

The current RDA for vitamin B-6 is 2.2 mg. for adult men and 2 mg. for adult women. However, the Optimum Daily Allowance for this nutrient *begins* at 25 mg. for both genders and goes up from there to 300 mg.

Certain foods could possibly interfere with B-6 absorption and utilization. A study published in *Nutrition Reports International* (30:483-91, 1984) examined the consumption of brans (wheat, corn, and rice) in 21 healthy subjects eating a controlled diet with or without them. It was observed by nutritionists at the University of Nebraska in Lincoln, that these different brans (especially wheat) adversely affected the availability of pyridoxine from other foods.

Hence, some moderate supplementation (25 mg. every two days) may be necessary in some cases.

Lengthy and excessive intake can do more harm than good, as the following case study demonstrated from a letter printed in *The New England Journal of Medicine* (311:986-87, 1984). A 34-year-old woman had taken a multivitamin providing 200 mg. of vitamin B-6 per day. After two years, she increased her daily intake to 500 mg. and took an additional 300 mg. no more than once a week. Soon she began experiencing sensations of electric shocks shooting down her spine when she bent her neck. She also developed progressive gait unsteadiness, which was worse in the dark. She also had numbness and paresthesias of both feet, gradually ascending to her hips. Then numbness of her hands, lips, and left cheek set in. She promptly discontinued all of her B-6 supplements and within several months she recovered from all of these unpleasant symptoms.

B-8 (BIOTIN): The Energy and Beauty Nutrient

Inside all living cells exist tiny "energy factories" called mitochondria. These extremely minute, sausage-shaped bodies produce a vital molecule, adenosine-triphosphate (ATP). This is the stuff that living cells constantly need in order to function properly. Another way to think of ATP is as a sort of basic "energy currency" being continually spent by living cells. ATP fuels every single thing we do. Cells that run short of it cannot perform their assigned tasks.

A single human cell contains 300 to 600 mitochondria. These cellular "power plants" depend on a little-known B vitamin, biotin, as well as other essential nutrients, in order to produce enough ATP. Biotin is necessary in the transformation of consumed carbohydrates, fats, and proteins into energy. All of these items are metabolized with the help of vitamin B-8 and then stored in the liver and muscle tissue in the form of glycogen. When needed, this principal carbohydrate reserve is readily converted into glucose, which the body then chemically "burns" as a fuel to produce physical energy.

When B vitamins are discussed in many books on general nutrition, short shrift or total lack of mention are usually given to biotin, which operates very discreetly within the human system.

Unfortunately, it just isn't one of the more glamorous nutrients like vitamins A, C, or E, which receive ample attention from journalists and health writers. As one health expert told me sometime ago, "Vitamin B-8 isn't sexy enough to grab headlines!"

Some health writers may tell you that biotin is essential to human health. And they might even point out that the state of health of your hair, skin, nails, bone marrow, and glands is quite dependent on biotin. But, as yet, I haven't found *any* of those few who mention biotin more than in passing, informing their readers just *why* this particular B vitamin is critical for the body's operating needs.

A crash course in one aspect of body biochemistry, therefore, seems to be in order here. Throughout the body, there exist (by last count in 1993) about 3,000 enzymes. Enzymes are nothing more than proteins which, in turn, are composed of individual chains of amino acids. There are 20 basic amino acids. Two or more amino acids become interconnected in specific links called amino acid chains. These chains then become arranged to form the various proteins and polypeptides found within the body. Each enzyme is composed of a very specific set of amino acid chains. All enzymes merely differ in the number and sequence of these 20 amino acids which are assembled into chains of varying lengths. For this reason, they all differ slightly from each other in appearance. Several amino acids are strung together like a string of pearls (the amino acid chain), which itself is wound together like a ball of yarn, with an indentation at one point. This is about how an enzyme would look under a. powerful electron microscope.

All 3,000 or more different enzymes are constantly being produced en masse by the human body. This is quite an amazing feat, but with one small drawback to it. Some of these enzymes lack a small portion of something to make them function as normal catalysts. What they are in need of is *coenzymes*. These special "enzyme helpers" come mostly from the B vitamin group, with some of them being produced within the gastrointestinal tract.

Biotin is one of these enzyme helpers, to a number of different enzyme systems. Without adequate amounts of biotin, the body's energy production will lag and its outward appearance will, in time, become rather scruffy looking. As with the other B vitamins covered in this section, biotin is interdependent on the rest of them. So, even if you get enough B-8, you may end up somewhat deficient in B-2, B-5, or B-6. That's why it's always a good practice to take a *complete* B-complex and some extra biotin on the side, if necessary.

Food Sources

Symptoms of biotin deficiency include manifestations of anorexia, nausea, vomiting, an inflamed and swollen tongue, gray pallor, depression, hair loss, dry and scaly skin, wrinkles, and brittle nails.

The best dietary sources for biotin are beef liver and kidney, egg yolks, soybeans, and brewer's yeast. Moderate amounts may be found in cereals like oats, barley, wheat, and rye, legumes such as beans and lentils, and nuts (almonds, cashews, and walnuts, among others). Most fruits, vegetables, and meats have very little biotin in them. The exceptions to this are cauliflower and mushrooms.

Recommended Daily Intake

A special report entitled "Vitamins and Minerals" issued by the editors of the *Harvard Health Letter* in 1995 stated that biotin was safe to take "at doses up to 10 milligrams."

B-9 (FOLIC ACID): Molecular Midwife, Oncologist, and Cardiologist All in One

Throughout this rather extensive section on the vitamin B group, occasional mention has been made of the fact that all of the nutrients comprising it are interdependent on one another. This certainly is the case with folic acid and B-12, as explained more fully under the Recommended Dietary Intake subsection.

Research by different teams of scientists working independently in America, Great Britain, and India in the 1940s eventually led to the near-simultaneous discoveries of vitamins B-9 and B-12, with mere months separating them in some cases. Originally, it took over *four tons* of spinach to isolate a few precious milligrams of folic acid! Such were the crude isolation techniques half a century ago.

The significance of folic acid in the human diet may be categorized in the following three areas of health importance: childbirth, cancer, and heart disease. Hence, the subtitle chosen for this particular B vitamin.

Birth Defects. For many years, around 100,000 babies a year born in mainland China routinely died of neural tube defects. Yet no one bothered to connect this with a B vitamin deficiency until sometime in the 1960s. In the United States an increase of one type of the same birth defect in South Texas finally brought national attention to the connection with folic acid deficiency.

There are two basic types of neural tube defect which occur very early in pregnancy. The first is anencephaly, a condition in which a major portion of the brain never develops. The other is spina bifida, a potentially crippling defect in which the spinal cord is improperly encased in bone.

An enlightening report appearing in a 1993 issue of the *Journal of the American Medical Association* provided nearly conclusive evidence that vitamin B-9 can prevent both kinds of birth defects. The study examined folic acid supplements in over 400 women who had previously given birth to babies with either neural tube defect.

Women in the study group who took daily multivitamin supplements containing a minimum of 400 micrograms of B-9 for at least a month before or a month after conception had a 60 percent reduction in their risk of such defects. (Prenatal supplements, however, usually contain much higher amounts—1,000 mcg. or more.)

In one of the largest previous studies, some 4,000 women enrolled in a Hungarian family planning program and expecting to get pregnant were given either multivitamins containing 800 mcg. of folic acid or trace element supplements (containing copper, manganese, zinc, and under 8 milligrams of vitamin C). Of the women who became pregnant, those who had taken the folic acid supplement for almost one month in advance and nearly a month after conception had a greatly reduced rate of neural tube defects. In fact, none of the women in the supplemented group gave birth to infants with such defects, while in the trace element group six cases were reported.

This discovery prompted the medical researchers to reach the conclusion that "all women planning pregnancy should receive a vitamin supplement containing folic acid." Similar studies, but not on as grand a scale, have offered equally strong evidence that vitamin B-9 combats birth defects, including, quite possibly, *genetic* birth defects.

In 1992 the U.S. Public Health Service recommended that all women of childbearing age consume 0.4 mg. of folic acid daily to reduce their risk of giving birth to children with such defects. In addition to fortified grain products, the same agency recommended that women should obtain this amount through food sources or a dietary supplement (such as a multivitamin) or a combination of both sources. In 1996 the Food and Drug Administration (FDA) issued a mandate to food manufacturers requiring them to enrich flours, pasta, rice, and cornmeal with folic acid, starting by January 1, 1998. The Centers for Disease Control and Prevention (CDC) in Atlanta applauded the FDA decision and noted that more than 4,000 fetuses are born with neural tube defects annually.

Beside the aforementioned neural tube defects, folic acid can also prevent cleft palate, low birth weight in premature deliveries, and even miscarriages. A pregnant woman should always keep in mind that when it comes to folic acid, she really is supplementing for two people—herself and her unborn child.

Cancer. Bruce Ames, who was "pushing toward a hard 68" at the time of a telephone interview with him in late 1996, certainly proved to be as much of a contradiction in some things as this author has in his own ways. Dr. Ames is a noted professor of bio-chemistry and molecular biology at the University of California at Berkeley. He has published almost 360 scientific papers and is one of the world's most frequently cited scientists in scientific literature.

Since 1983 he has been a staunch advocate of vitamin therapy for retarding the progress of cancer. He believes that vitamins A, C, and E and B vitamins such as folic acid hold the keys to cancer pre-vention. His work as a renowned molecular biologist has led him to conclude that cancer is caused by three major factors: smoking, chronic infections, and nutritionally-deficient diets. Smoking and infection generate huge numbers of free radicals (the latter does so when white blood cells make them to kill germs). In the body there are special enzymes that cruise up and down strands of DNA and repair most of the damage inflicted by such scavenger molecules.

However, these enzymes depend in large part on the presence of adequate amounts of B vitamins. "Breaks in your chromosomes from excessive free radicals eventually lead to cell mutations," he stated. "But folic acid (along with niacin) will prevent such chromosome breakage. People who subsist on junk food are really hurting themselves more than they could ever imagine. It would be nice to see everyone taking a multivitamin high in folacin every day. Then they would be doing themselves a big favor."

That's the good news coming from him; now for the bad news. Dr. Ames is convinced that chemical pesticides aren't as dangerous as the American public has made them out to be. He bases his conclusions on years of scientific research. And he is honest and forthright in this extremely controversial position, which he staked out some years ago in a major article in *Science* (221:1256-67, 1983). In that report, he noted that many edible plants had far more cancer-causing substances to be feared than the "miniscule residues left on food by synthetic pesticides." In fact, he thinks that if consumers would worry more about eating nutritiously than whether their foods are sprayed with pesticides or not, "they will undoubtedly be better off."

Several studies published in the medical literature suggest that high intakes of folic acid (also known as folacin and folate) might prove useful in the prevention of colorectal and cervical cancers. In a 1993 study that appeared in the *Journal of the National Cancer Institute* researchers looked at several thousand men and women and discovered that those with the highest folacin intakes (from both foods and supplements) had the lowest risk of developing intestinal polyps (colorectal adenomas) that eventually become cancerous. The scientists speculated that vitamin B-9 is somehow involved in the complex chemical process that "switches off" cancer genes.

A 1991 study from the University of Alabama at Birmingham provided evidence that women who are chronically deficient in folic acid have a much higher risk of developing cellular changes (dysplasia) of the cervix that often are forerunners of cervical cancer. But thanks in large part to widespread screening using the Pap smear, cervical cancer has become very preventable and even curable. In the Birmingham study, women with high amounts of folacin in their circulating blood plasmas had a much lower rate of cervical dysplasia, even when they were infected with human papilloma virus that is believed to be connected with this cancer in some way. The researchers believed that folic acid protects the genetic material of cervical cells, making it less vulnerable to this particular genital virus.

Other medical researchers at the same university in Birmingham studied 73 men who had been heavy smokers for a number of years. They were interested in looking for precancerous changes in the bronchial tubes of these men. Roughly 50 percent of the study group received oral doses of 10 mg. of folic acid and 500 mcg. of its augmenting nutrient, vitamin B-12, daily. The rest received placebos.

Four months later, there was a substantial reduction in the number of vitamin-supplemented patients who had abnormal bronchial cells. Smokers and those unfortunate enough to inhale such secondhand stench would do well to take a folic acid supplement every day.

Coronary Artery Disease. Heart disease currently ranks ahead of cancer as America's number one health problem. Until now cholesterol (particularly the LDL or "bad" kind) has been blamed as the major factor for causing this. But a mounting body of medical evidence points to an even worse culprit. Science reporter Ned Potter explained it in layperson's terms on a segment of the "ABC Evening News with Peter Jennings" on Wednesday, March 12, 1997. The new villain in promoting arteriosclerosis that eventually leads to heart attacks and coronary artery disease is called homocysteine. It is a short-lived by-product (a natural amino acid metabolite) of methionine (one of the essential amino acids the body needs on a regular basis).

Homocysteine comes from the consumption of meat (especially pork and pork-related items such as sausage and luncheon meats, and chicken), dairy products, eggs, and chocolate. According to the ABC report, "excess homocysteine in the system damages the inner linings of heart veins," which leads to fatty plaque buildup more quickly. Also mentioned was the fact that too much homocysteine leads to a narrowing of the carotid artery that feeds blood to the head and neck. In both cases, the tremendous harm done eventually "leads to a heart attack, heart disease, or stroke."

But as Potter pointed out, something as simple as "folic acid, one of the B vitamins, has been linked to decreasing dangerous levels of this substance" within the body. It has been calculated that close to 40 percent of the population is walking around every day with "elevated homocysteine levels in them, and totally unaware of it." Instead, "they are more concerned with their cholesterol counts, when their focus should really be on this instead."

While it was correctly noted that folic acid and vitamin B-6 cannot prevent arteriosclerosis directly, they certainly can "dramatically lower existing levels of this nasty amino acid" metabolite "in the blood of those individuals at highest risk for heart attacks and strokes." There is now available in most hospitals and clinics around the country "a new analytical technique for assessing homocysteine and folic acid levels, that's quicker and cheaper than older methods." Viewers were encouraged to start thinking in terms of their homocysteine levels and worry less about their cholesterol counts.

In a breakdown along gender and longevity lines, men over 65 and women over 70 years of age were more likely to be deficient in folic acid than those in middle age. Ethnicity also plays a role here, with African Americans being twice to three times as likely to have elevated homocysteine levels than whites or Hispanics. Interestingly enough, Orientals appear to have the least amount of homocysteine and the greatest presence of folic acid. Cultural differences obviously play a big role in determining the diets each group consumes.

Mental Retardation. Fragile X syndrome is a chromosomal deficit that is genetically inherited in males. It is second only to Down 's syndrome as an identified cause of mild to severe mental retardation. According to an article in the *American Journal of Medicine* (77:602-11, 1984), large doses of folic acid have improved the behavior of adult males and females who happen to be carriers of both syndromes. An interesting sidelight to this vitamin therapy showed that an average of 10 mg. of folic acid every day improved mental IQ and emotional behavior in prepubertal boys, but not in older children. Another study employed 250 mg. of folacin daily in subjects ranging in age from 8 to 13. Here again, improvements were observed in the younger ones but not the older ones.

Psychosis is a very common mental disorder in adult men and women. It is usually characterized by gross impairment of reality comprehension, being marked by delusions, hallucinations, verbal babbling, or disorganized and agitated behavior. According to nutritional therapists Eric R. Braverman, M.D. and Carl C. Pfeiffer, M.D., Ph.D. in their classic work, *The Healing Nutrients Within* (New Canaan: Keats Publishing, Inc., 1987; pp. 161-62), vitamins B-6 (pyridoxine), B-9 (folic acid), B-12 (cyanocobalamin), and the trace element zinc all seem be very useful nutrients in the natural treatment of psychosis.

Nervous Agitation afflicts tens of millions of Americans, teenagers, college-age youth, and older adults, but without any apparent evidence of mental disturbance. The respected British medical journal *The Lancet* drew attention to Vitamin B-9 as being extremely helpful to induce a state of calmness in a short article entitled, "Folic Acid and the Nervous System."

Miscarriage. Drs. Braverman and Pfeiffer (cited in the paragraph on Psychosis) wrote that "many women with histories of [spontaneous] abortion and miscarriage have been able to complete successful childbirth subsequent to folate supplementation." (p. 123).

Not long ago I met a woman at a book signing who gave her first name as Julie, and had an interesting tale to tell about how folacin helped her to achieve a normal birth after two previous miscarriages. A friend of hers was a distributor of nutritional and food products from a Colorado-based nutritional concern (see the Product Appendix).

This friend introduced Julie to several products that *collectively,* when taken together every day, gave her ample amounts of folic acid. Julie started taking 2 capsules each day and in the morning she also drank a glass of a milk substitute from whey, which is loaded with B vitamins. In the evening she had another glass. She kept this daily regimen up faithfully for "almost seven months during my third pregnancy in five years."

"And you know what happened?" she asked. I shrugged in apparent ignorance of the fact. She then called over her husband

Frank, who was pushing a baby stroller with a cute little infant girl in it. "This is the joy and pride of our lives," she beamed with obvious happiness.

Believing that her diet may have played as much of a role in this grand event as these supplements did, I questioned her at some length as to what she had consumed during this period of time. She mentioned a number of foods that are known to have some folacin content in them. But what really intrigued me was when she mentioned the testing that took place on two separate occasions within this time frame. In both instances, the tests showed *low* levels of folacin in spite of the fact that she was eating many folacin-containing foods. It was when she said that her doctor claimed "most prepared foods were already deficient in folacin" that she really got my attention. Under the Food Sources subheading the reader will find some valuable information regarding the shortage of folic acid in cooked or processed foods. It is, therefore, apparent that folic acid supplementation of some kind is *absolutely critical* for pregnant women in order to reduce the risk of possible miscarriages!

Sickle Cell Anemia. Sickle cell anemia is a hereditary, genetically determined blood disease that occurs almost exclusively in African Americans. (The disorder derives its name from the sickle shape of red blood cells in patients.) Folic acid therapy has been of considerable benefit to many who suffer from this disease. Note: Those with leukemia should ask their doctors about folic acid before taking any of it!

Vitamin B-12 Deficiency. High levels of folic acid can mask the symptoms of B-12 deficiency. Therefore, it is always advisable to take small amounts of B-12 every time folic acid is used in supplement form.

Food Sources

Most of us in our lifetimes have heard the old joke that starts, "I've got good news and bad news—which do you want to hear first?" It's just about that way when it comes to reporting food sources for folacin.

First, though, the good news. According to *Science News* (120:167, 1981) "up to 25 percent of the daily folacin requirement can be met by drinking five cups of green tea." Parsnips are also another rich source of vitamin B-9. (For those unacquainted with this vegetable, it looks like an anemic carrot, being creamy white in appearance, but is quite delicious when boiled, mashed, and sprinkled with melted butter, brown sugar, and cinnamon.)

Other nutritional sources of folic acid appear in the table below, which was adapted from one in Jane Brody's article, "The incredible, edible miracle cure," that appeared in *Family Circle* magazine, June 7, 1994.

Food Source	*Folacin Content (given in micrograms)*
All-Bran cereal (1 cup)	301
Asparagus, cooked	131
Black beans, cooked	128
Broccoli (1 spear)	107
Grape Nuts (1 cup)	402
Lentils, cooked	179
Orange sections	55
Orange juice from concentrate	109
Papaya	53
Pineapple juice, canned	58
Raspberries, frozen	65
Spinach, chopped, raw	82
Spinach, cooked	131
Total cereal (1 cup)	466
Wheat germ (1/3 cup)	108
Wheaties cereal (1 cup)	102
White beans, cooked	128

Now for the somewhat bad news. Shirley A. Beresford, Ph.D., an associate professor in the department of epidemiology at the University of Washington in Seattle, "estimates that as much as 50 percent of the folic acid taken nutritionally" through the diet "may be completely wasted." And Paul Hopkins, M.D., an associate professor of internal medicine and codirector of the Family Lipid Clinic in the Department of Preventive Cardiology/Cardiovascular Genetics at the University of Utah in Salt Lake City, declares that "nearly all forms of cooking and processing destroy the rather delicate vitamin." In fact, according to the new medical journal *Alternative & Complementary Therapies* (2(4):222, 1996), "Steaming and frying, two extremely common ways of preparing vegetables, can almost completely destroy the folic acid they may contain, and boiling for 8 minutes leads to a loss of 80 percent!"

Some years ago the folacin content of meals offered at 50 American colleges was carefully measured by nutritionists. It was discovered that nearly 75 percent of all meals served in the cafeterias of these institutions of higher learning failed to meet the government's RDA for this important nutrient.

Besides an obvious deficiency in the American diet of folacin due to processing and overcooking, there is another equally vexing problem when the same becomes reasonably available. Folic acid requires the presence of vitamins B-6 and B-12 in order to be converted into its active metabolite so that it can be readily absorbed into the bloodstream and become functionally active. A good percentage of the American population, however, are deficient in these other B vitamins. Therefore, it makes good sense to eat a variety of foods each day containing all three of the B group. Preferably, consume them raw or cooked as little as possible. Also, additional supplementation with a high potency B complex makes good sense.

Recommended Dietary Intake

Another term for folic acid is folacin. This name comes from the same root as *foliage*. This indicates that the vitamin is readily supplied by leafy green vegetables like spinach and kale, as well as the stalks and buds of asparagus and broccoli. The *ideal* nutritional therapy for dietary folate deficiency would be for everyone to consume just one fresh fruit or one fresh vegetable daily. According to Victor Herbert, M.D., "Such a diet would probably wipe nutritional folate deficiency from the face of the earth," according to what he wrote in "Folic Acid and Vitamin B-12," in *Modern Nutrition in Health and Disease—*

Dietotherapy, 5th ed. (Robert S. Goodhart, M.D. and Maurice E. Shils, M.D., eds. Philadelphia: Lea & Febiger, 1976; p. 242).

While Dr. Herbert may believe strongly in *food* sources for folic acid, he is just as adamantly opposed to nutritional supplements in general. For those not familiar with his decades-long tirades against the vitamin industry, he has fiercely lambasted such products in the media whenever an opportunity presented itself.

The government 's own RDA for folacin is 200 micrograms for men and 180 micrograms for women. (A microgram, or mcg., is one-thousandth of a milligram.) But now, more and more nutritionists and a few doctors are recommending intakes that are double that, or closer to 400 mcg. They believe that this is a more realistic and "significantly therapeutic" level of folic acid to ingest than the government's recommended lower amounts.

What 's ironic about this, though, according to Jeffrey S. Bland, Ph.D., a noted nutritional authority from Gig Harbor, Washington, is that while "more and more physicians and their families now take supplements, they still aren't recommending them to their patients." A random telephone sampling of 51 physicians in the Greater Salt Lake Valley, conducted by Anthropological Research Center in early January, 1997, revealed that an astonishing 57 percent used nutritional supplements to some extent within their own families, but that just a mere 9 percent felt justified in prescribing vitamins and minerals to their patients. Dr. Bland explained it this way: "They may feel comfortable using nutritional supplements themselves, but don't want to be criticized for practicing 'unscientific medicine.'"

Folic acid is one of those nutrients that works best in conjunction with other B vitamins to accomplish the greatest amount of good. Remember the dangerous homocysteine levels implicated earlier in coronary artery disease? According to Richard Podell, a clinical professor at the Department of Family Medicine at New Jersey's UMDNJ-Robert Wood Johnson Medical School, "one milligram each day of folic acid (2.5 times the RDA), 10 mg. of vitamin B-6 (5 times the RDA), and 0.4 mg. vitamin B-12 (8 times the RDA)" can reduce them in 90 percent of people carrying abnormal amounts of this amino acid by-product within them.

Older folks who depend on prescription or over-the-counter medications for different problems should understand that many of these drugs will cause folic acid deficiencies. For instance, sulphasalazine (SSZ), a drug often used by doctors to treat chronic inflammatory bowel disease and rheumatoid arthritis, has been shown to induce functional folic acid deficiency in a number of patients. SSZ inhibits an enzyme that converts one molecule form of folic acid to its absorbable form. SSZ thus inhibits intestinal absorption of the vitamin. So be sure to take extra folic acid if you happen to be on medication for some reason (see Product Appendix, p.381).

B-12 (CYANOCOBALAMIN): Its Biological Significance

This is undoubtedly the most potent of all the B group, and certainly a very powerful nutrient required by humans and other mammals. While other vitamin requirements are generally measured in thousandths of a gram, B-12 needs are always calculated in millionths of a gram (as in 1 *microgram*). "The vitamin B-12 molecule," according to Dr. Victor Herbert, a very orthodox nutritional expert, "is almost indestructible." Therefore, it would be fair to say that a little bit of this nutrient every *week* (as opposed to daily for other vitamins) goes a long, long way in providing nutritional benefits to the body.

In 1926 a couple of scientists found that pernicious anemia (PA) could be controlled by the ingestion of beef liver. Thereafter, a number of different laboratories were engaged in a feverish race to discover what factor in this particular animal organ meat was responsible for this. It wasn't until 1948 that other scientists finally isolated the substance that, in very tiny amounts, relieves PA. It was given the name of vitamin B-12.

Cyanocobalamin (the more correct chemical term for B-12) is a red crystalline compound whose complex formula contains two very important minerals—cobalt and phosphorus. Without the presence of a minute amount of cobalt, vitamin B-12 could not be synthesized by bacteria within the gastrointestinal tract. Cobalt also activates a number of important enzymes that help convert zinc into other compounds for stronger immunity and more rapid wound healing. Cobalt also stimulates the production of more red blood cells in the surface blood supply. Phosphorus, on the other hand, plays major

roles in the storage and release of energy as well as in the hardening of bones and teeth. It also occurs in nucleic acids in the nuclei
of cells; the important compounds of life, namely DNA and RNA,
contain a great deal of phosphorus.

The purpose of mentioning a few things about both minerals
here is to help the reader better appreciate their connection with
cyanocobalamin. Quite frankly, vitamin B-12 would be virtually
nonexistent without them. (More information on cobalt and phosphorus may be found under their respective individual headings in
the mineral section of this book.)

I am indebted to Mark N. Mead for some of the information that
follows hereafter. In early 1988 this biomedical researcher from
Greenville, North Carolina shared with me some of his own research
into this important B vitamin.

In herbivores, such as cows and sheep, cobalamins or B-12
compounds are produced by intestinal flora; the animals may also
get them by feeding on dung. Carnivores, such as lions and tigers,
must obtain B-12 from the flesh of other animals. As omnivores, we
humans can synthesize minute quantities of B-12.

But many scientists are inclined to believe that this amount is
insufficient for human needs, and instead advocate getting more B-
12 from animal flesh and organs. A few doctors, though, are of the
definite opinion that in people the normal B-12 requirements are
sufficiently met by bacterial synthesis in the colon. Still other nutritional authorities concur that some folks can supply this vitamin adequately through the millions of helpful microbes found in their
mouths and G. I. tracts. A 1978 study that appeared in the *British
Journal of Nutrition* (40(1):9) found that people who had followed
a strict vegetarian diet for 30 years showed no evidence of B-12 deficiency. The researchers concluded that "vitamin B-12 deficiency is
rare among vegans" (extreme vegetarians who exclude all foods of
animal origin from their diets).

Haptocorrin, a substance found in both saliva and gastric juice,
binds with the vitamin and protects it against stomach acid and possibly against bacterial degradation in the intestine. Saliva has a highly beneficial effect on B-12, as it renders the vitamin more usable by
the body's tissues. This supports the practice of thorough chewing,
since the amount of saliva increases the longer one chews. In the

small intestine, haptocorrin yields its B-12 molecule to what Mark Mead terms "the intrinsic factor," or a stomach secretion which facilitates intestinal uptake. This accounts for 99 percent of intestinal absorption.

Somewhere between 0.5 to 5 micrograms of stored B-12 are secreted into the alimentary tract daily, mainly in the bile. At least 65 to 75 percent is reabsorbed in the upper intestine (the ileum) by means of the intrinsic factor. This recycled B-12 is stored in the liver and kidneys. This efficient conservation, combined with the fact that vitamin B-12 stores for most Americans usually exceed the government's own Recommended Dietary Allowances (RDAs) by a thousandfold, helps us understand why strict vegetarians on low B-12 diets may take two or three decades to develop an evident deficiency of some kind.

Several physiological factors are important in the conservation of B-12, including adequate intrinsic factor activity and normal liver, gall bladder, and small intestine functioning. For instance, a reduced intestinal capacity to absorb B-12, due to overgrowth of bacteria or parasites, may promote B-12 deficiency. Intense stress can also compromise the body's digestive capabilities, so that absorption and utilization of B-12 become somewhat self-limiting. And stress can periodically bring on self-destructive habitual behaviors characterized by poor eating habits and abuse of alcohol, tobacco, and caffeine—all of which have some detrimental effect on B-12 balance.

The aging process of the body often takes its own toll on B-12. The older people get, the less ability they have to fully utilize the B-12 they may still have. Added supplementation of this vitamin is thought to help reverse some of those diseases frequently associated with aging.

Medications and major medical procedures can have a large impact on the body, depleting it of B-12. Some medications are known to interfere with B-12 metabolism and some lead to increased excretion of this nutrient. Surgery or radiation of the G.I. tract can adversely affect its ability to carry out the proper digestion of B-12. Antibiotics upset the balance of beneficial bacteria in the upper small intestine, allowing the unmitigated spread of unfriendly antibiotic-resistant bacteria and possibly inhibiting B-12 availability.

Toxic substances or environmental pollutants may, likewise, influence our B-12 reserves. Heavy metals can be absorbed into food and water from the use of aluminum cookware, lead plumbing, chemical fertilizers and pesticides, car exhaust fumes, and cigarette smoke, which is thought to promote B-12 deficiency. In general, toxic chemical substances tend to be more concentrated in fatty animal products and pose an increased demand on the liver, the central organ for storage of B-12.

Vitamin B-12 is quite useful for problems as diverse as substance addiction and mosquito bites to pernicious anemia and phobias. Evidence for this appears in the following sections.

Caffeine Withdrawal. Tens of millions of Americans are hooked on coffee and consume several cups of java every day. Still others may be drawn to this substance in cold form and get their daily "caffeine fixes" from the likes of caffeinated soft drinks. Many of those who patronize health food stores to purchase herbal energy stimulants are getting more caffeine than they might imagine.

This major xanthine alkaloid occurs not only in coffee, but also in black and oolong teas, guarana, kola nut, and yerba maté. Caffeine stimulates the central nervous system, mainly affecting the major portion of the brain known as the cerebrum. It also has a strong diuretic effect on the kidneys, stimulates striated muscles, and has a group of effects on the entire cardiovascular system.

The late Dr. William R. Maples, a renowned forensic anthropologist, once had a terrible addiction to coffee, but successfully overcame it with periodic injections of vitamin B-12 from his doctor. He was considered one of the world's most eminent scientists in his particular field. He authored *Dead Men Do Tell Tales,* in which he mentioned being able to determine the cause of death, age, gender, and ethnicity of a person by examining either a skeleton, a skull, or a mere fragment of bone. He was to forensic anthropology what Albert Einstein was to physics and mathematics or Hans Selye to epidemiology (the study of disease).

Typically, Maples worked on bodies that were beyond the skill of more widely-employed forensic pathologists. During his remarkable career, he found himself studying such notables as President Zachary Taylor, "elephant man" John Merrick, and assassinated civil rights leader Medgar Evers. In 1984, while working at the Peruvian Institute of Culture in Lima, he and other anthropologists matched the skull and remaining bones of Francisco Pizzaro, the Spanish explorer who conquered the Incas in 1532 and was slain in 1541 in a sword fight. He was also instrumental in helping to identify the remains of murdered Russian Czar Nicholas II and his family, which finally brought closure to a matter that had been surrounded by speculation and intrigue for a number of decades.

I met Dr. Maples several years ago at a scientific conference on forensic anthropology, where we enjoyed a long and pleasant chat one morning. He was intrigued with my work as a medical anthropologist in the areas of folk medicine and food therapy, as I was with his work in the science of forensic anthropology and, essentially, considerably decayed corpses. "You're lucky," I recall him saying with a laugh. "My work is, by far, more grisly than yours." Needless to say, you would have needed a pretty strong stomach that morning to have listened in on the morbid details of what we freely talked about.

Fortunately, not everything centered around badly decomposed bodies and the forensic pathological methods involved in identifying them. Maples brought up the subject himself of his past coffee-drinking habits. It wasn't unusual for him to have downed up to 15 cups of black coffee every day, especially when confined for long hours to his lab, examining human skeletal remains or a smelly corpse.

Finding himself becoming an insomniac and with a "jittery nervousness," he sought the advice of his physician, who recommended periodic B-12 injections. The doctor administered 100 micrograms of parenteral cyanocobalamin subcutaneously every day for one week, then weekly for one month, and finally every two months after that for one year. Dr. Maples' caffeine addiction disappeared to return no more.

"Just look at me now," I fondly remember him joking, while holding up a small glass of orange juice. "I've become a convert to healthier beverages—the kind of things you must write about!" We enjoyed a good laugh together over this bit of natural amusement.

Since then, based on what Dr. Maples had shared with me, I've sometimes recommended vitamin B-12 intake in the neighborhood of 2,000 mcg. for those addicted to coffee or chocolate. The success rate has been around 65 to 75 percent, though the group I've worked with has been relatively small in number.

Fatigue. Some doctors used to recommend B-12 for patients suffering from fatigue, but scientific studies didn't prove its effectiveness. Because of this it soon fell out of fashion and came to be viewed by the orthodox medical establishment as something bordering on nutritional quackery.

But in a 1987 issue of *The New England Journal of Medicine* (vol. 318, no. 26), researchers at Columbia-Presbyterian Medical Center in New York reported that they found that regular injections of B-12 dramatically boosted energy in 39 of 40 patients who showed no evidence of B-12 deficiency. (They probably suffered from an underutilization of this nutrient.)

A decade later more doctors are subscribing to the idea that this B vitamin does, indeed, have energy-boosting capabilities, and are prescribing it more often to some of their energy-deficient patients.

Insect Bites. In Boulder, Colorado in the 1970s, I was giving an herb lecture for a number of distributors affiliated with a large direct marketing supplements company. A woman named Betty Lane shared the following story with me about garlic and vitamin B-12.

Betty told me that mosquitoes were "a real big problem" in the mountain meadow where she and her husband resided in their self-built log cabin. She had always been susceptible to their bites and her husband reacted "even more violently" to them "and for days afterward" would usually be "sicker than a dog."

Sometime in 1973 a local ecological group suggested eating raw garlic and taking B-12 as perfect antidotes for mosquito bites. She said they added this to their regular herb and vitamin intake. "We later had an occasion to camp in an area literally swarming with mosquitoes," she continued. "I had no bites and my hubby had only three. But none of them itched the next day." She also stated that deer flies, which abounded in their meadowland at various times, would sometimes bite them, but "the itching lasts only a few minutes, not days as before, thanks to our garlic and B-12."

Ever since then they had been recommending it to many others. All those who faithfully tried it were astonished but quite happy with the success of both in keeping insect bites to a bare minimum!

Mental Illness. The use of major tranquilizers and other drugs to alter the body's biochemistry has enabled many mentally ill persons to function outside of institutions. Drugs, however, take their toll in time, sometimes substituting undesirable side effects for the original disease symptoms. Furthermore, such medications destroy the friendly bacteria that synthesize B vitamins in the intestines. Some of these potent psychiatric drugs have occasionally induced intestinal disorders such as celiac, Crohn's disease, or chronic diarrhea in small numbers of mental patients. Such individuals often show vitamin B-12 and folic acid deficiencies when tested.

Thankfully, not all psychiatrists depend on powerful synthetic drugs to do their work for them. Some, in fact, practice what is called orthomolecular medicine in some professional circles. These practitioners firmly believe that mental illness can be treated by altering the body's chemistry. They do it through the use of sound nutrition and vitamins and minerals that occur naturally in the body. In this way they are able to restore natural balance in a terribly imbalanced system. Orthomolecular means "correct molecule." So it stands to reason that these physicians can treat mental illness by providing an optimum molecular environment for the mind.

There are still quite a few doctors, though, who don't recognize that mental disturbances, especially in the elderly, can be early symptoms of a lack of vitamins B-12 and B-9 (folacin). Such deficiencies may be due to faulty diet or digestive disorders that inhibit the proper digestion, absorption, and assimilation of nutrients. It has been estimated by some psychiatrists that as high as 15 percent of all patients with senile dementia currently confined to institutions could be rescued by adding vitamin B-12 to the diet or giving it through injections. In 1965, one British psychiatrist made headlines in the *London Times* and other tabloids by recommending that *every single* patient then being admitted to mental asylums first be tested for deficiencies in B-12 and folic acid. While his idea was rather novel and obviously quite sound, it didn't help his public image or professional standing with his peers very much. Many, in fact, disparged him advocating this treatment!

Schizophrenia is a serious mental illness afflicting well over three million Americans. It hospitalizes more patients than heart disease, cancer, and arthritis *combined*! Without effective treatment these people hover in a kind of "Twilight Zone" betwixt life and death. Schizophrenia occurs more frequently in young men and women between the ages of 15 and 30 than in older people. Infants have even been known to be born with this disease in some instances.

Three Canadian psychiatrists, Abram Hoffer, M.D., Humphrey Osmond, M.D., and L. Kotkas, M.D., were pioneers in using moderate doses of B-1 (niacin), B-6 (pyridoxine), B-9 (folic acid), and B-12 (cyanocobalamin), along with vitamin C, in treating several thousand schizophrenic patients with almost complete success. If you know of someone suffering from mental illness and under psychiatric care, you should mention these nutrients to patient and practitioner alike. You would be doing them more good than you may know.

Nervousness. The human nervous system in many ways resembles a vast electrical network. The brain acts as the chief control panel for the ascending and descending tracts. The nerve cells can be favorably compared to tubes or batteries, while the nerve fibers resemble connecting wires. Impulses received and sent over the nerves are thought to be electrical in nature.

A single nerve viewed under a powerful light microscope yields some surprising finds. Deep within, you first find exceedingly fine filament structures called neurofibrils. In some ways they remind one of fiber optic filaments, only of a much finer material. On top of these you will find other threadlike filament materials known as axons.

Both of these are wrapped in a fatty protein substance known as myelin. This sheathing envelopes the neurofibrils and axons much like a plastic coating does the copper filaments inside an electrical wire.

This myelin sheathing is alternately layered with membrane composed of cholesterol, lecithins, phosphorus-containing lipids, and protein. The membrane is wound tightly around the axon in a variable number of turns, vaguely similar to what a baker might do to a jelly roll before popping it into the oven.

Vitamin B-12 is very critical to the maintenance of this nerve sheath. It insures that there will always be adequate amounts of fat and protein on hand to keep this double plasma membrane intact.

If holes or tears appear in it anywhere, then electrical impulses from the brain through the nerves are interrupted; the result can be external manifestations of unexplained nervousness fueled by emotional anxiety.

In the early part of March, 1997, I spoke on the phone with Lalana Lynne Island, who was 30 years of age. We chatted about different topics, including health-related themes. She said that at around age 24, "I was a bundle of nerves, and couldn't figure out why."

She consulted with several doctors, who performed different tests on her. It was finally determined that "my myelin sheathing was showing some wear and not being adequately replaced as it should have been."

One of the doctors involved in her care recommended that she take an oral vitamin B-12 supplement. "So, I started loading up on vitamin B complex," she continued, "including extra B-12. I stayed on this regimen for a couple of months, after which my body 'told' me I had enough, so I cut back on my intake for awhile. I felt a hundred times calmer and more relaxed than usual. It was a great feeling to have. When I turned 26, I had a lovely baby boy whom we named Stephan Conner Island (he's now 3 1/2). I probably couldn't have withstood the nervous strain of all this as well as I did, had it not been for my B vitamins," she testified.

Pernicious Anemia. Pernicious anemia (PA) is a chronic disease that tends to afflict persons in their 50s and 60s. It is of genetic origin and characterized by unusually large red blood corpuscles, inflammation of the tongue, and neurological disturbances such as limb stiffness, irritability, drowsiness, and depression. Calf liver was originally used to treat this disorder.

Doctors now know, however, that minute doses of vitamin B-12 (10 to 15 mg. per day) given by injection (intramuscularly) can relieve the problem. Additionally, 100 mg. given every month can prevent the recurrence of PA symptoms. Intramuscular administration of vitamin B-12 is effective in PA because it bypasses the stomach and the need for absorption; it isn't affected by the failure of the intestinal mucosa to secrete "the intrinsic factor" that Mark Mead had referred to nearly a decade ago. (This intrinsic factor is essential for the absorption of cyanocobalamin.)

Phobias. Agoraphobia is the most pervasive phobia. It is a disorder in which the afflicted suffer from unexplained "panic attacks." They have a dreadful fear of being in open spaces and, therefore, choose to remain in a safe and secure place, usually the home. They may also suffer from depression and loss of self-confidence, in part related to their inability to lead normal productive lives. In addition, they may manifest other undesirable mental and physical symptoms.

There is happy news for such unfortunate folks. Alternative-minded doctors working with nutrition therapy have found that it can be alleviated by supplementation with B vitamins. Agoraphobics do best when they take generous amounts of B-complex, and an additional 2,000 mcg. of B-12 every other day. (See Product Appendix, p. 381.)

Tumors. Mice were implanted with tumor cells and, starting 24 hours later, half of them received 8 daily subcutaneous injections containing 80 mg. each of vitamin B-12, L-ascorbic acid, and niacin ascorbate per kilogram of body weight in the area of the implant. Ten days after implantation, all 50 untreated mice had developed tumors, whereas only 2 of the 50 vitamin-treated mice had tumors; these tumors were much smaller in size and weight than those in the controls.

A mixture of vitamins C and B-12 had previously been found to completely inhibit mitosis in tumor cell cultures and in ascites tumors in mice. Interestingly enough, vitamin B-12 and vitamin C in the same doses given *separately* to mice had *no* effect. In in vitro experiments, noncancerous tumors weren't affected by the vitamin mixture. Treated mice surviving after leukemia or Ehrlich ascites tumor had no apparent toxic effects from the vitamin mixture, according to the September 1984 issue of *IRCS Medical Science* (12:813).

Both vitamin B-12 and folic acid are known to be valuable in the reduction of some malignant growths.

Food Sources

The following dietary sources for vitamin B-12 comprise the most complete list to be found in *any* recently published book on nutritional supplements. Don't take my word for it, go ahead and check it out for yourself. I am grateful to Mark N. Mead, a biomedical researcher, for some of this data, which he freely shared with me.

High (50-500 mcg/100 g)	Medium (5-50 mcg/100 g)	Low 0.2-5 mcg/100 g
Kidney, lamb	Kidney, rabbit	Barley-malt syrup
	beef	Whole-meal sourdough bread
Liver,		Shiitake (dried mushrooms)
Lamb		Cod
beef	Liver,	Flounder
calf	rabbit	Haddock
pork	chicken	Sole
		Halibut
Brain, beef	Heart,	Lobster
	beef	Scallop
Sea vegetables	rabbit	Shrimp
Wakame		Swordfish
Kekombu (kombu root)	Hawaiian tuna	Tuna, blue
	Oysters	Cow's milk
Blue green microalgae	Sardines	Cheese (regular)
Super Blue Green	Mackeral	Fermented cheeses (limburger)
	Salmon	Egg (whole)
Green microalgae	Egg yolk	Beef
chlorella	Clams	Lamb
spirulina	Crabs	Pork
	Indonesian tempeh	Miso
		Indonesian tempeh
	Seaweeds,	Sauerkraut
	hijiki	Pickles
	kelp	Tamari
	kombu	Natto
	alaria	
	nori	

Recommended Daily Intake

The Food and Nutrition Board of the National Academy of Sciences and the National Research Council issued revised Recommended Dietary Allowances (RDAs) for the American public in 1989. The Board was funded by grants from the federal government given to its two sponsoring organizations. The federal government accepted its findings and essentially approved them as being nutritionally sound and in the best interests of public health.

Below is a table showing the suggested amounts for vitamin B-12 intake (as measured in micrograms) for different age and gender categories.

Category	Age or Condition	B-12 (Mcg)
Infants	Birth-6 mos.	0.3
	6 mos.-l yr.	0.5
Children	1-3	0.7
	4-6	1.0
	7-10	1.4
Males and Females	11 and older	2.0
Pregnant Females		2.2
Lactating Females		2.6

Some medical doctors, though, have recommended doses a lot higher than those suggested in the foregoing table. Their thinking is that the increased amounts will do more good than harm, and the clinical evidence seems to support them in this. Sheldon Saul Hendler, M.D., for instance, informed his readers that up to 50 micrograms of vitamin B-12 could be taken each day in *The Doctor's Vitamin and Mineral Encyclopedia* (New York: Simon & Schuster, 1990; p. 71).

While most of those who advocate higher doses of B-12 stay in the range that Dr. Hendler does, there are some physicians who go quite a way beyond these fairly conservative limits. Take, for example, what H. Winter Griffith, M.D. wrote in his *Complete Guide to Vitamins, Minerals & Supplements* (Tucson: Fisher Books, 1988; p. 29) some time ago. Without coming right out and prescribing greater amounts of this important nutrient, he certainly worded things in such a way as to suggest that extremely large doses wouldn't hurt either: "There is a very low incidence of toxicity of vitamin B-12, even with large amounts up to 1,000 mcg./day."

A person would be perfectly safe in taking B-12 in a supplement surrounded with other B vitamins.

B-15 (PANGAMIC ACID): The Panacea Vitamin from Russia

In two decades of giving public health lectures (1977-1997), I've seen a lot of herbal and nutritional fads come and go. Among the more infamous ones have been devil's claw and blue-green lipped mussel from New Zealand for rheumatoid arthritis. There were even some old standbys from grandma's time that received "renewed life" among naive consumers when cleverly promoted by manipulative entrepreneurs. Does anyone remember Dale Alexander hawking his bottles of cod liver oil "for everything that ails you" at National Health Federation conventions?

Occasionally, though, something has come along that merits careful consideration, but still falls into a gray area so far as the Food and Drug Administration (FDA) and orthodox medicine and nutrition go. One that comes to mind is the subject of this section. It is called pangamic acid or vitamin B-15. All of the scientific research behind the many claims for it has come from the former Soviet Union.

This isn't to say that it's a phony nutrient by any means. In a number of countries (including England, France, Germany, Finland, Sweden, Pakistan, and India) it is still recognized as one of the B vitamins. Its legitimacy in these countries, however, is based in large part on Soviet research of the past.

One American researcher who looked into the Soviet work published on this subject noted that "nearly all of these studies suffer from methodologic flaws which seriously limit their probative value. Often patient populations and diagnostic criteria are incompletely described, and comparisons between treated subjects and suitably matched controls are lacking." Another author (also American) brought a similar complaint, stating that "the methodological laxness and wild-eyed enthusiasm of Russian clinical reports" cast a long shadow over the nutrient's ultimate value.

The Soviet studies declared pangamic acid to be the ester of dimethyl glycine and gluconic acid; the Russians eventually secured a

patent on this. Thus, N,N-dimethyl glycine (DMG), a normal intermediate in the metabolism of another B vitamin (choline), soon became
"the hottest substance to hit the ergogenic scene in recent memory,"
according to an article in *The Physician and SportsMedicine Journal*
(7(11):17, Nov. 1979).

Americans and Europeans went absolutely wild over it.
Pangamic acid was touted in the media as a powerful "oxygenator"
of body tissues, a superb aphrodisiac capable of delivering "flashy
brilliance" to orgasms, helping one to do yoga better, "mopping up
free radicals like mad," "saving people from the need for amputation
of gangrenous limbs," etc., etc.

Between sloppy Soviet research, news sensationalism, and
public clamoring for the stuff, pangamic acid inevitably started getting a lot of bad press through the scientific community. The charge
was led by the FDA (see *FDA Consumer*, Sept. 1978, pp. 15-16) and
the American Medical Association, among others. The U.S.
Government seized large quantities of pangamic acid from vitamin
manufacturers located in Hawaii, Oregon, Illinois, Florida, and New
Jersey. Individual health food store owners, who continued selling it
on their shelves, were threatened with intimidating actions that
included jail arrests and lawsuits.

Times have changed, however, and today the natural foods
and vitamin industries are extremely powerful, well-funded, and
politically connected. The FDA has become considerably weaker
and doesn't pack the punch it used to. Also, public attitudes
toward herbs and nutritional supplements have changed enor-
mously, and these products have become as mainstream as aspirin
or flu shots.

When I went to the former Soviet Union in the summer of 1979
with a delegation of other scientists for a couple of months of health
research, I had a chance to look at much of the published research
myself (with the aid of an interpreter, of course). I also spoke with
several of the scientists connected with a few of these original published papers. After careful evaluation and putting everything into its
proper perspective, I came away with this assessment, which I
believe to be an honest one: Pangamic acid *is* a nutrient of *some
kind*. Whether or not it's a true B vitamin, however, still remains to
be seen.

It is not the "magic bullet" or "potent pill" for every illness under the sun. Some, but not all, of the old Soviet research was done hastily and with poor attention paid to record keeping. But in all fairness to those who did the work with pangamic acid in that country, I must say without hesitation that their efforts were sincere and the double-blind studies were conducted as honestly as one could hope for under the circumstances they had to work in.

Pangamic acid cannot be totally dismissed as another scientific fraud. Granted that some hocus-pocus may surround it, but to dismiss it entirely would be equivalent to throwing the proverbial baby out with the bath water. I have interviewed many athletes in the former Soviet Union, in some of the former Iron Curtain countries of Eastern Europe, and especially in Pakistan and India, who've testified time and again to the remarkable strength-building properties of this highly controversial but curiously unique vitamin-to-be. There is something in Pangamic acid that still warrants our serious attention. Exactly what it is, I don't know. But it is some kind of life-giving factor that gives strength to the muscles, stamina to the heart, vigor to the nerves, and endurance to the body overall.

I don't mean to become guilty myself of sensationalizing something that has already been hyped way too much in times past. But I believe those who work in the nutritional sciences have missed a potentially huge find in this little nutrient, because of their past prejudices. It will take those of the upcoming generation to discover just what exactly makes pangamic acid so wonderful for strengthening the human body in times of great physical activity.

Food Sources

Some mainstream nutritional references, such as *Nutrition Almanac,* 2nd ed. by John D. Kirschmann and LaVon J. Dunne (NY: McGraw-Hill Book Co.., 1973) still carry information about pangamic acid.

In this particular case, four pages of interesting data are situated between Vitamin B-12 and Choline (two of the B group). This volume has become one of McGraw-Hill's all-time · best sellers, exceeding nearly two and one-half million copies sold!

Food sources mentioned for pangamic acid include brewer's yeast, whole brown rice, whole grains, pumpkin seeds, and sesame seeds. Ironically, the *best* source wasn't even mentioned by the authors of *Nutrition Almanac*. Legumes, especially lentils, are extremely rich in pangamic acid. I always wondered why wrestlers and body builders feasted on bowls of lentils before athletic events. It wasn't too long before I stumbled on the secret in the form of this very important nutrient. (A fairly balanced article to read about pangamic acid is entitled "The Life-Saving Banned Vitamin," found in *Prevention* health magazine, May 1968.)

Recommended Daily Intake

As much as I'm attracted to the obvious strength-imparting properties of this nutrient, I must play the devil's advocate here for a bit and take a decided stand *against* additional supplementation of this presumed vitamin. In his book, *The Doctors' Vitamin and Mineral Encyclopedia* (New York: Simon & Schuster, 1990; p. 355), author Sheldon Saul Hendler, M.D., cautioned his readers as follows: *"Don't* use any products labeled or related to 'pangamic acid' . . . or 'B-15.'"

When I was in the former Soviet Union, I had access to a book by Ya. Yu. Shpirt, M.D., appropriately entitled *Vitamin B-15 (Pangamic Acid): Indications for Use and Efficacy in Internal Disease* (Moscow: V/O Medexport, 1968). On page 7 the author mentioned regular clinical doses of 2.5 to 10 milligrams of pangamic acid being routinely given through intramuscular injections without any apparent problems. After speaking with several of the scientists connected with the original research into this nutrient, I became convinced in my own mind that it only had supplementation merit as an *injection,* but *not* orally consumed as an isolated nutrient.

This isn't to say, though, that pangamic acid shouldn't be taken every day or at least a couple of times a week. I firmly believe that it works best in whole food form. Call it a hunch or what you may, but I'm of the definite opinion that pangamic acid needs to be eaten in a meal in order for its full strength-giving abilities to be totally experienced. Barring this possibility from happening all the time, the second option would naturally be intramuscular injection. This is what some Europeans and Scandinavians still do. But people in South Asia seem to prefer to get their pangamic acid intake from cooked lentils, millet, rice, and beans.

Are we as Americans missing something here? I believe so. And it is because of scientific prejudice and pomposity that we have been thoroughly misled about pangamic acid in general.

B-17 (AMYGDALIN/LAETRILE): Nature's Own Chemotherapy for Cancer

The term laetrile was coined by Ernest T. Krebs, Jr. in the late 1940s as an acronym to describe a purified derivative of amygdalin laevo rotatory in polarized light that was chemically a mandelontrile. The Laetrile patented by Krebs and later successfully synthesized by an FDA-Johns Hopkins team in 1977 is spelled with an upper case L. It differs slightly from the more common, lower case version, laetrile, which is synonymous with amygdalin.

Amygdalin, however, is the principal constituent in Laetrile and is a naturally occurring cyanoglucoside. It can be obtained from various plant sources (vetches, clovers, sorghums, cassava, lima beans, acacia) and, most notably, the tiny seeds inside the pits of edible fruits and berries (apricots, peaches, plums, chokeberries). Amygdalin received legitimate status in the ninth edition of *The Merck Index* (Rahway, NJ, Merck & Co., 1976), a well-respected encyclopedic reference of chemicals and drugs, but only after years of considerable controversy surrounding it.

Amygdalin, under its more common name of laetrile, dominated news headlines from about 1977 to 1981. Two sides were fiercely pitted against each other in bitter confrontations. On one side were tens of thousands of cancer victims and alternative therapists, who believed that laetrile could really do something to help get rid of this dreaded disease. On the other side were scientists, doctors, and politicians who were equally determined that the public would never have access to what they viewed as a bogus remedy and potential poison.

But several things happened along the way that turned the tide very much in laetrile's favor. One precedent-setting case involved a then 58-year-old farmer from Wichita, Kansas named Glen L. Rutherford. In 1971 he was diagnosed with cancer of the rectum. When standard treatments proved ineffective, he went to alternative cancer clinics in Tijuana, Mexico for laetrile. Apparently it cured his cancer. On his return to his home state, he continued to get amygdalin from an illegal source who subsequently was arrested on account of the ban against it by the Food and Drug Administration (FDA). The feisty Kansas farmer went to the U.S. District Court in Kansas City and sued for an order prohibiting the FDA from interfering with his right to treat his own body in his own way.

"You [meaning the medical profession] set yourselves up as God and Jesus Christ all in one!" he barked out to the applause of an enthusiastic crowd at the federal government's first public hearings on the drug. "If I lost my laetrile, you would read my obituary in eight to ten months," he shouted with anger. "Give me the right to choose the way I want to die. It is not your prerogative to tell me how, only God can tell me that!" The courtroom audience hissed and loudly booed when physicians testified against laetrile and called it "sugar-coated cyanide."

A federal judge in Oklahoma City by the name of Luther Bohanon agreed with Rutherford and certified the man's class action lawsuit as meriting a ruling from the bench. His decision was to circumvent the FDA ban against laetrile and permit access to any cancer patients who wanted the substance. In his April 8, 1977 opinion, he stated that "many intelligent . . . citizens . . . have made a . . . decision . . . to employ an unproven and largely unrespected treatment in an effort to comfort, if not save, lives that orthodox [medicine] tells them have already been lost. They do so with an acute awareness of professional medicine's assessment of their choice. *Their decision should be respected!*"

The second setback for the laetrile opposition was a confusing series of statements issued by top officials at the Sloan-Kettering Institute in New York City, totally obfuscating its own research that supported amygdalin's anticancer properties. Considered by many to be one of the nation's premier centers for cancer research and treatment, it derived its name from Alfred Sloan and Charles "Boss" Kettering, two top executives of General Motors.

These men led the corporate movement in the 1940s to provide stepped-up private funding for medical and drug research. The Rockefeller family of Exxon Oil (formerly Standard Oil) fame became heavy investors later on. For over half a century Sloan-Kettering has tested thousands of chemicals and drugs provided by the pharmaceutical industry.

In 1972 President Richard M. Nixon was deluged with tens of thousands of petitions from ordinary citizens everywhere demanding clinical trials for laetrile. These demands were forwarded to his cancer advisor, Benno Schmidt, an investment banker and a vice chairman of Sloan-Kettering.

When Schmidt consulted all of his medical colleagues about laetrile, he found them vehemently opposed to it. But, interestingly enough, as he told reporters later on, "I couldn't get anybody to show me scientific proof that the stuff didn't work." Schmidt, therefore, encouraged Sloan-Kettering to test laetrile, hoping to put to rest once and for all the claims of its purported value. He got more than he bargained for in the process.

The task fell to one of the world's most respected cancer chemotherapy researchers, a Japanese scientist by the name of Kanematsu Sugiura. In 1972, when he began testing laetrile on rodents in his second-floor facilities at Sloan-Kettering's Walker Laboratories in suburban Rye, New York, he was a 55-year loyal employee and senior staff scientist. A fellow researcher from the former Soviet Union described the man's meticulous work this way: "When Dr. Sugiura publishes, we know we don't have to repeat the study for we would obtain the same results as he has reported." Put another way, Sugiura's reputation for absolute scientific integrity was unimpeachable.

What started out as routine testing ended up becoming a public relations quagmire for Sloan-Kettering. Dr. Sugiura expected laetrile to fail, but it *didn't*. In the first several tests conducted with mice having a genetic predisposition for tumors, he found that cancer spread in only 20 percent of those receiving laetrile injections, compared to a whopping 80 percent for untreated rodents. He reported these findings to his superiors, who called in other researchers to assist him in duplicating more of the same tests.

Again and again, the same results kept coming back: laetrile manifested *significant* effects against cancer! Totally frustrated by the same thing turning up in six separate experiments spread over a five-year period, the hierarchy of Sloan-Kettering decided not to report the positive findings in sworn testimony before a United States Senate committee investigating the merits of laetrile in July, 1977: "There is not a particle of scientific evidence . . . to suggest that laetrile possesses any anticancer properties at all."

Thus began the medical world's version of politics' Watergate. Sloan-Kettering officials fairly muzzled Dr. Sugiura and kept him away from the press. But in private with other respected scientists, he would declare that laetrile is "a useful preventive agent" and something that "really stops the spread of cancer." Someone in his lab (but not himself) leaked evidence of his positive research in support of laetrile to the outside press. An unsigned letter written on Sloan-Kettering stationery read: "Here are some of the results of Sloan-Kettering's continuing experiments with laetrile. Due to political pressure, these results are being suppressed. Please do your best to bring these important findings to the attention of the people." The letter was accompanied by photocopies of Dr. Sugiura's original hand-written lab reports, listing experimental results of the laetrile tests, day by day, mouse by mouse; included were Sugiura's summaries, as well as other supporting documentation.

Several other events of equal magnitude occurred separately within the same approximate time period. Dr. Chester Stock, Sugiura's immediate superior at Sloan-Kettering, told the *Medical World News* in August 1975 (more than a year after the Japanese researcher had completed six positive laetrile experiments): "We have found amygdalin (laetrile) negative in all the animal systems we have tested." Similar statements were made by other top-ranking officials as well. Dr. Lewis Thomas, president of Memorial Sloan-Kettering Cancer Center, allegedly told reporters: "Laetrile has shown after two years of tests to be worthless in fighting cancer." And Dr. Robert Good, president and director of the Sloan-Kettering Institute where Sugiura worked, said in his own press conference: ". . . There is no evidence that laetrile has an effect on cancer."

Not all institute employees, however, were willing to line up behind these confusing statements. One man, Dr. Ralph Moss, who was the assistant director of public affairs at Sloan-Kettering, held his peace for awhile as his different bosses continued massaging the media and the public with their statements. But when they reportedly hinted to nice and gentle Dr. Sugiura that he might have to take an "early" retirement (by then he was 85 and still working six full days a week) if he ever spoke the truth about laetrile, Dr. Moss had had enough. He convened a press conference at the Hilton Hotel in Manhattan on November 17, 1977, and came forward with the truth. He was promptly fired the next working day. He teamed up with Gary Null on WMCA's "Natural Living" program to inform the listening public and information-hungry journalists about the alleged deception at Sloan-Kettering.

Well, everything good seems to need a catalyst or two behind it to get things moving. Between the Sloan-Kettering public relations mess and Judge Bohanon's decision in favor of the Kansas farmer, there were enough other events to help the laetrile movement gain much greater momentum than it ever had before. Numerous journalists, politicians, and judges were favorably swayed in the other direction now. It wasn't too long until almost 30 states had passed independent legislation permitting the importing and medical use of laetrile within their boundaries. So, while most doctors and scientists and the FDA may have won the war over laetrile's lack of scientific proof, the public eventually won its hard-fought battle to gain access to something people truly believed would work in the prevention and treatment of cancer.

One of the things that really riled the opponents of laetrile was when its supporters started referring to it as vitamin B-17. According to *Clinical Toxicology* (17(1):94;1980), the reasoning behind this was the fact that amygdalin is abundant in trace amounts in many foods growing throughout tropical countries, where cancer rates have historically been much lower. Among the supporters who lined up behind laetrile's obvious nutritive value were some highly educated, scientific professionals who were well connected academically and politically. Two of these were the late Dean Burk, Ph.D. and the late Harold Manner, Ph. D. Burk was head of cytochemistry at the National Cancer Institute (NCI) for many years and one of NCI's original cofounders. Early on as the laetrile controversy started brewing and percolating on the back burner of public opinion, he entered the fray with calm dignity and announced with great confidence that "amygdalin qualifies as a vitamin by the very definition of one."

Next in line came Dr. Harold Manner, the controversial head of Loyola University's Biology Department in Chicago. I knew this man personally and met him a number of times at different National Health Federation conventions around the country during the 1980s, where we both spoke frequently. Dr. Manner considered amygdalin "a unique *vitamin* but not in the sense of what we know a vitamin to be." By technical definition, a vitamin is an organic substance, "present in minute amounts in natural foodstuffs, that is essential to normal metabolism." Furthermore, an "insufficient amount in the diet may cause deficiency diseases." That last part was what Manner took an exception to. "There exists little or no evidence," I remember him saying during one of several conversations we had together on the subject of laetrile, "to show that *without* adequate laetrile you're going to get cancer." But it certainly fit the rest of a vitamin's description of occurring in food and being necessary to normal metabolism. He regarded laetrile as "a unique nutritive factor for the immune system" that had yet to be fully understood.

Dr. Linus Pauling, the "father of vitamin C" and twice Nobel Laureate (the only man ever in Nobel history to win the same prize twice), supported the use of laetrile. His letter to this effect was published in the July 8, 1982 issue of *The New England Journal of Medicine*. "It is my opinion," Pauling wrote, "that there probably was a beneficial effect, including prolongation of survival" in laetrile therapy. He noted cancer patients treated with the substance and metabolic diet therapy survived an average of almost five months. He said that other studies had demonstrated that people with incurable cancer ordinarily survive for just under two months. He assigned nutritive properties to laetrile.

So, does amygdalin or vitamin B-17 "cure" cancer? Well, a lot depends on what it's taken with. Two examples of well-known screen actors serve to illustrate this. Steve McQueen developed a rare form of lung cancer due to smoking. He entered a Tijuana cancer clinic (Plaza Santa Maria Hospital) about 75 miles south of San Diego sometime in November 1980 for two months of alternative treatments that included lots of laetrile injections, massive amounts of coffee enemas, an array of vitamin supplements, and injections of animal cells. This regimen of "metabolic therapy" had been devised by the man in whose hands McQueen had placed himself, William Kelly, a Texas dentist whose license to practice in his home state had previously been suspended.

In the beginning things looked up for McQueen. After a month on this strict regimen, McQueen "looked and felt better" than he had in some months prior to coming there. "His attitude was very upbeat." Kelly, ever eager for media attention, scheduled a hastily arranged news conference to show off the "new" McQueen. At the same time, he and his staff claimed that the actor's tumor had "shrunk decisively." But just a month later, after an operation in Mexico to remove the same tumor, McQueen was dead.

Back in those days I was a regular speaker at the Cancer Control Society in Los Angeles and would regularly meet Kelly or some of his staff people. While I never cared much for the man's style myself, I will have to say in his defense that he wasn't to blame for McQueen's sudden health reversals. Once his patient started feeling better and x-rays showed a definite reduction in tumor size, McQueen went right back to his old habits of questionable lifestyle choices. "He was always a nervous sort anyhow," one of Kelly's staff people told me. "We strongly urged him to stick with our program for a few months longer, just to make sure the tumor didn't return. But, no, he wasn't going to sit in a Mexican clinic all day taking it easy. He said he was going to get out and 'live a little' and 'celebrate' his cure." The rest is history, as they say. McQueen failed to understand that when you go against the laws of nature, nature will come roaring back quite ferociously every single time! And that is what happened to him.

Contrast that with what happened to Fred MacMurray. He was a veteran actor of Walt Disney films and TV star of the long-running hit series, "My Three Sons." At age 69, he contracted throat cancer due to years of pipe smoking. He commenced radiation treatments at the urging of his doctors in February 1977 at St. John's Hospital in Santa Monica, California. The therapy lasted seven weeks. His radiologist at the hospital, Dr. Alfred Schmitz, spoke somewhat confidently, saying that the movie star's outlook "was good" that the cancer wouldn't return.

But come back it did within a very short time. This time the actor and his wife June flew to Hanover, Germany and consulted with Dr. Hans Nieper, a famous European doctor who treated patients using natural principles. (He had cured the wife of comedian Red Buttons of the very same type of throat cancer some time before this.)

Nieper's regimen for MacMurray included laetrile, a diet of organic foods, vitamins, minerals, enzymes, some medicinal herbs, and no red meat or alcohol. In place of the last two items, "lots of fish and organic carrot juice" were substituted. The fish was to be steamed or baked, *never* fried, deep-fried, or broiled. MacMurray was instructed by Nieper to drink carrot juice twice a day with a little cream in it.

He and his wife returned home where he spent several months at their ranch, leisurely resting up and having fun together. He soon put on weight, showed a healthy skin tone, and eventually tested negative for any further signs of cancer. Fred MacMurray lived for another 14 years after this, dying in November 1991 of pneumonia. Fred MacMurray worked in harmony with nature and was very cooperative with it in all aspects of his life. He took it easy and maintained a conservative lifestyle at all times. As a result, nature and Providence granted him many additional years of a wonderful life that was very fulfilling as a reward for his diligent efforts.

Food Sources

Amygdalin, as stated in the beginning, is a cyanogenic compound. When thoroughly hydrolyzed within the stomach by certain enzymes, amygdalin releases *very minute* traces of hydrogen cyanide, which some scientists believe accounts for its remarkably strong anticancer properties. According to a lengthy report in *Economic Botany* (30:395-407, 1963), there are about "200 species of plants from 45 families" growing in the Northeastern United States (and elsewhere) that contain amygdalin or closely-related compounds "capable of liberating hydrogen cyanide upon hydrolysis." This is the reference I worked from to present a variety of potential food and herb sources for amygdalin as found in the accompanying list.

Keep in mind that while elevated concentrations (anything over 100 parts per million) of hydrogen cyanide in an *isolated* form is certainly going to produce obvious health problems, nothing serious should ever occur when amygdalin in very *minute* amounts (somewhere between 15 and 43 parts per million) is ingested in food form surrounded by a number of other protective vitamins, minerals, amino acids, enzymes, sugars, and fiber. This is really the right way to take amygdalin instead of through pills or injections. At least this way, you know that the negative effects of hydrogen cyanide will be of extremely low impact upon the system. But, at the same time, this trace amount of hydrogen cyanide is always on patrol, making sure that cancer cells never develop or that existing tumor cells eventually meet a quiet chemical death within the circulating blood plasma.

The taste buds along either side of the tongue can readily detect vitamin B-17 in natural foodstuffs that are well chewed or swirled around inside the mouth for a few moments before being completely swallowed. The flavor thus yielded has a slightly bitter quality to it, signifying the presence of this presumed member of the B-complex group.

Plant Foods with Known Vitamin B-17 Contents
*(*Indicates higher amounts of amygdalin than usual, but not exceeding 100 ppm.)*

American mannagrass (cereal or salad/cooked vegetable)

Apple seed (snack/tea)

Apricot kernel, crushed (tea)*

Barley (cereal/breadstuff)

Bitter almond (snack/tea)*

Black cherry bark (tea)*

Black nightshade (fluid extract/tea)*

Borage (tea)*

Buttercup (salad/vegetable/tea)

Canadian thistle (salad/cooked vegetable)*

Cassava (cooked vegetable/stew)*

Corn (cereal/breadstuff)

European black currant (snack/preserve/juice)

Garden pea (salad/cooked vegetable)

Gram chickpea (soup/stew)

Hawthorn berry (tea/preserve)

Hyacinth bean (soup/stew)

Jimson weed (tea)*

Mexican tea (tea)*

Oats (cereal/breadstuff)

Passionflower (tea/fluid extract)

Peach kernel, crushed (tea)*

Peanut (snack/butter)

Perennial pepperweed (food condiment)

Plum pit, crushed (tea)*

Pyracantha bush (tea)*

Red clover (tea)*

Rye (cereal/breadstuff)*

Serviceberry (snack/preserve/juice)

Sorghum (molasses)

Sprouted seeds: alfalfa, garbanzo, mung, wheat (snack/salad or sandwich vegetable)

Sweet and sour cherry pits, crushed (tea)*

Watercress (salad vegetable)*

Wheat (cereal/breadstuff)

White clover (tea)

Wild cabbage (salad/cooked vegetable)

Wood sorrel (salad/cooked vegetable)

Yew bark (tea)*

Recommended Daily Intake

In the media heyday of laetrile of the 1970s, there was extensive information appearing fairly regularly in the medical literature pertaining to the potential harm that this substance could cause if taken in large enough quantities. Those opposing vitamin B-17 attempted to incite fear in the public mind by presenting unrealistic figures that they claimed represented legitimate human intake.

But it's one thing to overload small rodents with generous doses of laetrile and quite another to expect the same fatal results from large human beings. Take, for instance, the brief summary of a medical report that appeared in *Science News* (116:39, July 21, 1979). Researchers from Evanston (Illinois) Hospital and Northwestern Medical School gave varying doses of vitamin B-17 to rats that corresponded with the sizes of their individual tumors.

The result, of course, was the anticipated deaths in more than 50 percent of the rats they tested. The dosages ranged from 250 to 750 milligrams per kilogram of body weight per day for five days. The scientists conducting this fairly routine experiment drew some rather absurd conclusions, however, from their data. They argued that such high doses given to the rodents were "realistic in terms of human ingestion."

They would have been better off traveling to Tijuana first and visiting a few Mexican cancer clinics before making such a preposterous statement. At least then their educated ignorance wouldn't have been showing so much. Those familiar with the laetrile routinely administered by responsible therapists know that the normal range is usually *below* 250 milligrams as a rule. 'Nuff said on that!

B_T (L-CARNITINE): Nutrition for When You Get Older

It was G. Fraenkel who first stumbled across this vitamin-like nutrient in 1947, while in the course of investigating another B vitamin. Fraenkel was looking at the role of folic acid in the nutrition of insects, particularly the mealworm. (This small type of darkling beetle gets its unusual name from the short, cylindrical, and wormlike shape of the larvae; mealworms are used as food for such household pets as caged birds and tanked fish.) Fraenkel noticed that this tiny insect required a certain nutritional factor, present in the charcoal filtrate of yeast, which until then hadn't been recognized. To this factor he gave the name "vitamin B_T." The reason for the unusual designation is interesting in and of itself: the newly discovered nutrient behaved a lot like other B vitamins, while the $_T$ was appropriated from the first letter of the mealworm's scientific name, *Tenebrio molitor.*

If the mealworms were fed on a synthetic diet deficient just in vitamin B_T, they died in about a month. If this factor was added to the diet in very small increments, they grew to normal size (between 1/2 to 1 1/4 inches long). So consistent were his findings that they enabled Fraenkel to develop a technique for bioassay of vitamin B_T based on the rate of growth of mealworm larvae. Using this technique, he found there was a wide distribution of vitamin B_T in yeast, milk, liver, and whey, with particularly large quantities in muscle and meat extracts, which since have proven to be the most potent natural sources of vitamin B_T.

Fraenkel and his coworkers managed, with great difficulty, to concentrate large amounts of crystalline vitamin B_T in 1948. In collaboration with other scientists, he proved that vitamin B_T was identical with carnitine, a quaternary ammonium compound, which had been discovered in muscle in 1905. Carnitine, like so many other biological molecules, comes in two forms: L-carnitine (the active form found in body tissue) and D-carnitine (the biologically inactive form). The L- and D-forms have the same chemical makeup, but are mirror images of each other. To give you a better idea of what this means, stand in front of a mirror and look at your left hand; its mirrored image appears to be that of the right hand instead. There is also an equal mixture of both forms known as DL-carnitine. But due to possible side effects, consumers are strongly advised to use only the L-carnitine form and not the other two.

Six nutrients are required for the body to synthesize its own L-carnitine: lysine and methionine (a pair of essential amino acids), niacin and B-6 (two B-complex vitamins), vitamin C, and iron (a mineral). The synthesizing action takes place primarily in the liver and kidneys. In a study of adult rats the highest levels of L-carnitine were found in the heart, skeletal muscle, kidneys, and liver, with the lowest amounts showing up in the brain and blood serum, in that order. Hence, the prime uses for L-carnitine are in cardiac functions and the locomotion actions of the skeletal muscles.

The ranking of L-carnitine as a possible B vitamin is worth looking into more carefully. L-carnitine belongs to the same chemical family (quaternary amines) as choline, another B vitamin. Like choline, L-carnitine is an alcohol. And like other B vitamins, it contains nitrogen and is very soluble in water. Thus far, L-carnitine meets some of the qualifications for vitamin status. But, by strict definition, a vitamin is a substance essential to the body that can't be produced within the system and requires outside supplementation from the diet. In this sense then, L-carnitine doesn't measure up fully to all the criteria set for vitamins. But of all the amino acids, it is the most unusual in that it displays *some* behavior similar to the B-complex group. Therefore, it would be more proper to consider L-carnitine as an *auxiliary* B vitamin or a B-vitamin-like nutrient functioning in a subsidiary capacity instead of a main supporting role.

Deficiency of vitamin B_T may be categorized two different ways: those who are marginally deficient and those who are greatly deficient. Marginally deficient individuals are generally under 45 years of age and reach this state due to fasting, strenuous exercise, obesity, pregnancy, frequent sexual intercourse, or strict vegetarianism. Those who are greatly deficient in L-carnitine tend to be older as a rule (over 45) and suffering from a number of different disorders that include heart disease, high blood lipids, kidney disease, cirrhosis of the liver, malnutrition (manifested by underweight and extreme thinness), hypothyroidism (an underactive thyroid gland), and certain muscular and neurologic problems (such as muscular dystrophy and Reye's syndrome).

Following those body parts that have the highest concentrations of L-carnitine, we can trace this nutrient's usefulness for improving our health in several different ways.

HEART. According to *Postgraduate Medicine Journal* (72:45, 1996), "L-carnitine is found in high concentrations in cardiac muscle and serves several important physiological functions in the heart." This would include the prevention of myocardial infarction. L-carnitine also removes angina or heart pain.

According to *Cardiovascular Research* (29:373, 1995), "glucose utilization is markedly impaired in the diabetic heart." The result can be extreme fatigue, mental confusion, and belabored breathing. But with the addition of L-carnitine to the diet, fairly rapid recovery from these symptoms can be expected.

SKELETAL MUSCLE. According to *FEBS* (Federation of European Biochemical Societies) Journal (315:43, Jan. 1993), there is a significant decrease in skeletal muscle L-carnitine with increased age. But when prolonged administration of L-carnitine was given, levels of this vitamin-like nutrient became higher again in old animal models. And *The Journal of Clinical Nutrition & Gastroenterology* (8(1):28-29, Jan.-Mar. 1993) reported that old skeletal muscle lacking adequate L-carnitine eventually became weak, flabby, and fatty. But with consistent L-carnitine supplementation such symptoms were gradually reversed.

KIDNEYS AND LIVER. Italian biochemists presented convincing evidence that L-carnitine "significantly protects liver mitochondria against the damaging action of aging." Their report appeared in *Topics in Aging Research in Europe: Liver, Drugs and Aging* (7:104;108-09, 1986). (Liver mitochondria are small spherical or rod-shaped components found in the cell cytoplasms of that organ; they are the chief sites of energy generation within the liver. L-carnitine protects them from possible damage by free radicals and xenobiotics.)

Data presented in *Biochemical Medicine and Metabolic Biology* (43:163-174, 1990) shows that L-carnitine can stimulate the kidneys into action to remove ammonia toxins from the circulating blood plasma more quickly, so that there isn't a buildup that could lead to ammonia poisoning. Ammonia is a constant by-product of protein degradation, which comes from the frequent consumption of cooked red meat and from overexercise. L-carnitine works to reduce ammonia levels by increasing its incorporation into urea, which is subsequently excreted in the urine.

BRAIN AND BLOOD SERUM. L-carnitine influences the levels of certain neurotransmitters (such as GABA and taurine) in brain tissue. It is believed that vitamin B_T can help delay the progress of Alzheimer's disease and senility to some extent.

Food Sources

As an anthropologist I have been fascinated for many years with the incredible muscular strength and massive bone size of Late Paleolithic hunters and gatherers living close to the Ice Age. The Neanderthals of 50,000 years ago and the Cro-Magnons of 35,000 years ago consumed an exceptionally high proportion of wild game, which was very rich in L-carnitine. They were in the habit of roasting or consuming raw certain internal organs of such animals, like heart and liver, which were very high in iron and certain amino acids. Likewise, they foraged a lot for leafy greens and tuber vegetables that were rich in B-complex and vitamin C. All of this helped to produce *additional* L-carnitine within their remarkably powerful bodies.

Since they were wanderers, more than anything else, they weren't cursed with the debilitating effects of agriculture and animal husbandry, which is to say that they ate no cereal grains, eggs, or dairy products of any kind. And since their food processing was minimal at best, they weren't subjected to highly refined or overcooked foods as we are today. With the dramatic increase in food technology has come a severe reduction in public intake of L-carnitine.

It has been estimated by one scientist, R. Elwyn Hughes of the University of Wales, author of *L-Carnitine: Some Nutritional and Historical Implications* (Basel: Lonza Ltd., 1993; p. 33), that Late Paleolithic people consumed an average daily intake of 400 mg. per person of "nutritional carnitine base" components. This is compared with a puny 120 mg. daily per person for modern humans.

I have prepared the following table to show the L-carnitine contents of certain foods. It shows that animal foods are generally much better sources of this vitamin-like nutrient than are most plant foods. I have drawn my data from several sources for this: *FASEB Journal* (6:3381, 1992), *L-Carnitine (Vitamin B$_T$)*, 2nd ed. (Basel: Lonza Ltd., 1992; p. 7), and *The Analysis of Prehistoric Diets,* Robert I. Gilbert, Jr. and James H. Mielke, Eds. (New York: Academic Press, Inc., 1985).

Food Items	Total Content of L-Carnitine mg/100 grams of raw food
Sheep (mutton)	210
Lamb (meat)	78
Beef (meat)	64
Pig (meat)	30

Rabbit (meat)	21
Chicken (meat)	7.5
Fish (meat)	4.0
Cow's milk	2.0
Wheat germ	1.0
Eggs	0.8
Chicken liver (meat)	0.6
Bread	0.2
Avocado	0.2
Asparagus	0.2
Cauliflower	0.1
Peanuts	0.1
Cabbage	0
Orange juice	0
Barley seed	0
Spinach leaf	0
Potatoes	0

Of the previously mentioned nutrients (lysine, methionine, ascorbic acid, niacin, pyridoxine, and iron), lysine forms the backbone of the L-carnitine molecule. Since cereal grains such as corn, wheat, and rice are known to be very low in this essential amino acid, people consuming lysine-deficient diets are usually at highest risk for L-carnitine deficiency. Complicating this even more is lysine's sensitivity to heat: frying, baking, or toasting are known to destroy this delicate amino acid. Cooking foods at high temperatures is almost guaranteed to result in marginal lysine levels. So it stands to reason that processed foods can only provide marginal sources for L-carnitine biosynthesis. Light and heat also affect vitamin C, another L-carnitine cofactor.

Recommended Daily Intake

As we become older our bodies require more L-carnitine. For instance, it is now medically recognized that the infertility in the sperm of older men can be significantly improved with the addition of an L-carnitine supplement (300 mg., four to five times a day).

Eating foods rich in L-carnitine obviously makes good sense. But for those who are dedicated vegetarians for religious, cultural, economic, or health reasons, consumption of animal flesh is not an alternative. Also, cooking meat for any length of time is going to reduce some (but not all) L-carnitine content.

This is where dietary supplementation comes into focus. The *Physician's Desk Reference* (Montvale, NJ: Medical Economics Data, 1990) suggests 600 mg., 1 to 2 tablets three times a day or 1,800 to 3,600 mg. every day. In their classic work, *The Healing Nutrients Within* (New Canaan: Keats Publishing, Inc., 1987; pp. 308-09), authors Eric R. Braverman, M.D. and Carl C. Pfeiffer, M.D., Ph.D. mentioned that some of their patients took L-carnitine within the 500 to 600 mg. range three times a day to successfully correct heart arrhythmias and elevated triglycerides.

One teaspoon of brewer's yeast every day is also going to give you some L-carnitine. Mix it in with milk or juice to mask the taste.

Vitamin C

The Discovery of Vitamin C in Ancient and Modern Times

Writing some years ago in the consumer health magazine *Let's Live,* founded in 1939, (vol: 46, no. 8, p. 140), authors B. F. Hart, M.D. and Shirley S. Lorenzani, Ph.D. made this singular statement: "It can be said safely that vitamin C is the most versatile therapeutic agent known to man." From all that we know about it now, their remark certainly rings true. It is just because of this extreme healing and bolstering versatility that vitamin C "is required in greater amounts than all the other vitamins" combined, according to two Nigerian biochemists writing in the *Journal of Agricultural and Food Chemistry* (24:354, 1976).

Although ascorbic acid was discovered by the Hungarian biochemist Albert Szent-Gyorgyi, Ph.D. in 1927, its unofficial presence (or lack thereof) goes back to more than 3,500 years ago. Szent-Gyorgyi may have isolated the "energy" molecule with its unique six-carbon atomic structure to which he gave the name hexuronic acid, but the Egyptians knew that their slaves didn't thrive without plenty of fresh greens and fruits loaded with vitamin C.

Szent-Gyorgyi went on to prove that what he had found in working with orange juice, cabbage juice, and adrenal glands was, indeed, vitamin C. It was only a short step from this find to the actual synthesis of ascorbic acid. In 1937, he was awarded the Nobel prize for his contribution. There probably wasn't any equivalent award in the times of the pharaohs, but some of them were probably very grateful to the unnamed physicians who recommended that slaves be given more garden vegetables and fruits when it became apparent that they were tiring too easily from only minimal physical labor.

Information along these lines may be found in the Ebers Papyrus, one of the world's oldest medical texts, believed to have been compiled around 1550 B.C. Besides listing a number of things good for overcoming fatigue—one of the sure signs of low levels of vitamin C in the blood—this medical scroll also included a surprisingly accurate description of the circulatory system, correctly noting the existence of numerous blood vessels throughout the body and the heart's function as the center of the body's blood supply. The Ebers Papyrus was acquired by George Maurice Ebers, a well-known German Egyptologist and novelist, from certain bedouin tribesmen in 1873, who, it is believed, pilfered it from an ancient royal burial tomb.

Szent-Gyorgyi eventually bequeathed the name of ascorbic acid to his new vitamin discovery, as mentioned in the January 7, 1933 issue of *Nature* journal. He picked this scientific name because it emphasized the antiscurvy (or antiscorbutic) properties of the vitamin, hence *ascorbic*. Of course, now we know that it does a lot more than just prevent scurvy.

Interestingly enough, it is through the recorded history of scurvy that we can at least trace back for many centuries the "hidden" presence of vitamin C.

How Vitamin C Cured Scurvy, the Nutritional Plague of Centuries

Scurvy is probably the first disease ever to be associated with a dietary deficiency of some kind. It is marked by a weakening of the capillaries, which causes hemorrhages into the tissues, bleeding and sponginess of the gums, loosening of the teeth, anemia, edema, a brawny hardening of the muscles of the calves and legs, and general debility.

For many, many centuries scurvy was a serious health problem in many of the colder parts of the world, where fresh produce wasn't available in the wintertime. It was especially common among sailors in the distant past when only nonperishable foods could be stocked aboard ships. The ancient Phoenicians encountered this problem, but found ways around it. These seafaring people established numerous colonies all along the shores of the eastern Mediterranean. Two of their greatest cities were Tyre and Sidon, occupying what is now the coast of Lebanon.

By 1250 B.C., they were well-established navigators and traders of the entire Mediterranean world. They sailed to the edges of the known world at that time, trading from the Iberian Peninsula (Spain and Portugal) to the Dardanelles (a strait northwest of Turkey). Some historians are of the strong opinion that the Phoenicians even sailed to Cornwall in Southwest England in search of tin, and around the horn of Africa to the East Indies seeking exotic spices. There is some archaeological evidence, however meager, that a few Phoenician ships might even have reached the eastern coastline of South America and, quite possibly, retrieved hardwoods from the Brazilian rain forests.

While never contributing anything original themselves, these traders of the high seas bequeathed to Western civilization a lot of what they borrowed from other cultures that they came in contact with through their frequent business dealings. We don't know exactly when or where it was in their history, but early on some of their sailors became sick with a strange malady that we now know to be scurvy. The first indication of this approaching "plague" (as a few ancient medical manuscripts referred to it) was a pale and bloated complexion in the Phoenician navigators. This was invariably followed by a general listlessness and an aversion to any kind of physical activity. Soon there followed, according to one Phoenician record which was recently found and translated by scholars, "putrid breath of our crew, whose bodies were covered with large, discolored spots, and whose legs swelled like small melons."

How it was that they came by the secret of dried greens as an essential part of their seafaring rations, we will probably never know for sure. It could have been the Egyptians, Greeks, Persians, Hebrews, or some other more distant culture that first mentioned this idea to them. Or they may have incorporated several ideas from other people into one lifesaving technique. Needless to say, the idea enabled them to go longer distances without fear of this awful plague striking any of their navigators ever again.

The plan was so simple, it's surprising no one came up with it sooner than they did. Before embarking on any maritime expedition of considerable distance, it was mandatory to bring on board adequate supplies of *dried* leafy vegetation that were securely stored so as to be kept dry at all times. The "leafy vegetation" mentioned in these few ancient sources was never specified. It has generally been assumed, however, by historians and other scholars that it had reference to edible grasses, which were probably dried and ground into powder before being hauled on board, and more common leaf vegetables such as lettuce or cabbage. They, too, were probably dried in similar fashion and stored in clay jars or rough, wooden containers until needed for use.

These types of leafy vegetation would supplement regular fare of dried meat or fish, fruit such as figs or dates, and fresh drinking water or wine brought along for quenching the sailors' thirst. Just how such dried vegetation was reconstituted, though, remains a mystery. We can only conjecture how it may have been done. The ship crew may have built small fires on board in some iron contraptions and then heated water for simmering some of these dried greens in. Or, they may just have been crushed in a mortar with a stone pestle and the green powder thereof then mixed in with some water or wine and drank that way.

It should also be kept in mind that the Phoenicians docked at enough foreign harbors from time to time to allow them to replenish their food supplies. It is very possible that they made sure of bringing on board adequate amounts of fresh produce to give them enough ascorbic acid to prevent further recurrence of the plague they dreaded so much, namely scurvy. In time, their far-flung city states became overrun by other empires and the Phoenician civilization was entirely swallowed up into the various cultures of its different conquerors. What is really amazing about all of this, though, is that the simple Phoenician dietary cure for scurvy was eventually lost to the world.

Let us now fast-forward our historical narrative many centuries later to the time that the Iberians (Spanish and Portuguese) and Britannia ruled the ocean waves. Standard fare for those times on board all sailing vessels was dry biscuits, salt beef, and salt pork, which hardly contain any ascorbic acid. This diet was fairly routine for anyone who sailed around the time Columbus discovered the Americas (1492) and continuing on down to the last half of the nineteenth century. As a result, thousands of sailors died like flies. In fact, to go to sea meant almost certain *nutritional* death for many men, without a vessel ever having to engage in any type of combat.

In the event the reader may think I'm exaggerating the mortality statistics, let me cite just one example of many to confirm my facts. Vasco da Gama was a famous Portuguese navigator of the late fifteenth and early sixteenth centuries, who opened the sea route between Europe and India by way of the Cape of Good Hope. On his first epic voyage, made between July 8, 1497 and sometime in July 1499, he took a fleet of four vessels manned by a crew of 160. In this interval at least *100 sailors died of scurvy*. Most of these deaths occurred between the end of August, 1498 and January 8, 1499, when his severely weakened expedition finally managed to reach Malindi, a town in the coast province of Kenya. Unfavorable winds caused the Portuguese to take almost three months crossing the Arabian Sea, leaving them with scant supplies and virtually no food containing any vitamin C. Multiply these deaths by those suffered on the long sea voyages of many dozens of other Portuguese, Hispanic, and British navigators and it is fairly easy to see how such staggering losses could easily run into the thousands, if not tens of thousands!

It didn't take the Dutch very long, however, to catch on to the fact that something was missing from the diets of their sailors and was badly needed to curb this dreadful nutritional deficiency. They soon figured it out and began carrying citrus fruits and juices on board every one of their ships; as a result they cut their mortality rate to zero and scurvy disappeared forever from their vessels. But because the other three great maritime powers despised the Dutch (and vice versa), common knowledge of this nutritional factor remained known to only a few for several more centuries.

Deaths from scurvy became so unbelievably high for Britain during the eighteenth century that more British sailors were dying from ascorbic acid deficiency during wartime than were actually killed in battle!

Another grim example serves as a reminder of what happens when simple knowledge is set aside because of national pride and cultural prejudice. British Admiral George A. Anson undertook a voyage around the world in the ship Centurion between 1740 and 1744. He started with six ships and nearly 2,000 men, yet only the main flagship returned. Well over *one thousand* sailors died from— you guessed it—scurvy! This became such a national embarrassment that a British naval surgeon by the name of James Lind determined (or was ordered by the King of England) to seek the cure for this disease. He went on board the ship Salisbury and there performed his classical experiment on the 20th of May, 1747 with citrus fruits and plenty of green vegetables. The results were truly astonishing and nothing short of a real miracle: Those fed these foods didn't get scurvy; and those who were given regular ship's fare to begin with got it, but then saw a total disappearance of their sufferings once they began eating the same vitamin-C-rich foods their companions had been subsisting on. All of this is brilliantly portrayed in Lind's *A Treatise on the Scurvy* (London: A. Millar, 1753).

Again, the fickle finger of fate intervened and more British sailors continued dying. It took Dr. Lind seven years to finally publish his scientific results. But the British admiralty and numerous other physicians whom they consulted with refused to even give the good doctor's classic experiment a fair hearing. Nearly another half-century had to pass before lemon juice was finally prescribed to all British sailors in 1795, thereby earning them the perpetual nickname of "limey."

But Lind's efforts weren't entirely in vain. They had a prompt and profound effect upon a close friend of his, one Captain James Cook, one of the very first explorers to completely circumnavigate the globe. His lengthy voyages led to the discovery and exploration of New Zealand, Australia, and the Hawaiian Islands, where he was later killed by unfriendly natives. Cook wasn't just content with Lind's recommendations, for he also insisted upon absolute cleanliness and extreme hygienic measures aboard ship. This was something entirely new for his crew and unprecedented in those dirty times of infrequent baths or hand washings. He sent some of his crew ashore at every opportunity to gather all manner of greens, even grasses just as the ancient Phoenicians had done many centuries before; these were prepared, served, and eaten on his strict orders. He employed the ingenious technique of insisting that his officers eat this food in front of the men, whereupon they deemed it more than suitable and ate their fair share without raising much of a fuss. By these clever methods Captain Cook was the first (other than the Dutch and Phoenicians) to demonstrate that prolonged ocean voyages didn't really need to result in scurvy if a little dietary common sense was used along the way. His first voyage from 1768 to 1771 and his second from 1772 to 1775 conclusively demonstrated that scurvy could be prevented.

So some of the health wisdom of the ancient seafaring Phoenicians finally was rediscovered in the likes of men such as physician Lind and explorer Cook. While it would remain for Szent-Gyorgyi to actually isolate and name ascorbic acid properly a few centuries later, full credit must go to these others who found the "food cures" for one of mankind's worst deficiency diseases.

The Only Thing Wrong Was Subclinical Scurvy

Here is a real medical horror story to make your hair stand on end and make you vow never to become a hospital patient, no matter how serious your health problem may be. It actually happened to one woman and was reported in detail in the March 28, 1977 issue of the *Journal of the American Medical Association* (JAMA). If someone on the medical staff at the facility she kept going back to hadn't inquired about her eating habits, the chances were very good she might have died in surgery when doctors opened her abdomen for the seventh or eighth time to find out why she kept bleeding internally. I've greatly condensed her bizarre case history to make it more readable and save space.

Sometime in April 1967, a 48-year-old woman visited her physician complaining of excessive menstrual flow for a year and abdominal pain for about five weeks. Her abdomen was severely distended, but no evidence of blood-containing tumors called angiomas could be found. He figured she had endometriosis, hospitalized her, and a couple of days later cut her open, only to discover a large quantity of blood in her abdomen. The decision was made to remove her uterus, her ovaries, and her appendix, just in case they might have been contributing to this internal hemorrhaging.

Four months later, she was readmitted with the same symptoms. This time another doctor decided it was a bowel obstruction and cut her open again to straighten out a small twist in her colon. In doing so, he noticed a number of places oozing blood and surgically removed some of these and cauterized the rest.

One year and one month later, this same patient was readmitted a third time with identical symptoms: excessive internal bleeding, cramping pain, and abdominal distention. She requested an entirely different surgeon, who stuck a diagnostic needle into her abdomen and, you guessed it, found blood. He put her under the knife again and found unclotted blood, along with many cysts, all over the inside of her belly. The surgical team removed the cysts, drained off the excess fluid, and stitched her back up.

In November 1968 and January 1969 she again suffered the same problems. A battery of tests was run to help doctors understand what could be causing her trouble.

Nothing seemed to make enough sense, though, from the data generated by all of these tests to form a reliable diagnosis. So, another operation took place, which drew out considerable blood that had been floating around in her abdomen. Since her spleen contained blood tumors, it was removed this time and she was sewed up again. Then the same tests were repeated all over again—bone marrow tests and every imaginable test of blood function that her doctors could think of. Everything checked out as being normal. She went home and left doctors scratching their heads in total ignorance.

In May 1969, she was readmitted for the same thing, and this time had her pancreas removed since it appeared to the doctors to be "acting up." In June 1970 a similar surgical procedure was repeated for the sixth time for the same identical reasons. After that, she was immediately discharged.

In March 1971, guess who came back to where for more of the same pain and anguish ? By now it had moved from being multiple déjà vu to what may have seemed to be sadomasochism. But the woman clearly wasn't deriving an ounce of pleasure from all of the physical, mental, and emotional pain being inflicted upon her by various doctors. After a thorough psychological investigation had been conducted on her by a competent psychiatrist, doctors even ruled out a possible Munchausen syndrome. This woman certainly wasn't returning for repeat treatments of an apparent acute illness and giving false information to make it seem all the more plausible.

But there were no more proverbial straws for doctors to grasp at, even though the same symptoms were clearly being manifested for the umpteenth time. By now, none of the hospital surgeons even dared running the risk of a seventh exploratory operation. And yet the poor woman was begging for help.

It was left up to a hospital dietician, who, quite by accident, overheard some of the physicians discussing this bizarre case over lunch together. The dietician went to the patient's room and inquired if she ever ate any fresh fruits or vegetables. The dietician was astonished to learn that the patient almost *never* consumed such items. This was reported back to her equally amazed doctors, who ran a nutritional blood analysis on their puzzling patient.

The results came back indicating that her circulating blood plasma was almost totally devoid of vitamin C. They promptly prescribed 1,000 mg. of ascorbic acid daily and instructed her to go on taking that much for as long as was necessary. For several years everything went fine, until one day in 1976 when she showed up again at the hospital with the same symptoms. The doctors on call that day, after reviewing her medical records, asked her if she had been faithfully taking her vitamin C. The woman shamefully admitted she hadn't been doing so for some time. Her blood tested out again as being virtually free of any vitamin C.

This time doctors explained the need for her to diligently consume vitamin C every day in terms of life and death: take it and you'll live; don't take it and you'll soon die! This made a believer out of her at last, and they never saw her again with her old symptoms after that. Two of. the doctors from the California hospital where this strange event unfolded made these observations in their *JAMA* report: "The salutary outcome (of this case) can be interpreted in terms of the vascular effects of vitamin C. Deficiency leads to formation of defective ground substance in collagen, the support material of vascular structures. Serious deficiency leads to vascular disruption and bleeding. Moreover, if superimposed on vasculature already flawed, bleeding eventuates more readily. *This process, however, is reversible* . . . Subclinical scurvy should be considered whenever bleeding develops in an angiomatous (blood-tumor-forming) patient."

Imagine all of the suffering, sorrow, and economic costs that could have been saved if someone had had the good sense and judgment to inquire of the patient's diet on the very first visit and then ordered her to take plenty of ascorbic acid. Just think how crippled for life she became with having so many of her important internal organs removed for something as ridiculously simple as a vitamin deficiency disease. An investment of just a few dollars per month in vitamin C could have prevented all of this from ever happening. Imagine how many hundreds of thousands of people who visit clinics or hospitals every year might be cured easily and painlessly with a small investment of pocket change in a nutritional supplement that has proven to be one of the greatest health blessings to mankind in the twentieth century.

Vitamin C Fights Scurvy Fatigue

You would think, with all of the emphasis being placed on healthier diets these days, that people would be consuming more of those citrus fruits and leafy green vegetables that are rich in vitamin C, and that because of this there would be virtually no evidence of *outright* scurvy.

In some ways this is true, but in other ways it isn't. Yes, more people are eating oranges and drinking orange juice, thanks to massive advertising campaigns conducted by the Florida Citrus Growers Association and the Sunkist Corp. of California. But because of the pasteurization process of all commercially sold orange juice in America (that invariably involves heat), very little vitamin C remains in the finished product.

If that isn't bad enough, consider what happens to fresh produce intended for restaurant salad bars. There is nothing to worry about, of course, in terms of vitamin C loss due to heat, since refrigeration keeps everything cool, crisp, and green-looking for awhile. In this case, according to *Science News* (136:255, 1989), it's the excessive use by farmers of nitrogen fertilizer that's going to cut down the vitamin C content quite a bit in such salad produce. A soil scientist with the US DA 's Agricultural Research Center in Beltsville, Maryland compared chard grown under two different types of farming techniques. Chard grown without fertilizers had 81.4 mg. of vitamin C per 100 grams of leaves, whereas the same quantity of heavily fertilized plants yielded just 54 mg. The same research also pinpointed nitrogen as the cause of a vitamin C decline in green beans and kale. Elsewhere, it has been observed that the "gassing" of tomatoes, bananas, and other produce to improve and hold their colors for longer periods of time actually diminishes their vitamin C content *drastically!*

So what we have here is an unbelievable irony taking place with consumer dietary practices: A greater percentage of the American public are eating more of those foods known for their high ascorbic acid contents, but, in fact, are actually getting *far less* vitamin C than is generally supposed.

Besides these factors, there are also the "junk food" and "fast food" problems to contend with. Foods high in sugar quickly remove vitamin C from the body. And foods cooked in hot grease of *any* kind not only have their *entire* vitamin C content destroyed, but the saturated fats themselves bind up whatever vitamin C remains in the blood so it can't be fully utilized as it should.

All of this has created a unique kind of *subclinical scurvy* that is usually quite difficult for most doctors to detect with ordinary diagnostic measures. There generally aren't the extreme symptoms manifested that plagued sailors centuries ago. But there is one common problem that seems to have surfaced more in the last few years in this country. That is a general malaise of public fatigue that is evident everywhere you go.

Put in plain terms, Americans these days are more tired for longer periods of time than their parents or grandparents before them were. This generation and the younger one coming up appear to run out of steam sooner every day than their forebears did. We live in a nation of exhausted citizens whose "get-up-and-go" seems to have "got-up-and-went" before the day is done. We can't blame all of this on lack of sleep, stress, the rat race, or modern technology. In fact, probably a good 40 percent of it is due to *insufficient vitamin C* in the circulating blood plasma of 70 percent of Americans between the ages of 15 and 55.

And yet, to all outward appearances, they look healthy enough. Their gums, tongues, breath, skin, and muscles don't suggest any kind of obvious scurvy at least. But beneath the facade of presumably good health lurks what some health experts have determined to be subclinical scurvy. The only outward proof of it that keeps surfacing all the time is fatigue, fatigue, fatigue!

The best solution for this lack of necessary vitality when it's needed the most is ample supplementation of vitamin C on a *daily* basis. I have been recommending upward of 1,500 to 3,000 mg. every day for those who can't seem to muster enough energy to finish the day out. And most of those I've been thus advising in the last few years usually eat at least two good meals a day and consider themselves fairly health-conscious in terms of their diets. Still, they find their reduced vigor to be inadequate for accomplishing everything they've set their minds to doing each and every day. And they're frustrated as can be by this, not really knowing what is happening to them.

In many instances their own health care providers are just as baffled by this creeping lassitude as their patients are. Tests are run, diagnoses made, and numerous things prescribed, but still the weariness remains. The obvious "energy-draining diseases" have already been ruled out: no hypoglycemia, no yeast infection, and no herpes. So, what's left to diagnose as a probable cause for all this listlessness?

The answer may surprise you as it did me when I first started investigating this mysterious phenomenon a few years ago. Thinking it may have been overlooked candidiasis or herpes simplex in many of those who contacted me for free advice, I started suggesting vitamin C with the idea in mind that at least it would be able to arrest any such infection hidden deep inside the body.

Imagine my own pleasant delight when some of those I had passed that recommendation on to reported back later on how much better they felt after taking a good brand of vitamin C *and* increasing their daily intake of *organically* raised fruits and vegetables that are high in ascorbic acid content.

I remember speaking with a woman by phone on a radio talk show I did in Chicago some time ago. She called in complaining of constant lethargy. I mentioned in passing a new product which had helped many others in similar situations to experience more vim and vigor once they had begun taking two capsules every morning.

I noted that most of its herbal ingredients were relatively high in vitamin C, which I felt was a definite plus in terms of energy delivery. Dick Drewery, the show host, gave the woman my address off the air in the event she wanted to write to me later on. Several months passed before a letter came bearing a Winnetka postmark. The woman writing identified herself as the one with whom I had spoken sometime before on "Drewery at Night." She said she had contacted the company (see Product Appendix), obtained some of this product, and had been using it faithfully ever since. "Thanks to your information, I now have more energy than I've had in years." She had also been eating more citrus fruits and leafy greens as well, which certainly was a wonderful testimony of the energy-producing capabilities of vitamin C.

A phone call to my home one night shortly after appearing on the Chicago talk show to discuss the many health benefits of vitamin C came from a middle-aged fellow residing in Kenilworth (near Winnetka). He was calling to share with me his own success involving vitamin C. He had gone to a nearby health food store on my advice and purchased some chewable vitamin C tablets. He said he didn't like swallowing pills that much, and so opted for something chewable instead. He chewed one of these 250 mg. tablets every couple of hours on an empty stomach whenever he felt a need for a *little more* energy. He reported feeling slightly more vigorous about 20 minutes after chewing one of these tablets. He said that while the effects were rather subtle, "it did make some difference in the way I felt afterward."

There are three different ways of getting vitamin C for energy-boosting purposes: from fresh produce consumed raw or else juiced in a whole food machine; from an herbal combination; or from a chewable tablet. The point here is that ascorbic acid in *different forms* really can make a difference in that type of puzzling fatigue that is most often attributed to a mild case of subclinical scurvy. Ascorbic acid may not always work as dramatically as energy-producing products are hyped to do. In fact, as in the case of the gentleman from Kenilworth, vitamin C is usually more modest in its initial impact upon an energy-drained system. But once the ascorbic acid does take effect, it makes a world of difference in how you feel after that!

Antisocial Behavior Corrected with Vitamin C

The next time you're on a major freeway somewhere in metropolitan America and an angry truckdriver behind you swears at you or an irritable career woman lays on her horn beside you indicating she wants to cut in, ask yourself if that person doesn't need a healthy dose of vitamin C.

In the two decades following the actual isolation of vitamin C by Szent-Gyorgyi in 1928, some important nutritional studies were published in the medical literature by American, British, and German psychiatrists and biochemists relevant to ascorbic acid levels in patients experiencing a variety of psychological disorders. Several interesting findings emerged from the collective works of F. Plaut, M.D., O. Altaman, M.D., J. Monouni, M.D., Donald G. Kemp, Ph. D., P. Berkenau, M.D., and others during this period. First of all, brain, blood, and spinal fluid levels of ascorbic acid were considerably lower in those manifesting mental diseases of some kind and in the elderly. Secondly, and more important for our purposes here, was the substantial improvement in many of those formerly exhibiting psychotic behavior when given a mere 300 milligrams per day of ascorbic acid in tablet form. (It should be observed here that in those times, such an amount was considered quite high, but by today's standards that dosage would be regarded as rather low.)

Evidence like this lay mostly dormant in the medical literature without much attention being paid to it until the start of the 1970s. At that time some within the scientific community went back and began reevaluating the old reports from several decades before, deciding for themselves that they warranted additional follow-up research to either sustain or disprove those earlier claims about vitamin C helping to improve behavior in people with social and mental problems.

The first significant study in this promising direction was completed in 1970 by the Department of Internal Medicine at the University of Iowa and was partially funded by the United States Army Medical Research and Development Command. The study was conducted with the permission of the warden and volunteer inmates of the Iowa State Penitentiary. Prisoners were gradually deprived of vitamin C in the food they ate until blood tests showed extremely low levels of this vital nutrient. At this point, inmates became more unruly and cranky than usual, also exhibiting bouts of depression, hysteria, melancholia, hypochondriasis, increased fatigue, and lassitude. But when vitamin C was reintroduced into their diets through citrus fruits and juices and fresh vegetables, these same inmates eventually became more well-behaved and tolerant toward others. This report appeared in the April 1971 issue of the *American Journal of Clinical Nutrition* (24:455-64).

During this decade a small group of psychiatrists, committed to treating antisocial behavior with nutritional therapy more than with drugs, utilized vitamin C a lot in treating their mentally disturbed patients. Dr. Jordan Scher's work with alcoholics at the Methadone Maintenance Institute in Chicago and Drs. Alfred Libby and Irwin Stone's work with heroin addicts in California were typical of such pioneering efforts. While a full complement of nutrients was usually employed for such treatments, vitamin C always occupied a very central position in such endeavors, These psychiatrists discovered several remarkable things happening to their recovering alcoholics and addicts while on high ascorbic acid intakes (between 2,500 and 8,500 milligrams daily):

- Vitamin C decreased withdrawal symptoms.
- Vitamin C reduced hangover symptoms.
- Vitamin C detoxified the body of drug and alcohol residue.
- Vitamin C had "a moderating and tranquilizing influence on the behavior and emotional states" of recovering alcoholics and addicts.
- Vitamin C *removed* much of the further craving for alcohol and illicit substances such as heroin, methamphetamines, and marijuana.

Much of this research was published in various issues of the *Journal of Orthomolecular Psychiatry* throughout the middle to late 1970s.

The quiet work of the unassuming Barbara Reed also took center stage and received considerable publicity in the media in the last half of 1977. For some 14 years this woman had been working in criminal rehabilitation. At the time her star of fame ascended into public relations heaven, she had been the Chief Probation Officer in the Cuyahoga Falls (Ohio) Municipal Probation Department for about five years. In an exclusive interview in the *Wall Street Journal* (June 2, 1977), she blamed much of the criminal behavior she had seen in juvenile delinquents and adults on junk foods fed to them "from babyhood on." Sugary foods were the real culprits, she felt, in robbing the body of valuable vitamins and minerals, such as ascorbic acid. With little or no nutrients for stabilizing behavior, it was no surprise to her that such individuals had turned to a life of crime and violent behavior.

But when she started changing the diets of several hundred offenders and putting them on a highly nutritious diet, there was "a definite change in attitude and appearance" in nearly all her subjects. One of them, she told the reporter from the *Journal,* was a 20-year-old man arrested for criminal damage, destruction of property, and discharging a firearm. He was placed on a special diet rich in vitamin C foods and high in protein. His depression soon vanished and he became "optimistic, cooperative and realistic."

About three weeks later Reed went before the United States Senate Select Committee on Nutrition and Human Needs and explained in considerable detail her experience with 318 offenders. Of these, "252 required attention as to their diet and vitamin needs." She then outlined for committee members certain aspects of what she referred to as "my anticrime diet." For our purposes here, only the vitamin C part is mentioned: fresh citrus fruit (oranges, grapefruits, tangerines, and nectarines), citrus juices (orange and grapefruit) that were frozen, canned, or bottled, cooked potatoes (white or sweet), fresh tomatoes and tomato juice (canned or bottled), and dark-green (bell peppers, parsley, spinach) and orange-yellow (carrots, squash) vegetables.

This prompted former Senator Robert Dole of Kansas (the Republican candidate for the U. S. Presidency in 1996) to inquire: "Mrs. Reed, I wonder how many of these success stories are because of your diet and how many are because they may have been receiving special attention [from you], someone caring about their rehabilitation?" Barbara Reed responded to his question this way: "I've been in this field for 14 years. I was giving people a lot of loving attention before without nearly the results as now. *The two work hand in hand* . . . but, I just don't think probationers heard what we were talking about when they were so disconnected with reality that they couldn't remember what had been said. Now they do remember and it makes a big difference." In wrapping up her Senate testimony, she concluded: "Never before has the court had such a tool for working with the many ill people who find themselves in court. We wonder what the results would be if this method could also be applied to all those sentenced to jail."

One study that was published just a year after Reed's testimony would have satisfied her in this respect. The report by M. E. Ware on the effects of ascorbic acid on the behavior of institutionalized juvenile delinquents appeared as a chapter of *Ecologic-Biochemical Approaches to Treatment of Delinquents and Criminals,* edited by L. J. Hippchen (New York: Van Nostrand & Reinhold, 1978). Ware tested both ascorbic acid and niacin on 45 adolescent males. They were selected because of extreme antisocial behavior, even bordering on violence sometimes. Subjects were randomly assigned to receive either the two vitamins, a placebo, or no medication during the six-week trial period. Those receiving vitamins C and B-3 showed a 32 percent decrease in antisocial behavior; those receiving a placebo demonstrated a 15 percent decrease; and those receiving no medication manifested a mere 9 percent decrease. Such differences were considered to be "statistically significant," indicating the merits of vitamins C and B-complex *together* in greatly minimizing, if not actually curbing, destructive and unfruitful behavior.

Another person called to testify before the same Senate Select Committee on Nutrition that Mrs. Reed had appeared before was Dr. Carolyn Brown, the executive director of "The Growing Mind," a California center for treating delinquent children. She said, "There is a direct connection between juvenile delinquency, disturbed children and nutrition. I have seen plenty of clinical evidence that nutritional therapies can play a significant role in helping these children. A diet free of chemicals, low in refined carbohydrates, free of synthetic foods, with a judicious and individualized program of nutritional supplementation (that includes adequate amounts of vitamin C and B-complex)—together with the avoidance of foods and chemicals to which children may be allergic or hypersensitive—can be a critical factor in reversing the personal decline of many of the children we have worked with."

The extensive research conducted by Stephen Schoenthaler, Ph.D. during this same decade with vitamins C and B-complex also needs to be cited in passing. At that time he was an associate professor of sociology and director of the Criminal Justice Studies Program at California State University at Stanislaus. In his first study, Schoenthaler monitored 276 youth in a Virginia juvenile detention center after major food changes had been instituted at the facility. The cafeteria began offering menus higher in fiber and fresh vegetables and fruits high in vitamins C and B-complex, and reduced the sugary desserts and foods with chemical additives. Following the changes, the number of reported behavioral problems among inmates fell 48 percent. There were also reductions in assaults, threats, insubordination, and hyperactivity.

Testing further, Schoenthaler set up similar studies at 12 juvenile correctional facilities in Alabama, California, and Washington, D.C., involving more than 8,000 youngsters. The results: a whopping 47 percent drop in overall trouble after improvement in the nutritional program. Additionally, a parallel series of standard psychological tests indicated noteworthy behavioral improvement among the institute populations.

The question now needing an answer was why did these positive changes occur? Schoenthaler wondered if they were "due to the elimination of things from the diet, such as the sugars or food additives," or, perchance, was it because some basic and vital nutrients were absent from these young people's diets?

To find out once and for all, he carefully analyzed the diets of 328 institutionalized offenders in New York, Oklahoma, California, Virginia, and Florida. He found that the youths who behaved the worst selected foods that tended to be significantly lower in two key nutrients— vitamin C and members of the B-complex group (B-1, B-2, B-3, B-6, and B-9). Four minerals (calcium, magnesium, zinc, and iron) were also sorely missing from foods these children liked to consume often.

"These specific deficiencies were the most clearly correlated with behavior problems," Schoenthaler observed. "An individual who was low in the vitamins especially was found to have a 90 percent likelihood to commit serious crimes within the institution. By contrast, a person who wasn't low in any of these vitamins or minerals had a less than 50 percent likelihood of becoming a troublemaker."

But Schoenthaler's inquisitive mind just didn't stop with these satisfying results. If such apparent nutritional deficiencies were a causative factor in antisocial behavior, what would happen, he wondered, if a vitamin and mineral supplement high in ascorbic acid and B-complex were given and the diets left unchanged?

"We knew the improved diet had a positive effect and we now wanted to know if a nutritional supplement strong in vitamins C and B-complex and some supporting minerals could do the same job by itself," he stated.

Three institutions in Oklahoma, California, and Florida were selected for a three-month supplement test. Menus were left the same. Participants received a one-a-day supplement that emphasized ascorbic acid and many of the essential B vitamins previously mentioned and included moderate amounts of some minerals.

The results were astonishing, even to Schoenthaler! In Oklahoma, there was a 43 percent drop in behavioral problems among the 23 individuals who participated; in California, among 17 individuals, there was a 37 percent improvement; in Florida, 16 youths participated and registered significant improvements in standardized psychological tests. According to sociologists, behavioral changes started to be observed in many individuals within 24 to 48 hours. Of the 40 subjects 22 remained out of trouble during the entire study period, including the worst offender among them, a youth whose record listed 26 serious incidents during the prior 2 months.

The implications are enormous from Schoenthaler's patient and careful work in the turbulent 70s. His work confirms that vitamin C, B-complex, and key minerals play critical roles in human behavior. With as much violent crime as is now going on among many youth gangs in America, it would certainly pay for those involved in dealing with such problems to seriously investigate and start using inexpensive vitamin C and B-complex tablets every day. Not only would the crime rate be drastically slashed, but an entire generation of budding criminals might eventually grow into healthy and responsible citizens, thereby making their respective communities better places to live.

(I am very much indebted to my long-time friend, Martin Zucker of Hollywood, California, for bringing to light Schoenthaler's impressive research on this subject.)

The question now arises, "About how much vitamin C each day is necessary to maintain your cool?" Put another way, how much ascorbic acid should you be taking to prevent some type of *serious* antisocial behavior from occurring in you? Several orthomolecular psychiatrists and psychologists who emphasize nutritional therapy in their practices and with whom I conferred for their input on this matter suggested a *minimum* daily intake of not less than 200 mg. of vitamin C. Nutritionists will tell you that eating your choice of just five fruits and vegetables every day will easily provide you with this much ascorbic acid. My therapist informants noted that anything below 100 mg. of vitamin C a day is going to make a person tired, cranky, despondent, and, as one psychiatrist abruptly stated, "temperamental as hell!"

Stop the Wheezing and Sneezing

Just about every one of us knows somebody who has had a critical medical problem of some kind and gone from doctor to doctor in hopes of finding a solution for it. Ultimately, such individuals sometimes turn to alternative health care specialists as a last resort, in desperate hope that something along more natural lines of treatment might save them from their dilemmas. Cancer is probably the one disease that causes the most of these "doctor-hopping" experiences to take place.

I know someone who went through the "medical gristmill" because of her asthma, and then repeated her trial-and-error routine with a number of holistic practitioners. She asked that her real name not be used, so I will assign the pseudonym of Jill to identify her in my short narrative. I will spare readers the intimate details of her visits to seven different orthodox medical doctors in search of drug relief for her chronic asthma. Nothing they prescribed really helped, so she turned to what seemed the next most logical procedure—alternative medicine. I will let "Jill" tell her own story from this point, though I've obviously edited somewhat for brevity's sake.

"My first visit was to a licensed massage therapist, who rubbed, slapped, pinched, pulled, thumped, and whacked my skin so much that I felt afterward as if I'd been in a fight with someone and had been unable to defend myself. But I still wheezed a lot in spite of that rough ordeal.

"A well-intentioned friend at the travel agency I work at suggested I visit her chiropractor, saying how much relief she obtained for her own allergies after several spinal adjustments. I paid a visit to Dr. B——— and he jerked my neck sideways twice until I thought I had a whiplash, cracked my back in rapid succession until I wondered if I would ever be able to stand again, and adjusted my pelvis more fondly than I wanted him to. After that, he pronounced me 'cured' and directed his receptionist out front through an office intercom to 'Send in the next patient, please.' He then interlocked his fingers together, reversed his hands, and gave them a powerful cracking pop so as to be ready for his next unlucky victim. I paid the $65 for his three minutes worth of treatment and left feeling humiliated and frustrated at the same time.

"Then there was Dr. Aye Ching (pronounced I Ching), the acupuncturist. After poking and prodding my body with his bony fingers, he pronounced as the problem for my asthma that my 'kidneys are deficient in yang energy and my liver had too much old chi power in it.' He then proceeded to place a number of needles of various lengths and thicknesses in my left ear and all over my back as I laid semi-naked on top of a cushioned table in one therapy room. An ointment of some kind was rubbed over a portion of my skin and a match lit to it. The next thing I knew small parts of my back were ablaze with herbal moxa and I could distinctly smell burning flesh. When he finished I had several permanent scars for life. And to add insult to injury, my asthma still persisted.

"Another time I visited a homeopathic specialist on the recommendation of another—you guessed it—helpful friend. This fellow gave me four or five vials of different material and told me which ones to take when and how often. I followed his advice for several days until I broke out in hives. Alarmed by this unexpected side effect, I frantically phoned him. He reassured me there was nothing to worry about, that it was just the 'old poisons coming out' with the new ones he was having me put into my system. Several more days of this and I checked myself into the local hospital where a dermatologist gave me immediate relief for my severely inflamed skin with a bunch of medicated creams. He wondered aloud if I had accidentally burned myself with kerosene or something. I was too ashamed to tell him what had *really* caused it.

"I finally lost it when I screamed at another friend to 'get the hell away and leave me alone,' after she mentioned seeing an iridologist for my complaint. I quickly made amends by apologizing and then broke down in tears and sobbed 'Why can't someone tell me something simple that will work? Am I so bad to deserve all of *this?*' "

Help finally came to Jill in a most unusual way. "One day I was driving down the Pacific Coast Highway just north of San Diego a couple of miles," she related, "and was 'channel surfing' on my radio trying to find something interesting to listen to. I flipped the radio over to the AM side and immediately got a talk show segment then in progress on XTRA, the all-sports radio station down this way.

"Some doctor whose name I never caught was discussing a condition of one of his patients, a well-known tennis star. I gathered from the gist of things that this guy was into sports medicine or something like that. Anyhow, he was telling listeners how his patient used to suffer from chronic asthma, just like I did at the time. And the doctor claimed that his big-name tennis star was actually *cured*—that's the exact word he used over the air—by taking megadoses of vitamin C every day.

"I couldn't believe my ears when I heard this. It was truly a godsend right out of the clear blue sky! I couldn't wait to find myself a health food store. I bought a 1,500-milligram strength of *esterified* vitamin C with rosehips, found a drinking fountain, hurriedly unscrewed the bottle cap, and took four tablets right then and there.

"As I continued up the road to a luncheon business conference of local travel agents, I waited in anticipation to see what would happen next. I was startled but extremely pleased when for the next six hours I *didn't* have anymore recurring wheezing, breathing resonance, or periodic rapid heart beating. *It was truly heavenly to be able to breathe normally again without reliance on my medications!*" (She had been regularly using an inhaled steroid, beclomethasone diprorionate, as well as taking cromolyn, a well-known antiasthmatic drug, every day.)

Jill has been free of asthma now for several years ever since she's been taking eight 1,500-mg. strength tablets each day (four in the morning and the other four in the evening). Medical research has shown of late that ascorbic acid does, indeed, strengthen the lungs of those suffering from bronchial asthma. It is known that vitamin C concentrates certain prostaglandins, which exhibit hormone-like actions, that dilate the bronchial tubes. As little as 500 mg., in fact, can stave off exercise-induced asthma for those suffering from milder versions of the same problem.

How to Stop Heart Attacks and Strokes

In the early 1950s, Dr. G. C. Willis made the national and international medical communities sit up and take notice with some rather provocative published research. He showed that ascorbic acid was vital in the maintenance of the integrity of the arterial walls of the heart (known as the intima). Any social (stress), emotional (anger), or dietary (excessive meat or fried and deep-fried foods intake) factors disturbing this vitamin C metabolism would invariably result in arterial wall injury with subsequent fatlike deposits occurring thereafter. In his landmark paper, Willis concluded that acute or chronic vitamin C deficiency in guinea pigs produced atherosclerosis and closely simulated the human form of this pervasive disease.

A year later Willis and his fellow coworkers studied the actual progression and retrogression of atherosclerotic plaques in living patients by a serial x-ray technique. The study demonstrated quite clearly a definite reduction in atherosclerotic plaque lesions in the group of ascorbic acid patients that was not observed in the non-vitamin-C-supplemented controls. Based on these studies, Dr. Willis confidently announced that "massive doses of parenteral ascorbic acid may be of therapeutic value in the treatment of atherosclerosis and the prevention of intimal hemorrhage and thrombosis."

Considerably more work on a worldwide scale followed his pioneering research. Toward the end of the 1970s, cholesterol in general was no longer the implied villain in heart disease. The catchphrase that then started popping up with regularity at every medical symposium and journal concerned with heart disease and was relayed by an eager media to the listening and reading public was lipoproteins—the "good" cholesterol (high-density lipoproteins) versus the "bad" cholesterol (low-density lipoproteins). In a way, these lipoproteins are as different from each other as some of the big names in professional wrestling—heroes like Hulk Hogan and Randy "Macho Man" Savage going up against culprits like The Junkyard Dog or Brutus Beefcake.

Lipoproteins are those large globules of fat and protein which transport cholesterol through the bloodstream. They range in molecular weight from 200,000 all the way up to 10 million and from 4 to 95 percent fat; the higher the density, the lower the fat content. The low-density fractions are especially rich in triacylglycerols and cholesterol esters, which chemically harden on contact with blood vessel walls. But the high-density fractions have very minimal amounts of these materials and, therefore, don't accumulate like the others do.

Think of the high-density lipoproteins (HDLs) as good wrestlers; they come into the ring (the circulatory system) and toss the bad guys or low-density lipoproteins (LDLs) out. The HDLs cruise around in the circulating blood plasma. When they spot a Junkyard Dog or Brutus Beefcake, they quickly put these bad LDLs into chemical "headlocks," "armlocks," or full "body grips," before hauling them off to the liver where they are soon hustled into the digestive tract and finally excreted from the body altogether.

But if the bad guys prevail (due to low ascorbic acid levels) then the gradual result over many years is atherosclerosis of the heart or even brain stroke due to a fatty blood clot. Evidence for vitamin C preventing fatty plaque buildup in the heart and possible stroke may be seen in a remarkable study that was published in the May 8, 1992 issue of the medical journal *Epidemiology*. A research team headed by Dr. James E. Enstrom, an epidemiologist with the School of Public Health at UCLA, examined dietary and supplemental sources of vitamin C regularly consumed by 11,348 men and women around the country. These individuals were original participants in a major government study of dietary intake and health known as the First National Health and Nutrition Examination Survey.

The participants' diets were first investigated in the early 1970s through personal interviews. They were asked to recall what they had eaten over the last 24 hours and how often they had consumed various foods in the preceding 3 months. They were then followed for an average of ten years to see if any relationships existed between dietary intake and causes of death.

The researchers divided the participants into three levels of daily vitamin C consumption: below the recommended amount of 50 mg. a day from foods alone, more than 50 mg. from foods alone, and more than 50 mg. from foods plus supplements.

How much vitamin C was consumed by the supplement users—and for just how long—was never specifically determined. Dr. Enstrom and his people noted that most supplement users took a multivitamin tablet, the type that generally contains 50 to 100 mg. of ascorbic acid.

Data gathered from 8,000 surviving participants in 1982 to 1984 suggested that those who took concentrated supplements of vitamin C took an average of 800 mg. of vitamin C daily, at least at the time they were questioned.

The researchers discovered that as vitamin C intakes increased from below to above the RDA, there was a noticeably steady drop in overall deaths and particularly in deaths from heart disease and stroke among both men and women. The protective effect of vitamin C was especially apparent among men. Those at the highest level of vitamin C consumption experienced an almost 50 percent lower death rate from cardiovascular diseases. For women, there was a 35 percent lower rate associated with high levels of vitamin C intake.

Dr. Enstrom and his coauthors at UCLA, Linda E. Kanim, a research associate, and Morton A. Klein, a technical consultant, observed that the large drop in cardiovascular death rates since the late 1960s added validity to their findings. The decline in deaths from heart disease, heart attacks, and strokes invariably coincided with large population-wide increases in the consumption of supplements containing vitamin C.

Enhancing Male Virility

Men who are smokers may laugh at the idea of trading in their smokes for a sack of apples or carrots, but it might just be the virile thing for them to do. Fairly recent studies have shown that low vitamin C levels, exacerbated by cigarette smoking and a diet low in fruits and vegetables, could very well lead to damage to the genetic material in sperm and lead to birth defects and childhood disease.

In the first research of its kind, biochemist Paul Motchnik at the University of California at Berkeley studied the semen of ten men on diets containing varying amounts of vitamin C. For the first two weeks of the study, diets were supplemented with 250 mg. of vitamin C per day, more than four times the RDA. On that regimen, damage to the sperm's DNA, or genetic material was minimal, Motchnik claimed. But one month after the men lowered their intake of vitamin C to 5 mg. per day, considerable damage was evident.

Another piece of fascinating research that appeared in the *Journal of the American Medical Association* (JAMA) (249:2747, May 27, 1983) would suggest that by swallowing 1,000 mg. of vitamin C daily, a man could restore his fertility in just four days. It certainly sounds implausible. But Earl B. Dawson, Ph. D., in company with other medical colleagues then working at the University of Texas Medical Branch in Galveston, demonstrated that this could very well be possible in men with infertility secondary to nonspecific sperm agglutination.

At a meeting of the Federation of American Societies for Experimental Biology in Chicago that year, Dawson reported on a study of 35 male patients who couldn't impregnate their wives because more than 20 percent (an average of 37 percent) of their sperm clumped together, as demonstrated by microscopic studies of semen samples. The men's serum ascorbic acid levels averaged 0.2 mg. per deciliter of blood, which is considered borderline by the U.S. National Nutrition Research Council, in contrast to a normal level of 0.6 to 0.8 mg. per deciliter of blood. Semen levels of the vitamin averaged 4.2 mg./dl.

The test subjects were subsequently given a one-month supply of pure ascorbic acid in 500 mg. gelatin capsules. By self-report, the 15 subjects who returned for reevaluation at the end of one week followed the researchers' instructions to take one tablet every 12 hours. The results were nothing short of amazing: Mean serum ascorbic acid levels of the men had risen to 1.3 mg./dl; their semen was "supersaturated" with vitamin C at an average level of 12.7

mg./dl. Most important of all, however, was that the average per-centage of sperm that agglutinated had dropped to 14 percent, well below the 20 percent considered the dividing line between fertility and infertility.

Ten of the men returned at the end of two and three weeks for further tests. Researchers noticed that by the close of the second and third weeks, serum ascorbic acid levels had leveled off at 2.5 mg./dl, while semen levels held steady at the original first week plateau of 12.7 mg./dl. Both of these levels remained the same until the entire study was finished. Better still, sperm agglutination had decreased to 13 percent by two weeks and to just 11 percent by the end of the third week.

Throughout the study, Dawson and his team confirmed statisti-cally significant, continuous increases in percentage of normal sperm, sperm viability, and sperm motility. They also observed a profound decrease in precursors of spermatozoa.

Prior to Dawson's experiment, physicians had for a long time been dispensing 60-day supplies of ascorbic acid to would-be fathers with nonspecific sperm agglutination. Dawson and his col-laborators reported that pregnancy occurred in the wives of each of a dozen men whom his group placed on the 60-day vitamin C reg-imen in 1979. "The wives of eight subjects who were not given the vitamin preparation, however," he recalled, "didn't become preg-nant." So, the message to men (and especially those who smoke) is this: If you want to have children, start taking 1,000 to 3,000 mg. of vitamin C every day! (See Product Appendix, p. 381.)

Put Some Passion Back into Your Lovemaking

As people get older their glandular energy starts to flag, resulting in a gradual diminishing of their physical actions. Among the aspects that experience slowdown in both men and women is sexual vitali-ty. In an intimate relationship one or both may not quite have what it takes to make an intimate event satisfying and worthwhile.

During the approximate five years (1992-1996) that I served as editor of *Utah Prime Times,* a monthly seniors' newspaper, I had occasion to interview different individuals who were 70 years or older about their particular lifestyle and health practices. Two of the questions put to each of my respondents were: "Are you still able to enjoy sexual fulfillment from your partner or spouse? If so, what have you been doing to keep your sexual vitality alive and well in your advanced years?"

I put these questions to Jack and Elaine LaLanne, Gypsy Boots, and Art Linkletter and wife on different occasions. While each of their answers was somewhat different, a common thread connected them all: They took a lot of vitamin C on a regular basis.

Jack LaLanne has been a fitness pioneer, promoter, and progressive thinker for most of his 82 years. He's been labeled by the media as the "Godfather of Fitness" or an "evangelist of exercise as Evangelist Billy Graham is of religion." But he thinks of himself more as a "physical culturist" instead.

LaLanne and his wife were in Salt Lake City on May 27, 1992 to address Senator Orrin Hatch's fifth Annual Conference for Seniors at the Little America Hotel. He told me at that time, "Fitness is the king and nutrition is the queen of good health, and together they make a magnificent kingdom!" I remember seeing him years ago on his nationally syndicated television program dedicated to health and fitness; it was called "The Jack LaLanne Show." He was doing aerobic exercise long before it became cool and fashionable to do. His show ran for 25 years.

In a small press room at the hotel away from the noise of the huge gathered crowd in the adjacent ballrooms, I had a chance to carefully inquire about some of the more intimate activities in the LaLannes' private lives. Jack told me that he and Elaine had been using "vitamins C [3,500 mg.], E [800 IU], and L-carnitine [500 mg.] on a daily basis" for many years "to keep our sexual health alive and well!"

My interview with Southern California's legendary exercise and vegetarian guru Gypsy Boots appeared on the front page of the May 1994 edition of the seniors' newspaper I then edited. Born Robert Bootzin on August 11, 1911 to Russian Jews in San Francisco, he developed a love affair with Mother Nature at a very early age. "I used to sleep out in the open whenever I could when I was just knee-high to a grasshopper," he recalled with a hearty laugh. "I fell in love with her [Mother Nature] so much that I quit school when I was 13 and went to the school of life experience instead. I slept all over creation—in Sonoma Valley haystacks, under fig trees in Vacaville, in grape vineyards at Lodi, in the orange groves of Orange County, and under the date palms near Indio. You name a place and I've probably slept there outdoors at some time in my life. It's been a wonderful romance with Nature and I!"'

I've known this man for many years, meeting him first at holistic health conventions back in the late 1970s where I was a featured speaker. "What do you eat or take," I specifically asked him, "to make yourself so vibrant and alive?"

"I eat lots of figs, dates, grapes, apples, oranges, and berries. These things give me tremendous energy and keep my system clean. But I find that it's the *raw* nuts and seeds that I'm forever chewing that really gives me my sexual vitality. Why shouldn't they, since they contain life-bearing elements within them?

"I also take 3,000 to 6,000 mg. of vitamin C every day, along with ginseng product. That stuff works great with ascorbic acid when I'm in the mood and being passionately aroused. I also chew a raw clove of garlic whenever I eat large slices of black (dark rye) bread. I'll wash it down with some buttermilk or kefir."

In the same year that I spoke with Gypsy Boots, I also interviewed Mr. and Mrs. Art Linkletter. He is a well-known television personality, having hosted a daily show bearing his name for many years. But he is probably best remembered for his book, *Kids Say the Darnedest Things,* which is a collection of witty and remarkable things kids said to him over the airwaves on a variety of topics. He came to Salt Lake City early in June 1994 to be the featured speaker at Senator Hatch's Seventh Annual Conference on Seniors.

The Linkletters confided that they still managed to keep "the flame of romance and love in all of its wonderful dimension, brightly burning on the home front"—and in the bedroom, too. They attributed much of their marital bliss in this direction to their faithful consumption of vitamins A, C, E, and zinc on a regular basis. She sometimes would add calcium and iron to her regimen, while he would increase his intake of potassium "when the need seemed apparent." They were quick to point out that "without these supplements, a good diet, a positive mental attitude, and healthy emotions, we probably wouldn't be as satisfied in our marriage as we are."

Indeed, it does appear that vitamin C, in combination with other useful nutrients already mentioned, certain herbal formulas and plenty of *live* food (Raw oysters, anyone?), the lovemaking process will be kept healthy and vibrant for many decades to come! (See page 383 of the Product Appendix for specific brands of supplements capable of inducing greater physical passion.)

Curtailing Birth Defects

In 1978, when I had just started writing my first monthly column for *The Herbalist* magazine and making some of my first public speaking appearances with Nature's Sunshine, Inc. (a Utah-based networking health products company), I had a chance to meet and interview Dr. Robert S. Scott, then an assistant clinical professor of obstetrics and gynecology at the University of Southern California.

He had been recommending large doses of ascorbic acids to over a thousand of his patients with outstanding results. He started each of them on 1,000 mg. of vitamin C three times a day, and gradually worked it up to about 10 grams (10,000 mg.) daily. By his own admission this was way more than what most women were then getting during their pregnancies. (The RDA of vitamin C was only 60 mg. per day at the time.)

The many wonderful results he saw because of this were nothing short of astonishing! "I have never, never seen a deformed baby of any kind that I've delivered from those mothers on my vitamin C program. The babies have always come out healthy, pink, squalling, and as full of life as you would ever want a newborn to be. And rarely have I ever seen any stretch marks. In fact, come to think of it, I can't remember the last time I did."

Other research elsewhere in the world has backed him up on this. In 1980-81, a British pediatrician at the University of Leeds in England by the name of Richard Smithells, M.D. decided to run a nutritional experiment on "high-risk" women—those who had previously had babies born with birth defects, but who planned to become pregnant again. He had one group take vitamin supplements high in vitamin C and two B vitamins (riboflavin and folic acid) for one month before and two months after becoming pregnant, give or take a few weeks either way. Another group took no supplements whatsoever.

He discovered that there were almost ten times more defective babies born among the women without the benefit of vitamins. But, as expected, there was *only one* of the 178 women taking his prescribed vitamins who had a malformed infant. A follow-up study conducted by N. Habibzadeh, M.D. in the same school and published in the *British Journal of Nutrition* (55:23-35, Jan.-Feb. 1986) confirmed the Smithells findings.

Tolerating Heat and Cold Better

There is no question at all that body temperature regulation is affected a lot by what you take into your body as well as what you put on your body in the way of fabric covering. The following experiments were randomly selected to show the reader that vitamin C can make a world of difference in how your own body reacts to hot summer or frigid winter weather.

A common heat-induced malady is prickly heat. During the Second World War, this malady caused nearly universal distress among our soldiers in the South Pacific theater of action. The intense itching, paresthesias, and burning interfered with concentration and sleep, while secondary infection of excoriated areas at times caused temporary disability. The same skin disorder in milder forms occurs widely in America during the long, hot summer months, especially in infants.

R. I. Stern, M.D. began investigating the use of vitamin C to relieve prickly heat sensation way back in the beginning of 1951, as reported in the *Journal of the American Medical Association* (145:175). He discovered that 300 to 500 mg. of ascorbic acid daily gave dramatic relief to most patients. The itching cleared and the rash subsided, usually within 30 minutes, and these effects lasted for 6 to 24 hours. Although he didn't analyze the blood or urine for vitamin C initially, he indicated that none of his subjects exhibited the usual signs of clinical deficiency.

In his report Stern cited an experiment conducted by two other doctors the previous summer in Coachella, California (a desert-bordering community). They tested the effect of vitamin C on patients with prickly heat. Adults received 500 mg. daily by mouth and infants (8 pounds and under) were given 100 mg. Itching was promptly relieved and the rash cleared up in every single case. Yet none of these people showed signs of clinical deficiency either.

G. A. Poda, M.D. explored the possible use of vitamin C for heatstroke and heat exhaustion in an article that appeared in the *Annals of Internal Medicine* (91:657, Oct. 1979). Following a heat-stroke in 1951, one of his patients, a salesperson, subsequently would become weak and shock-like if the temperature rose to more than 85° F. Since air-conditioned cars weren't common then, he couldn't conduct his sales work. Dr. Poda administered 100 mg. of ascorbic acid three times daily to his patient. Even though temperatures hovered between 90° and 105° F., the man was able to drive his non-air-conditioned car and resume his regular work hours. Heat intolerance returned only when he forgot to take his daily allotment of ascorbic acid.

In 1970, a professional tennis player who had had heat exhaustion discovered that he couldn't teach nor play the game of his love between 10 a.m. and 4 p.m. Following Dr. Poda's advice, he started taking 500 mg. of vitamin C once or twice daily, and was able to resume his daily tennis routine without further interruption.

Vitamin C also helps the body to endure cold climates much better by inducing a type of chemical warmth within the system. In the first controlled human experiment of its kind, Japanese scientists demonstrated in 1967 that regular amounts of ascorbic acid can keep you warmer in the winter. Specifically, they administered 200 mg. of the nutrient every day for about 2 1/2 weeks to 20 healthy medical students whose diets furnished about 80 mg. of vitamin C daily during the testing period.

By measuring the temperature of their skin at room temperature (68° F.) and 40 minutes after exposure to cold (41° F.), M. Nakamura and his fellow coworkers showed conclusively that skin temperatures in those receiving the vitamin C supplement decreased less after cold exposure than they did for the control group.

They noted that acclimatization to cold increased as the blood ascorbic acid level rose and that a concentration of at least 1.0 mg./dl in the blood is essential for maintaining an adequate resistance to cold. The Japanese researchers concluded that "ascorbic acid seemed to enhance the resistance to cold by raising the body temperature and the basal metabolism rate." Their report appeared in the *Tokyo Journal of Experimental Medicine* (92:207-19, Jun. 1967).

The work of S. D. Livingstone, which was published in the *Journal of Applied Physiology* (40:455-57, Mar. 1976) and the British medical journal *Lancet* (2(7980):319-20, Aug. 7, 1976) is also worth noting in passing. By carefully studying the impact of frigid temperatures on military personnel following their tours of duty in the Arctic, he was able to recommend vitamin C supplements with military rations for outdoor operations in bitter cold conditions.

A team of Russian scientists led by V. M. Krasnopevtsev reported to the Fourth International Symposium on Circumpolar Health, which was held from October 2-7, 1978 in Academic City, Novosibirsk in Siberia, that a large quantity of vitamin C and B-1 were needed for effective adaptation in extreme northern climates.

There is adequate human evidence to show a definite relationship between the body's vitamin C status and its tolerance of heat and cold. The clinical data strongly suggests that this nutrient is operative at both ends of the thermal spectrum. Vitamin C stimulates sweat-gland activity to help cool the body down, while it enhances cold tolerance by increasing cold-induced vasodilation of the blood vessels.

Linus Pauling and the Common Cold

The late Linus Pauling (who died in 1994 at the remarkable age of 93) was the only person in history to ever win two unshared Nobel prizes. He earned his first Nobel Prize for chemistry in 1954 and his second, the Nobel Peace Prize, in 1962 for his staunch support of a nuclear test ban treaty. He almost earned an unprecedented third Nobel Prize for medicine, but was eclipsed in these efforts by James D. Watson of the U.S. and Francis Crick and Maurice Wilson of Great Britain. Pauling and the other trio were in a neck-to-neck race right down to the finish line to see who would be the first to discover the correct structure of DNA (deoxyribonucleic acid), the premier trophy in the world of biology. In one of life's strangest ironies, Watson and Crick used Pauling's own classic textbook *The Nature of the Chemical Bond* as their most important reference book to help them toward their great discovery. Because of his twin backgrounds in physics and chemistry, Pauling had already covered a good portion of the research in this particularly exciting field. But his problem was that he didn't go far enough, whereas the others did, thereby beating him out of a triple crown in Nobels by just a few months!

Strangely enough, though, it isn't for these grand scientific accomplishments that Pauling is best remembered, but rather for something very controversial and medically unorthodox to say the least. In 1970 he wrote a simple book with a very plain title, *Vitamin C and the Common Cold* (San Francisco: W. H. Freeman and Co.)

The book took off and became an overnight health bestseller. The author immediately fell from grace in the scientific community with his claim that large doses of vitamin C can fight the common cold. How dare a chemist—not a real nutritionist—suggest we get a nutrient from pills instead of food? Doctors were also livid over Pauling's brash statement that megadoses of ascorbic acid could cure cancer. The media, of course, eagerly reported this heated controversy.

On the one side stood the world's most decorated chemist, a true scientific celebrity and public hero then in his early 70s, who advocated the *daily* consumption of between 1,000 and 2,000 mg. of ascorbic acid for "the suppression of the disagreeable manifestations of the common cold" (p. 86 of Pauling's book). His opponents at the other end of the spectrum, coming mostly from the fields of medicine, nutrition, and biochemistry, believed that these ideas were "preposterous, virtually unproven, and potentially bad for people's health." But, as the *Los Angeles Times* pointed out in a lengthy article on Pauling in its Sunday, June 2, 1985 edition (part IV, p. 1), ". . . It turns out that some of his . . . ideas about vitamins are correct, as recent evidence suggests. [This is] another footnote in a long, illustrious career, forcing his critics to concede that Linus Pauling was at least partly right after all."

Pauling's interest in vitamin C began in 1965, when "he and wife Ava began taking three grams [3,000 mg.] of Vitamin C a day." According to Pauling, "they not only felt better, but they found they no longer caught colds." From that moment on Linus became an ardent champion of the world's most popular nutrient, earning him the moniker, "Mr. Vitamin C Man."

A short while after this, he was invited to speak at the dedication of a new medical school in New York City. As he recalled some years later of this particular incident: "I had only about ten minutes to speak. In order to say something medical, I mentioned that Vitamin C would help stop you from getting the common cold."

Sitting in the audience was a doctor who was then a professor of pathology and medicine at Columbia University. Soon after returning to the West Coast, Pauling continued, "I received a letter from this physician, Victor Herbert, M.D., asking me if I had even one study that supported my idea.

"I wrote back saying that I hadn't really checked the literature. But after several months I finally did check into the matter and found four papers on the subject. I made photocopies and sent them to him. But all he tried to do was find fault with them."

Pauling declared that the whole episode "made me so damned mad, that I decided to sit down and write a book setting things straight. That's how this little best-seller was born," he declared in a firm voice, while at the same time hefting a copy of his *Vitamin C and the Common Cold*. With that book, the battle was on and the war would become quite fierce at times in the ensuing years.

But what of vitamin C—is it really *that* good for the common cold, or was Pauling's theory just that: a theory with no proof? A quarter-century later, evidence largely tends to confirm what the old gent believed. Harri Hemilä, Ph.D., of the University of Helsinki, Finland, analyzed the results of 21 controlled studies on vitamin C and the common cold in 1993.

He discovered that ascorbic acid intake didn't influence the likelihood of a person catching a cold—hand washing probably does a much better job of that. But each of the reports "showed a decrease in the duration or the severity of symptoms," according to Hemilä's article in the *Scandinavian Journal of Infectious Diseases* (26:1-6, Jan. 1994). People taking 1,000 mg. of ascorbic acid had a 19 percent decrease in cold severity, according to Hemilä. Those who took 2,000 to 6,000 mg. of vitamin C daily benefited from a 29 percent decrease in symptom severity. While this figure may not promise complete relief from symptoms, Hemilä explained, it did help lessen the misery of a cold, nevertheless.

Pauling's book made such an overwhelming impact with the public that even doctors began reconsidering their former positions on ascorbic acid. Linus told me in the summer of 1982, when I had a chance to interview him, that he had recently been to a party given by the dean of a university. "This professor of medicine took me aside and quietly whispered in my ear, 'Linus, you'd be astonished how many of the doctors in this very room take large doses of vitamin C based on your book's recommendations, even though they won't ever admit it in public.'"

Taking vitamin C in the amounts previously suggested before, during, and after the cold or flu season won't hurt you. In fact, these amounts of ascorbic acid will greatly minimize the symptoms in the unlucky event you contract either. At those levels—between 1,000 and 6,000 mg.—there is nothing to worry about.

But in this crazy world of ours, nothing is ever certain if you're trying to help others, as the following true news item from the January 14, 1984 *Arkansas Gazette* (p. A-1) goes to show. "Victoria Kokoras, 30, a sixth grade teacher, who outraged some parents by giving chewable vitamin C tablets to her students with cold symptoms, was suspended by the school board in Peabody, Massachusetts, for two days with pay. This prompted the teacher to declare to reporters: 'If I were a parent, I would be a lot more concerned with the pounds of candy I've seen kids eat and not with the vitamins I've been giving some of them.'"

Stunning Action against Infection

I met Frederick Klenner, M.D. of Riedsville, North Carolina in July 1985. He had then been practicing general medicine in the same community for 46 years. During much of that time ascorbic acid in large amounts was his favorite and most successful treatment for many kinds of infectious diseases. "When I've reached my half-century mark of practice," he joked, "then I'll probably hang up the stethoscope for good."

Dr. Klenner first became attracted to this nutrient quite a few years ago when he read of the experiments performed by Dr. Claus W. Jungeblut at the College of Physicians and Surgeons, Columbia University. This researcher reported that ascorbic acid was used successfully in experiments with monkeys to protect the animals from poliomyelitis and to prevent paralysis after they had been injected with particles of this virus.

Dr. Klenner showed me a well-worn and wrinkled copy of his first paper on the subject that appeared in *Southern Medicine and Surgery* (Jul. 1949): "Ascorbic Acid Treatment of Poliomyelitis and Other Virus Diseases." He said, as he handed his personal copy over to me, I'll spare you the time of having to read it, Dr. Heinerman, by summarizing what I said there and what the journal editors *wouldn't* let me put in." I nodded and he continued.

"I've probably cured—you heard it right, c-u-r-e-d," he said, slowly and methodically spelling the word out for greater emphasis, "more cases of infectious diseases than just about any doctor in America. I'm not saying this to be bragging, but I've treated literally thousands in this community and from elsewhere, who've flocked to my office over the years once word got out that this 'country doctor' here was 'doing something right,' and making people well again.

"In every case of the many diseases I treated and cured, I've always used both oral and intramuscular injections of vitamin C, never one form alone. The degree to which body tissue gets thoroughly saturated with vitamin C is of the utmost importance. Many years of practice have taught me one thing: that deficiency in this vitamin predisposes an individual to infection and a severe attack of whatever else happens to invade the body at that time.

"Remember way back in 1948 to 50, when American kids were taking such a heavy beating with polio? Many of them ended up in iron lung machines just to help them breathe better. Countless others were permanently crippled and had to get around with the assistance of heavy metal braces that clanked whenever they took a step forward. Well, I treated hundreds of young polio victims by giving them intravenous injections of 2,000 mg. of vitamin C every two hours for one day, then every six hours for the next two days. Every single patient recovered successfully within three to five days.

Some of the national media guys heard about this through the grapevine and came down here looking for a story. But I wouldn't give them any and sent them away empty-handed. That 's probably why I wasn't written up a lot and didn't become rich and famous like you" (pointing to this author). We had a laugh together over this one.

Here is a list of the many different infectious diseases that Dr. Klenner has treated in almost a half-century of medical practice:

allergies (food & environmental)	influenza
	measles
ankylosing spondylitis	mononucleosis
asthma	mumps
burns	polio
cancer	rheumatoid arthritis
chicken pox	sepsis
cold sores	(pus-forming, hospital-induced blood infection)
fever blisters (see cold sores)	shingles
	tetanus
hay fever	viral pneumonia
hepatitis	yeast infection

At the time I spoke with this lovable North Carolina sawbones, he had no real idea of just *how* vitamin C worked inside the system to help get rid of infections. But a few years later, I came across an explanation of the way in which ascorbic acid so nicely accomplishes this remarkable medical feat. An Arizona State University study published in the April 1990 issue of the *Journal of the American College of Nutrition* (9:150) had what I had been looking for through the MEDLAR and MEDLINE computer data banks. (These are information retrieval systems located at the National Library of Medicine in Bethesda, Maryland, containing tens of thousands of medical related topics from all over the world.)

When a 1,000 mg. tablet of vitamin C is consumed, it quickly floods the bloodstream with this vital nutrient, *increasing body temperature* ever so slightly. Once body heat is "turned up" a bit, the immune system rapidly kicks into action, cranking out more white blood cells and other substances with which to battle and handily defeat any infectious viruses or bacteria that may have invaded the body.

Cancer and Vitamin C

Linus Pauling, the man who finally gave vitamin C the nutritional respect it had sorely lacked for years, obtained his doctorate in chemistry from Caltech (California Institute of Technology) in Pasadena in 1925. From there he went on to the Institute for Theoretical Physics in Munich, Germany, where he began to apply quantum mechanics to the problem of the structure of molecules and the nature of the chemical bond. In 1927, he returned to America and began a long, distinguished, and very productive career at Caltech as a teacher and researcher.

In 1923 this son of a Portland, Oregon pharmacist married Ava Helen Miller in a simple ceremony. He was to say many times throughout their 58 years of married bliss, "I married her because she was simply the most beautiful and most intelligent woman I had ever met." He confided to this author in a short interview in the spring of 1985 that "the most rewarding thing that has ever happened to me was marrying Ava." He prized her more than both of his Nobel Prizes put together.

In 1965 they both began taking about 3,000 mg. each of ascorbic acid on a daily basis, convinced that it was good for their health. Unfortunately, though, life offers no lasting guarantees and periodically deals some of us fatal ironies. This was the case for the Paulings and one of Linus' major collaborators, as the evidence will show.

Commencing in 1971 and concluding in 1976, Pauling teamed up with Ewan Cameron, M.D., who was then chief surgeon at the Vale of Leven Hospital in Loch Lomondside, Scotland, to conduct an extensive research project on 1,100 terminal cancer patients. One thousand of them served as controls, while the remaining hundred were placed in an ascorbate treatment group. They received their daily allotments of vitamin C by intravenous infusion (usually 10,000 mg. daily for about 10 days) and also orally.

At the end of the research project *all* 1,000 of those patients *without* the benefit of vitamin C were dead. But nearly 20 percent of the ascorbic acid group were still alive in spite of their terminal cancer. It was noticed that 90 percent of the 100 patients treated with vitamin C lived 3 to 4 times as long as the untreated ones, while 10 percent of that 100 lived 20 times as long as the controls. Beside this, the vitamin C patients had far less pain, were more optimistic and cheerful, and led more productive lives than the controls. (Those desiring to read the complete medical report, "Supplemental Ascorbate in the Supportive Treatment of Cancer: Prolongation of Survival Times in Terminal Human Cancer," should consult the *Proceedings of the National Academy of Science,* 73:3685-89, Oct. 1976, under the Medical Sciences section.)

A short time afterward, both men collaborated on a best-selling book called *Vitamin C and Cancer* (San Francisco: W.H. Freeman & Co., 1970), which gave to the public for the first time hard medical evidence that ascorbic acid can really assist in the treatment of cancer, even when it's diagnosed by doctors as being medically untreatable! But they were realistic enough to admit that vitamin C *isn't* any kind of special anticancer wonder drug. Rather, they opted for the more conservative approach that this nutrient works against cancer by bolstering the body's natural protective mechanisms in a number of different ways. Dr. Pauling told me in a second interview a few years later that he believed vitamin C to be an important catalyst for the formation of prostaglandins, which are now known to definitely control tumor growth.

Over the next decade and a half, however, a set of triple ironies occurred that reflected badly on the therapeutic merits of vitamin C, at least on the surface. Ava Pauling died rather quickly from cancer in December 1980 at the age of 77, which astonished everyone who knew her, most of all her own husband, "Mr. Vitamin C." Several years later Dr. Cameron died of lung cancer, being a lifelong chain smoker. He had always been embarrassed in front of others on account of his nicotine habit, according to H. L. Newbold, M.D. in his book, *Vitamin C Against Cancer* (New York: Stein and Day, 1979; p. 33). To Newbold, who once paid Cameron a visit in the hospital where he worked, the doctor's "smoking seemed extraordinary to me" in light of the man's great interest in cancer and his judicious consumption of ascorbic acid.

Then in early January 1992, the great Vitamin C master himself learned he had prostate cancer. He received treatment with a hormone-blocking drug, flutamide, as well as taking huge megadoses of vitamin C, both of which managed to delay the inevitable, but only temporarily. On Friday, August 19, 1994, at the remarkable age of 93, the renowned Linus Pauling breathed his last breath, as he too, fell victim to cancer.

While such facts may not be good selling points for ascorbic acid as a potent weapon in the war against cancer, they don't change the respectable body of medical evidence that ultimately supports such a claim. Always bear in mind that nutrients alone cannot do a decent job of cancer prevention or regression; they require the definite assistance of other factors that are mental, emotional, and social. Ava Pauling, being a shy, somewhat retiring personality by nature, came under a great deal of stress during the decade of the 1970s, when the medical and scientific professions fiercely persecuted her husband in print, over the airwaves, and through public debates, and he vehemently retaliated with nearly equal vengeance. Upon her death, Linus' whole world caved in around him, burying him for several years in a great deal of sorrow and self-pity. It was only through the combined and strenuous efforts of his sons and daughter that he managed to climb back out of his emotional "black hole"; but the damage had already been done in terms of wrecking his immune system. And Dr. Cameron's disgusting social habit finally proved to be too much for his body to adequately handle.

So, when taking daily doses of vitamin C to ward off cancer or treat an existing malignancy, just remember that the mind must be at peace, the heart filled with joy, and the body free of harmful addictions in order for this nutrient to be of any lasting value to you.

Lose Weight Fast with Ascorbic Acid

In all of the consumer health books dealing with the specific benefits of individual nutritional supplements, I have never once seen any mention made of using ascorbic acid to help obese people lose weight more quickly. Perhaps it's because no one has ever thought of using vitamin C for this major health problem. Or maybe the authors of such published works were unfamiliar with some of the medical research that has been done in this area already.

The study by G. J. Naylor and associates, entitled "A Double Blind Placebo Controlled Trial of Ascorbic Acid in Obesity," which appeared in the October-December 1985 issue of *Nutrition Health* (4:25-28) is fairly typical of what I mean. Grossly overweight women were instructed to take three grams (3,000 mg.) of ascorbic acid each day for 1 1/2 months (6 weeks). As a result they lost *more* weight than another group of severely obese women who were given a placebo instead. Only general dietary advice was given to both groups; *no* emphasis was placed on specific exercises or particular food selections that would obviously contribute to weight loss.

It is believed by some scientists that ascorbic acid may work in a couple of different ways in this respect. For one thing, vitamin C contributes to the process of thermogenesis, which is the *physiologic* action of heat production within the body. In other words, vitamin C is thought to "reset" our individual "fat thermostats" that are located in those regions of the body containing adipose tissue known as brown fat. Brown fat is nothing more than thermogenic tissue that is composed of cells containing numerous small fat droplets; this is situated between the shoulder blades (the interscapular region), in the thymus gland, and around the lymph nodes (the mediastinal region). When we 're young this brown fat chemically combusts ("burns") or converts regular fat into energy fuel for the body to run on. But as we grow older, these regions of brown fat tend to shrivel, which means considerably *reduced* "burning" of ingested carbohydrates and proteins. The end result of all of this extra material being constantly crammed into the system is that it has nowhere to go except to accumulate as unwanted body mass. Hence the emerging problems of an expanding girth and greater weight gain. But *daily* and *consistent* intake of 3,000 mg. of vitamin C will keep what little brown fat remains within the body functioning properly so that most consumed carbohydrates and proteins are regularly "burned" (as they should be) and weight gain doesn't happen—at least not in an accelerated way.

The other intriguing role of ascorbic acid in helping to curb obesity is in the prevention of viral infection. In this case, it prevents not just any virus, but a certain one in particular: a *fat* virus! Medical research presented at a biology meeting in New Orleans on April 8, 1997 tends to support this interesting paradox. A virus extracted from obese patients and then injected into normal-sized animal models made them become fat. The findings thus far are only preliminary and the evidence, at best, circumstantial, but it is, in the words of one medical researcher, "very tantalizing and promptly warrants additional research."

A *minimum* daily intake of 1,500 mg. of ascorbic acid is recommended to ward off infection by this newly discovered fat virus. This, of course, can be increased to 3,000 mg., if warranted.

Vitamin C Foods for Detoxification

Vitamin C is required in far greater amounts than any other vitamin that I know of. This is because it performs a wide number of varied functions on primary and secondary levels of biological importance. These can range from antioxidant protection to slow the aging process, to delivering relief in cases of prickly heat sensation, from reversing gangrene to controlling hypertension.

Even something as common as periodontal disease (the chief cause of tooth loss among people over 35) may be curtailed to a great extent with dietary *and* supplemental sources of vitamin C. Whatever its many functions may be, know this about ascorbic acid—it performs them in a very capable fashion.

One of the *chief* jobs which this nutrient does exceptionally well is to detoxify the body. Believe it or not, each of us, every single day of our lives, breathes, touches, eats, drinks, and wears poisons of some kind. These can range from city smog, soaps, and perfumed deodorants to junk or fast foods and colas or soft drinks, not to mention the many different types of synthetic fabrics we fashionably adorn ourselves with. Pollution is all around us in some form: from carbon monoxide in the air we inhale to growth hormones in the chicken we eat with lip-smacking relish. This is only the tip of the proverbial iceberg, however. What about all of those internal poisons we constantly generate because of agitated feelings and mental stress? Doesn't it seem reasonable to assume that the *extra* adrenaline, hydrochloric acid, and numerous hormones cranked out by the body when it is in a highly-charged state of excitement wouldn't somehow poison the bloodstream, since they're not needed in such great abundance?

This is where ascorbic acid enters the picture. It is a potent detoxifier that counteracts and neutralizes the harmful effects of these many different forms of pollution, whether environmental, dietary, social, or emotional. It accomplishes this seemingly impossible task quite efficiently by first "disarming" and then "packaging" or containing all of these toxins. One writer has referred to the process as "complexing," but I prefer my own terminology here because it more broadly defines what vitamin C does, though in lay terms.

After rendering such poisons relatively inert and bundling them up, vitamin C then assists in their final elimination from the body. This is effectively done by increasing the processes of urination and bowel movements. For a long time now this nutrient has had a wonderful reputation as being the best nutritional friend the kidneys and bladder and colon ever had.

Obtaining as much vitamin C as you can from food sources is obviously the preferred way to go. A convenient method for remembering the best sources of vitamin C is to divide them into three categories: excellent, good, and fair. I've arranged them in the table below for better visual perception.

Ascorbic Acid Foods

Excellent (100 mg./100 gm)	Good (50-99 mg./100 gm)	Fair (30 to 49 mg./100 gm)
broccoli greens	cabbage	asparagus
Brussels sprouts	cauliflower	lima beans
collards	chives	Swiss chard
black currants	kohlrabi	gooseberries
guava	orange pulp	currants
horseradish	lemon pulp	grapefruit
kale	mustard	limes
turnip greens	beet greens	loganberries
parsley	papaya	melons (especially cantaloupe)
sweet peppers	spinach	okra
dandelion greens	strawberries	tangerines
rose hips	watercress	potatoes
acerola cherries		turnips

There are also some very good herbal sources of vitamin C: bladderwrack, burdock root, cat's claw bark, licorice root, prickly ash bark, queen's delight root, red clover blossom, slippery elm bark, sheep sorrel herb, and turkey rhubarb root. But since vitamin C is extremely heat sensitive, this means that capsules, tablets, and teas are out, since they require some type of friction or heat to render them in these forms. Alcoholic-based tinctures and extracts also greatly diminish ascorbic acid content in such herbs.

But there is a way to take these herbs every day (other than in raw form, which isn't practical for some of them) so that the vitamin C content is perfectly preserved. This is in two types of beverages that have been *cold* extracted with purified water. They are Essex Botanical (a dietary drink supplement) and Hoxsiac (an herbal drink). (See Product Appendix, p. 380.)

Gavriel Harel, the present owner, and his late father carefully consulted the extensive research work of Renee Caisse and Harry

Hoxsey before they started manufacturing both beverages. Renee Caisse discovered her formula from an old native Indian medicine woman in 1922 while working at a northern hospital in Hilleybury, Ontario. Hoxsey's grandfather noticed one of his prized Percheron stud horses casually munching in a region of pasture that contained a number of flowering plants and shrubs. Each of them went on to create a particular formula of vitamin-C-rich herbs that have helped, literally, several million people overcome just about every kind of disease imaginable.

This isn't to suggest that these herbal formulas are some kind of magic potions for instant recovery (though some folks would like to believe that). But they are healthy elixirs rich in ascorbic acid, which can assist the body in eliminating most of the poisons it accumulates regularly.

For general detoxification I usually recommend one cup of the Essex Botanical Dietary Supplement in the morning and one cup of the Hoxsiac Herbal Drink in the late evening (usually after 6 p.m.). For more aggressive detoxification, though, where malignant health problems may exist, I advise doubling or even tripling these amounts, with an interim administration sometime in the midafternoon. These beverages should always be taken about 20 minutes *before* eating a meal, so that the body has a chance to process them without interference from ingested foods. Both beverages store well in a dry, cold place without any light. They come in dark amber glass bottles (32 oz. size) and contain *no* sugar, yeast, preservatives, color, or flavor. For some, an acquired taste may require a little bit of patience and forbearance.

New Forms of Ascorbic Acid

On March 11, 1995 I attended a highly interesting meeting in Anaheim, California. It was the Second Conference on Vitamin C, in conjunction with the Natural Foods Expo West going on at the same time. This conference brought together leading investigators and clinicians to present new findings on the biochemistry, epidemiology, nutrition, and pharmacology of ascorbic acid. I came away loaded with enough material to write an entire book on the subject, let alone some pages in this text.

A review of *esterified* vitamin C was given by one presenter. He noted that the word *ester* is a chemist's term to describe a particular chemical bonding configuration. Thus, esterified vitamin C means that several ascorbic acid molecules have been linked together in a certain way to form one large molecule.

The advantages of the esterified form go way beyond simply bonding several ascorbic acid molecules together. Some of these were highlighted by the presenter. He correctly noted that non-ester forms are more quickly eliminated from the body. He gave evidence to show that about 73 percent of ingested ascorbic acid is removed from the system in less than 24 hours, whereas just 5 percent of the ester form is eliminated during the same period. Most forms of ascorbic acid create uncomfortable effects within the stomach due to their high acidity. Some buffered forms of vitamin C can partially alleviate this. Esterified C, on the other hand, is pH neutral–neither acidic nor alkaline. Hence, it is the most agreeable form, especially for those with sensitive digestive tracts.

Vitamin C enhances calcium absorption just like vitamin D does. The esterified C is nearly always bonded with calcium, so the consumer is getting double supplement benefits instead of just from the vitamin itself. Thus, when an esterified and calcium-bonded vitamin C is used, the consumer is getting the maximum benefits of *both* nutrients, as well as improving the absorption of the mineral.

I was equally intrigued with the data on time-released forms of ascorbic acid. Their purpose, we were kindly informed, was to insure that much of the vitamin C would get by the G.I. tract without being absorbed and could reach more specific parts of the body that desperately required this nutrient in generous quantities. *Total* saturation of the circulating blood plasma in timed increments was essential to keep the immune system active, infection in check, and the body in a ready state of sound health at all times.

Another speaker mentioned that the human body can transform ingested ascorbic acid into numerous metabolites that may have physiological actions quite different from those of vitamin C itself. These metabolites—whether manufactured in the body or else ingested along with supplemental vitamin C—could influence how this particular nutrient is transported and utilized. One example given was that of dehydroascorbate, the oxidized and transportable form of ascorbate. Both with and without enzymes, it can be metabolized or modified in numerous body tissues into tinier fragments, like threonate, xylonate, and lyxonate. The level of these metabolites in the blood plasma may not rise significantly, however, until megadoses of vitamin C are administered, which obviously leads us to consider the various dosage ranges that are available for consumer health needs.

How Much Is Enough?

The question of "How much is enough?" for daily ascorbic acid intake was cleverly stated in the syndicated cartoon *B.C.* by Johnny Hart, which appears in over 1,500 newspapers throughout North America. In one panel which ran in the comic section of the June 22, 1990 edition of the *Salt Lake Tribune,* the main Stone Age character B.C. was casually leaning over the top of a large, round rock with the words "Vitamin Store" written on the front of it. Another unidentified caveman was on the other side asking, "Can a person take too many vitamins?" To which B.C. responded, "I suppose it's possible." Then the customer asked, "How can I tell when I've taken too much vitamin C?" B.C. answered with an air of obvious indifference: "When the doctor asks you to step inside and *unpeel* for a checkup."

From all the information I've read by various nutritional and medical authorities, it appears that there is *no* clear consensus on just how much ascorbic acid should be ingested each day from supplemental sources. There are as many varying opinions on this topic as there are on the topics of religion or politics, it seems.

To give you an idea of just what I mean, consider the following differences. The standard RDA (Recommended Dietary Allowance) is 60 mg. for adults every day. However, the Harvard Medical School Health Publications' *Vitamins and Minerals* (Boston: Harvard Medical School, 1995; p.26) suggests 100 mg. daily for smokers. Sheldon Saul Hendler, M.D., Ph.D., a nutritional advisor to the U.S. Olympic Committee and the American Association of

Retired Persons (AARP), suggests somewhere between "a daily intake of 250 milligrams to 1,000 milligrams (1 gram) of vitamin C," in his book, *The Doctors' Vitamin and Mineral Encyclopedia* (New York: Simon & Schuster, 1990; p. 93). Interestingly enough, his recommendation pretty much coincides with that of the Alliance for Aging Research, a Washington, D.C.-based organization. However, the National Institute of Health believes that less than this—200 mg. of vitamin C a day—is all that's necessary for maintaining good health.

Even those who've fought together as supposed allies on behalf of ascorbic acid in the trenches during the hotly contested vitamin C skirmishes that raged throughout much of the 1970s and 80s couldn't reach a joint agreement on an ideal daily intake for adult consumers. In 1985 *Healthview* newsletter interviewed both Dr. Linus Pauling, then Chairman of the Board of the Linus Pauling Institute of Science and Medicine in Menlo Park, California, and his cofounder, President and Scientific Director of the same facility, Dr. Arthur B. Robinson.

Dr. Pauling was first asked the question, "How much vitamin C should a healthy person take?" He very enthusiastically responded: "I would recommend between one and ten grams (1,000 to 10,000 mg.) or more a day, taken regularly, not stopping ever." He then went on to clarify the "or more" part of his answer by adding that "20 to 40 grams (20,000 to 40,000 mg.) a day" may be necessary for some.

This clearly irked Dr. Robinson and he wasn't at all afraid to speak his mind on the matter, even if it meant disagreeing with his boss and the man who signed his paychecks every month. "Dr. Robinson, how much vitamin C do you feel a healthy person should take?" came the same inquiry.

Pauling's colleague and collaborator replied: "Everyone should certainly take the 50 to 100 mgs. necessary to meet their vitamin requirements. [However], in my opinion, it is safe and may be of value to take up to 500 mgs. of vitamin C daily as has been recommended by many health food authorities for thirty years. But, to take 10 grams or more a day, as Pauling [here] recommends, is of no known benefit, and may be seriously harmful [to human health]."

This, along with other apparent disagreements they obviously had in the past, enraged Pauling. He abruptly terminated their long friendship and severed the professional relationship between them. Since Robinson had been given a tenured position at the Institute, he sued Pauling, who then countersued for "defamation of character" in publicly disagreeing with him. A nasty, five-year court battle ensued, resulting in Pauling paying Robinson a settlement of $575,000.

Since there really doesn't seem to be a clear answer to this question, I will referee the matter from this end and help the reader arrive at what I believe to be a prudent and practical approach to this thorny issue. *A lot depends on your own health circumstances at the time.* To illustrate what I mean, consider this: Food-derived vitamin C can increase the absorption of certain medications into the body.

This discovery came about quite by accident. A Canadian medical researcher in Toronto, David Bailey, Ph.D., was asked to conduct a study to determine whether it was safe to take the blood pressure drug Plendil with alcohol. To make the study results more legitimate, he wanted to mask the taste of alcohol so his subjects' reactions would be purely physiologic, rather than influenced by any preconceived expectations of how they would respond if they knew what they were imbibing. Many beverages were tried to disguise alcohol's taste, but grapefruit juice was the only one that did the trick.

As it turned out the alcohol had no effect. But the subjects' blood levels of Plendil were higher than anybody had ever seen before. Apparently, something in grapefruit juice, besides its obvious abscorbic acid content, changes the rate at which an enzyme in the intestine breaks down Plendil, thereby permitting more complete absorption by the system. That same enzyme is also responsible for controlling the absorption rate of several other drugs. That is how the connection between grapefruit juice and a variety of medications was made.

According to the March 1997 issue of *Tufts University Health & Nutrition Letter,* the following drugs mix extremely well with grapefruit juice and the juice increases their rates of absorption into the body:

Drugs Affected by Grapefruit Juice

Type	Generic Name	Trade Name
Sedatives	Triazolam	Halcion
	Midazolam	Versed
Antihypertensives	Felodipine	Plendil
	Nifedipine	Procardia
Antihistamine	Terfenadine	Seldane
Immunosuppressant	Cyclosporine	Sandimmune

The daily stresses that each of us must cope with in life usually demand *more* vitamin C intake than we are accustomed to getting. Animal studies have shown this to be so. Primatologists (scientists who study primates) who took blood samples of vervet monkeys in the wild noticed that they only required 0.5 to 0.7 mg. of ascorbic acid per kilogram of body weight every day to ward off symptoms of scurvy. But when captured and put in a lab or zoo environment, their ascorbic acid needs soared dramatically— to 3 to 8 mg./kg/day. In another study, *uncaged* guinea pigs only needed 1.5 mg./kg/day to prevent scurvy. But when put into captivity these needs climbed to 16 mg./kg/day, and went even higher than this—to 50 mg./kg/day—for recovery from surgery and anesthesia.

Hence, we see that stress is a critical factor in determining daily human vitamin C needs. Much earlier in the text, under the subsection dealing with antisocial behavior and vitamin C, I provided a table of incremental increases of ascorbic acid for various age levels, commencing at 1,000 mg. and reaching a high of 3,000 mg. Along with several other given nutrients, the plan is intended to help cope with anger, meanness, contempt, selfishness, stinginess, violence, anxiety, fear, depression, and other forms of mental and emotional stresses that would clearly be construed as antisocial in nature. An average daily intake of 2,000 mg. of *supplemental* vitamin C would appear to be of definite assistance in managing individual stress.

Besides these stresses adversely affecting the mind and heart, there are also the dietary stresses we willingly impose on our bodies each day by what we carelessly eat and drink. Way too much sugar in some form is still consumed by tens of millions of Americans on a daily basis through poor food, beverage, and snack selections. The impact of all this sugar is felt in the adrenal glands first and usually brings about a quick drain of energy that leaves the unsuspecting person wondering what happened. The answer, of course, is that this excess sugar in the circulating blood plasma just emptied the adrenal glands of most of the vitamin C that the body likes to accumulate in that particular region.

When this occurs, there is an unexpected drop in physical energy. Fatigue then sets in, which can't reasonably be justified. The adrenal glands restrict their production of adrenaline, a potent stimulant that increases heart rate, the force of muscle contractions, and the conversion of stored carbohydrates (glycogen) into energy-producing glucose. Without adequate vitamin-C-generated adrenaline, the body's physical responses to external challenges are momentarily delayed. Brain output is likewise affected, requiring a few extra seconds for memory recall instead of the normal instantaneous response.

Those familiar with hypoglycemia will recognize in the foregoing descriptions symptoms that are disturbingly similar to those associated with low blood sugar. Hypoglycemics who've been placed on 3,000 mg. of ascorbic acid daily report feeling a lot better physically and mentally within a matter of days. This is because high concentrations of vitamin C have been rebuilt within their adrenal glands.

Orthomolecular physicians, naturopathic doctors, chiropractors, and holistic nutritionists who work with vitamins and minerals a great deal often prescribe megadoses (amounts above 10 grams or 10,000 milligrams) for those difficult diseases that stubbornly resist conventional antibiotics: influenza, mononucleosis, viral pneumonia, asthma, cancer, ankylosing spondylitis, rheumatoid arthritis, and serious bacterial infections. In doing so, they've discovered that maximum relief of symptoms is achieved, the course of the disease itself is generally shortened, and the greatest reduction in complications is obtained.

Ordinarily such high doses of ascorbic acid in healthy individuals are very apt to produce diarrhea. But according to Robert F.

Cathcart, M.D., writing in *The Journal of Orthomolecular Psychiatry* (10(2):125-26, 1981), "I discovered the sicker a patient was, the more ascorbic acid he would tolerate by mouth before diarrhea was produced. At least 80 percent of adult patients will tolerate 10 to 15 grams [10,000 to 15,000 mg.] of ascorbic acid fine crystals in one half-cup water in four divided doses per 24 hours without having diarrhea. The astonishing finding was that almost all patients will absorb far greater amounts without having diarrhea when ill. This increased tolerance is somewhat proportional to the toxicity of the disease being treated. Tolerance is increased some by stress (e.g., anxiety, exercise, heat, cold, etc.)."

In spite of what other vitamin C proponents have stated, I have never been an advocate of megadosing—that is, amounts of 10 grams (10,000 mg.) or more. For one thing, "a high ascorbic acid intake is antagonistic" to the copper status of men and can reduce such levels of this important trace element, according to *The American Journal of Clinical Nutrition* (37:553, Apr. 1983). Individuals who've formed calcium oxalate kidney stones should *always* limit their supplemental vitamin C intake to just 1,000 mg. daily, unless they're working with a health care professional sufficiently knowledgeable in nutritional therapy. Since only about 80 percent of ingested vitamin C is ever absorbed, this means a good 20 percent is routinely passed off in the urine. Mathematically speaking then, about 2 of every 10 grams taken is flushed down the toilet! (See *International Journal of Vitamin Nutrition Research* [47:383-88, 1977] for the complete report "On the absorption of ascorbic acid in man.")

A much wiser approach than megadosing would be to take a specific amount of vitamin C every four days instead of every day (unless a cold or flu or a disease like cancer prevails, which then would necessitate *daily* supplementation). In an experiment of nutritional significance, healthy subjects were divided into two groups: Group I was given ascorbic acid in a 240 mg. dose every four days, while control Group II got 20 mg. three times per day. But when blood samples of both groups were taken, it was noticed that Group I maintained blood levels of vitamin C very similar to the levels of Group II.

This led the team of researchers to report the following in *The American Journal of Nutrition* (37:537, Apr. 1983): ". . . It appears that *periodic* supplementation [wasn't] detrimental [to Group I]. Therefore, individuals do not need to consume ascorbate daily to remain in good status as long as they ingest adequate ascorbate over a period of days." This has *always* been my own belief and one that seems to make more sense (according to the evidence just given).

Most animals have the capability to manufacture their own ascorbic acid and don't require the nutrient in their diets. A few, though, such as the guinea pig, the red-vented bulbul (an Asian bird), the fruit-eating bat from India, two kinds of fish (rainbow trout and Coho salmon), and, of course, human beings, are unable to produce their own ascorbic acid. Therefore, it must be obtained from a number of different food sources as well as supplemented, when it comes to our human needs.

Vitamin D
THE SUNSHINE NUTRIENT THAT COULD SAVE YOUR LIFE IN MORE WAYS THAN ONE

Unlike Any Other Nutrient

Of all the many nutrients listed throughout this book, vitamin D is exceptional in two ways. For one, the *best* way to get it has absolutely nothing to do with food at all. By just exposing yourself to 30 minutes of sunlight every day, you provide your body with the daily RDA intake of 5 micrograms. The sun triggers your skin to produce "provitamin D," which is converted to active vitamin D in the liver and kidneys. But you need not worry about getting megadoses from sunlight, since the body has a built-in mechanism to prevent this from ever happening. Exposure to sunlight during summer months is said to provide enough vitamin D to last throughout the year.

One would think that with all the sunlight there is in the world, there wouldn't be any shortages of vitamin D from this primary source. But the fact of the matter is there are *frequent* sunlight-derived vitamin D deficiencies going on around us that we never realize.

- Cold, northerly climates can create a 2- to 4-month deficiency of sunlight vitamin D.
- City smog, heavy fog, or burning smoke can filter out more sunlight vitamin D.
- Sunscreens are a *big* culprit since they block ultraviolet rays and inhibit vitamin D production.
- Dark skin can screen out as much as 95 percent of the ultraviolet rays. African American children are more prone to rickets than white children simply because their skin pigment limits the amount of vitamin D produced during exposure to sunlight. Recent blood sampling of Hispanic Americans and whites in Phoenix, Arizona revealed that the former had 30 to 50 percent *less* vitamin D in their systems than did their fair-skinned counterparts.

- Sunlight doesn't penetrate dense fabrics such as wool or denim very well. Loosely woven materials like silk and rayon or plant fabric such as cotton permit greater ultraviolet ray penetration.

- Ordinary window glass blocks ultraviolet rays, too. Sitting near a sunny window will *not* boost your vitamin D production at all. This means that housebound or institutionalized folks won't be getting any vitamin D to speak of.

- Aging compounds the problem further, even when warm weather is present. The skin of elderly people is far less efficient at making vitamin D than is the skin of younger adults. Research has indicated, for instance, that the skin of an 80-year-old has just half the ability to manufacture the vitamin as the skin of a 20-year-old.

The other way in which vitamin D appears to be so unique is its twin functions not only as a vitamin but also as a *hormone!* A hormone can be broadly defined as any type of chemical substance produced in the body by an organ (in this case, the skin) which has a regulatory effect on the activity of a specific organ or organs or cell types. As a micronutrient, Vitamin D is required for the absorption and metabolism of calcium and phosphorus from the small intestine for depositing in bones and teeth; for bone mineralization; for improving kidney absorption of calcium; for preventing excess urinary loss of calcium and phosphorus; and for maintaining serum calcium and phosphorus levels. In addition, vitamin D maintains and keeps nerves, skin, heart, and muscles healthy by regulating the level of calcium in the blood and assisting in the regulation of normal blood sugar. Sunlight activation of vitamin D in the skin is quickly metabolized to an active form which then acts on distinct target tissue with feedback control occurring at the site where it was first made; in this case, vitamin D' s behavior very much resembles that of a hormone.

Bone Up on D to Avoid Broken Bones

If you happen to be a woman past menopause and believe you meet the adult RDA of 200 I.U. daily by eating vitamin-D-rich foods (which few people do anyway), you're *still* not getting enough of this nutrient to minimize bone loss from your hips and, quite possibly, reduce your risk of a hip fracture somewhere along the way. That' s no small thing to ignore. Hip fractures occur in 300,000 people a year and cause complications that end in death for one in five of them.

The vitamin D/hip bone connection was discovered by Bess Dawson-Hughes, M.D., chief of the Calcium and Bone Metabolism Laboratory at Tufts University' s USDA Human Nutrition Research Center. She looked at some 250 Boston-area women who consumed 100 to 125 units of vitamin D a day, a typical amount for adults in the United States, she said. All were in their 50s and 60s, ages at which low vitamin D intake becomes particularly problematic since our skin's ability to manufacture the nutrient diminishes as we grow older. Of course, women 50 and older are also the group at highest risk for hip fractures because of the menopause-related thinning of their bones.

To half of the women, Dr. Dawson-Hughes gave daily supplements that contained 100 units of D so that they came up to the 200-unit RDA mark. To the other half she administered 700 units, bringing their total to about 800 units a day, or four times the RDA.

The result: At the end of two years, the women taking just 100-unit supplements of the vitamin every day lost more than twice as much bone from their hips as the others, 2.5 percent as opposed to only 1 percent. "The difference may sound small," Dr. Dawson-Hughes notes, "but if you reduce bone loss by half, you can delay by many years the time it takes to reach the point at which a fracture is likely to occur."

It should also be added that all the women participating in Dr. Dawson-Hughes' study took calcium supplements—500 mg. each—*with* their vitamin D, which put them a step ahead of women at large by practically doubling their consumption of the mineral to more than 1,000 mg. a day.

Where to Get Your Vitamin D

I was riding a subway from Manhattan over to the borough of Queens in an April 1996 visit to the Big Apple. I couldn't help but periodically glance over to the matronly-looking woman beside me with hands and arms exposed to the elbows. She had one of the worst cases of psoriasis I believe I've ever seen. A number of reddish, scaly patches nearly covered one forearm and the underside portion of the other one.

I leaned over, introduced myself and whispered that I knew of a food cure that would treat this disorder for her. She promptly accepted my advice and proceeded to hunt around in her purse for a pen and piece of paper to write my recommendation down on. I told her: "Just eat one-half of a 15-ounce can of mackerel or a small can of sardines every day for four months. You'll discover that your psoriasis will automatically clear up." I forgot the incident after that and wasn't reminded of it for several months, until one day I received a cute thank-you card in the mail from her. Inside, a grateful patron of my free counsel had inscribed:

> *Dr. H-:*
>
> *Your fish cure worked wonders for my skin. The rashes are all gone! I did just like you said to do. But, I must confess, the number of alley cats hanging around our garbage cans must have tripled during this time! Thanks ever so much. Your friend, 'The Fish Lady from Queens'*
>
> */s/ Ruth Goldschmidt*

A businessman from the Chicago suburbs wrote to me recently about his own success with vitamin D. "It's been nearly 30 years since I suffered my first and only heart attack," his letter began. "It was then that my doctor suggested I incorporate into my daily diet a regular allotment of lox and bagels, but without the cream cheese. He said that the fish used for the lox was rich in vitamin D. He felt that I should have at least ten ounces of lox per week in order to prevent another heart attack from occurring. Almost three decades later, my ticker is just fine and I haven't had another close brush with death since then, thanks to my lox."

Other fish that are high in vitamin D are herring, swordfish, cod, sea and striped bass, and flounder. Certain non-fish staples include generous amounts of the nutrient, too—chicken livers, egg yolks, fortified milk, and some fortified, prepared, and packaged dry cereals.

Too Much of a Good Thing May Not Be Good

Science News (141:295, 1992) carried a report about overdoing your intake of vitamin D. It pointed out that if a person is *regularly* eating vitamin D-fortified foods (milk and cereal) and consuming some kind of fatty fish and eggs on a frequent basis, then additional supplementation generally isn't required.

But where such may be necessary for deficiency-linked health problems, a safe amount taken every *other* day would be a vitamin A and D combination (see Product Appendix, p. 381) that gives the consumer 10,000 I.U. of A and 400 I.U. of D.

Vitamin E

THE VITAMIN THAT MOVED FROM THE HEALTH FRINGES INTO THE MEDICAL MAINSTREAM

From Quackery to Respectability

Probably no other vitamin has had quite the staying power that vitamin E seems to have. Its move from the extreme fringes of health care to the very center of orthodox medical care would have stunned early researchers, who were mocked for their faith in its benefits. Among the pioneers were two Canadian doctors, Evan Shute and his brother Wilfrid, who treated heart patients with vitamin E in the late 1940s at their clinic in London, Ontario. Both were soundly denounced throughout the North American medical profession, which then focused on a healthy diet as the best source of all nutrients.

I spoke a short time ago with Denham Harman, a University of Nebraska medical professor, who is now an octogenarian. He provided the theoretical framework that explained why vitamin E worked against scavenger molecules called free radicals in the 1950s. "If you'd been around with me at that time," he recalled by phone, "then you'd realize this work was being ridiculed to the hilt. People paid no attention to us. Our research largely went ignored by doctors and press alike until the late 60s and early 70s. It was extremely difficult to get any money to do our work with."

But then the whole environment changed within just a couple of years. The hippie movement brought with it a national public craze for health foods. All of a sudden vitamin research became a very hot topic of media discussion and scientific interest. Eventually vitamin E found its way into regular medical care after much research had been published in accepted scientific journals with regard to the nutrient's many positive health benefits. Additionally, a growing consumer interest in preventive health care has helped boost its popularity. Before long, say some vitamin manufacturers and purveyors of health supplements, this vitamin has a good chance of becoming a permanent part of the nation's diet. Vitamin

E is certainly one that has hung in there for a long time to get what comedian Rodney Dangerfield claims he still lacks from his audiences—"a little respect!"

Stay Young with Vitamin E

Juan Ponce de Leon and the proverbial "Fountain of Youth" are virtually inseparable and quite synonymous with each other. This Spaniard began his long career of exploration in 1493 as part of Christopher Columbus' second expedition to the New World. In 1508-09 he explored and settled Puerto Rico.

Royal orders to search for new lands, combined with a strong belief in the legend of the Fountain of Youth on Bimini Island in the Bahamas, led him at the age of 53 to the discovery of Florida in the spring of 1513. The region was named Florida because it was discovered at Easter time (in Spanish, *Pascua Florida*). After landing near the site of what is now St. Augustine, he coasted southward, sailing through the Florida Keys and ending his search near Charlotte Harbor on the west coast.

Unfortunately, Ponce de Leon never found the legendary springs that flowed with the magical waters guaranteeing eternal youth for anyone who frequently drank or bathed in them. But in a strange twist of fate the Spanish explorer and his crew *already had* the means of youthful restoration within their grasp but never realized it. They partook of various kinds of nuts and sunflower seeds they brought with them or else found growing wild in the Florida interior, according to ship records. Yet none of them understood at the time that these things were rich in vitamin E.

So far we've discussed vitamins A and C in their roles as potent antioxidants. But vitamin E works in an entirely different manner than these other two nutrients do. A double-blind study done on old or middle-aged mice and reported in the May 1996 *Proceedings of the National Academy of Sciences* found that high intakes of vitamin E supplements (equivalent to a human dosage of 400 I.U. per day) assisted in protecting brain tissue and the immune system against age-related oxidative damage by slowing the decline of certain proteins that play a role in cellular transport and metabolism. These proteins are found in all mammals' cells, suggesting people could reap the same benefits as the mice did.

Referred to as band 3 proteins, they are located primarily in the brain and white blood cells, and are involved in cell respiration, acid base balance, and cell membrane structure. These particular proteins aid in the transport of chloride, fluoride, ammonia, and other negatively charged ions through cell membranes.

Damage to band 3 proteins from scavenger molecules missing their electrons is prevalent because the proteins are intertwined throughout the cell's membrane. This permits exposure to these crazy molecules or free radicals, as they're known, from both inside and outside the cell walls. In the study, vitamin E, a fat-soluble antioxidant, was able to penetrate and protect the fatty cell walls where band 3 proteins are located. The study was conducted by researchers affiliated with the University of Arizona College of Medicine and with the Veterans Affairs Medical Center in Tucson.

As one medical investigator in Tucson explained it to me over the phone one day, "Damaged cells eventually pile up more quickly than the body's own systems can remove them. Our research indicates that vitamin E can expedite this process, thereby slowing the aging process somewhat." He momentarily paused before adding this final qualifier to his previous statement: "But vitamin E can *not* indefinitely postpone it. Everyone's going to get older, sooner or later. That's just a fact of life."

The University of Arizona study also concluded that 400 I.U. of vitamin E—the amount determined to be protective against damage—is greater than the amount consumed in a normal low-fat diet. According to the researchers, this suggests the need for supplemental vitamin E in order to fully achieve the desired results.

How Antioxidant Vitamins Defend Body Cells

Plenty of research in the last decade has shown that antioxidants like vitamins A, C, and E act as chemical messengers, intercepting free radicals before they have a chance to damage cells. Two recent studies made public in the early part of 1997 shed some light on how such protective mechanisms work.

In one study, researchers from Keele University in England examined how this trio of vitamins collaborate to get rid of these highly reactive molecules, whose harmful effects arise from their readiness to grab an electron from another normal molecule. The scheme the chemists have proposed works something like a bucket brigade at a fire scene, with the dangerous chemical property being passed from one molecule to the next.

First, vitamin E reacts with the free radicals, restoring them to their less harmful state. This reaction, though, turns vitamin E into a potentially damaging radical itself, which the vitamin A factors called carotenoids (from beta carotene) then inactivate. Finally, vitamin C repairs the resulting carotenoid radicals, and the water-soluble vitamin C radicals eventually are flushed out of the system.

This protective mechanism may help us understand better the puzzling results of clinical studies indicating that beta carotene supplements boost the incidence of cancer in smokers. The now famous Beta Carotene and Retinol Efficacy Trial, funded by the National Institutes of Health, was halted early because of this very finding.

According to the British researchers' proposed scheme, smokers tend to be low in vitamin C, so they don't have enough ascorbic acid to scavenge carotenoid radicals. Giving smokers supplements of beta carotene (carotenoids) only adds to the radicals in the body. Beta carotene originally showed great promise in the laboratory, but its effect was radically different in human beings. The full report of how these antioxidants defend body cells appeared in the January 22, 1997 *Journal of The American Chemical Society.*

Thinning Your Blood for Stroke Prevention

Several decades ago a British physician by the name of John Yudkin, M.D. reported in the prestigious British medical journal *Lancet* that when fat and sugar are consumed in the same meal together, they promote *greater* platelet aggregation. Blood cells become greasier and stickier, causing them to form into clusters similar to bunches of grapes. This aggregating action not only slows blood flow through the body like a massive traffic snarl on a California freeway or the

New Jersey Turnpike at job quitting time, but it also can form dangerous clots that may be life-threatening.

Warfarin, which *The Merck Index* 9th ed. (Rahway, NJ: Merck & Co., 1976) cites as a potent rat poison (entry # 9700) has been the favored drug of doctors' choice to prevent such coagulation from happening. But now there is a much safer, more nutritious alternative in the form of vitamin E. According to *Science News* (148:175) for September 9, 1995, this nutrient binds itself to the site on the same enzyme where vitamin K normally attaches to start the blood clotting cycle. In doing so, vitamin E promptly halts coagulation and thereby helps prevent clot formations that could trigger fatal heart attacks or crippling strokes.

A really good blood-thinning duo is vitamin E (400 I.U.) every day paired with ginger root (4 capsules daily with a meal). The gingerol in the spice root thins the blood, preventing platelets from clumping. The second phase of clotting is the attachment of the platelets to a vessel wall. This is where vitamin E's role comes into play. The nutrient can help ward off that initial adherence by covering blood platelets with a nonstick coating of sorts that makes it more difficult for them to latch on to the wall. This action of vitamin E may be compared to greasing an indoor rock wall that athletes like to scale in order to test their mountain-climbing skills. They may *try* hard to get up with the aid of ropes and pulleys, but they're not going to be able to grab or stand on any jutted projections to help pull or boost them upward.

This combination was used on 100 patients for almost 2 years. The 42 men and 58 women were given a daily dose of ginger alone (4 capsules). Half of the group also took 400 I.U. of vitamin E per day. At the end of the experiment, those getting both herb and nutrient together fared a lot better, with only 2 cases of blocked arteries compared to 21 cases in the ginger-only group.

Keeping Your Immune System Healthy

Some European medical data suggests that vitamin E can correct the age-related decline in immune function that predisposes elderly people to infections. Investigators from the Czech Republic discovered that nursing home residents who took 400 I.U. of vitamin E and 1,000 mg. of vitamin C on a daily basis had fewer viral infections and were less likely to die from influenza. Similarly, researchers at Tufts University found that when elderly people took 200 to 800 I.U. of supplementary vitamin E per day, they had an improved response to hepatitis B immunizations and tended to have fewer infectious diseases.

Man's Hernia Healed

Over the years I've had literally hundreds of people write or call me after reading one or several of my books on folk medicine or food therapy. Both my address and home phone number (probably the best publicized one in the entire nation) are given in the back of each volume for readers to contact me with any health questions they may have.

When they do so, I always act responsibly by letting them know at the onset that I am *not* a medical doctor, just the Ph.D. kind. Still, they seek my advice and counsel, which is always carefully phrased in a way that *never* suggests outright medical treatment, though the information offered might be regarded as prescriptive in nature by some.

The following letter represents one such case and is used here with the writer's permission.

Saturday, October 5, 1996

Dear Dr. Heinerman:

I have spoken to you on three separate occasions. And each time, you have helped me better deal with my condition as well as improve my spirit.

The last time we spoke was on Thursday, August 15, when I was visiting my family in Philadelphia. On that occasion you suggested that I start taking slippery elm tea [2 cups daily], in addition to the horsetail [2 capsules daily], calcium-magnesium supplement [2 tablets daily with meals], zinc tablets [two 50 mg. divided between two meals daily], and the Rex's Wheat Germ Oil [1 tablespoon of veterinary-strength pure, unrefined vitamin E oil; see Product Appendix].

On August 15, you made it clear that in addition to taking these remedies for a torn hernia that I [should] begin to wear a truss. You specifically suggested that I contact the Brooks' Appliance Company [310 East Michigan, Marshall, MI/616-781-3993]. I want to express my sincere gratitude for this advise [sic] you gave me. I have been wearing my Brooks Appliance and using the Rex's [Wheat Germ] Oil and other things faithfully since September 10 and this has aided in the improvement of my condition.

I appreciate the time you have taken to speak to me on the telephone. I want to thank you again for all the information and help you have provided. Your [health] books [from Prentice Hall] are a constant source of information and comfort to me. Thank you once again.

/s/ Gary L. Herlich
2428 Caminito Ocean Cove
Cardiff, CA 92007

Reducing Cataract Risk

Millions of people suffer oxidative stress of their eyes every day of their lives without knowing it. This is. primarily true of those engaged in occupations that demand considerable exposure of their eyes to light and oxygen. Computer screens and photocopy machines in air-conditioned workplace environs provide the ideal setting for eye damage by free radicals.

A number of different studies have demonstrated that inadequate intakes of vitamins A, C, and E are generally associated with a greater incidence of cataracts as people get older. In order to reduce personal risk of cataract formation, medical tests have shown that *consistent* supplementation of vitamins A (10,000 I.U.), C (1,000 mg.) and E (400 I.U.) every day is necessary.

More recent data, as reported in the November 1996 *Harvard Health Letter,* suggests that vitamin E (400 I.U.) and beta carotene (10,000 I.U.) can help lower the cataract formation and reduce a person's chances of ever incurring macular degeneration.

Energy Success in a Big Way

In 1983 the tennis world was set on its ear with the stunning performance of a sixteen-year-old newcomer by the name of Aaron

Krickstein. In the third round of the U.S. Open he handily defeated tennis dynamo Vitas Gerulaitis. This incredible win made the American teenager the youngest player at that time to ever attain a top-10 ranking.

Reporters noticing the athlete's seemingly boundless energy asked him what he took or did for it. He replied that he started every morning by taking 400 I.U. of vitamin E, one tablespoon of wheat germ oil, a multiple vitamin-mineral supplement, and 1,000 mg. of ascorbic acid. The Grosse Point, Michigan teenager began this vitamin regimen in 1982 on the advice of his coach, Nick Bolletieri, who told him: "Kid, if you want the energy to win, you'll need to get in shape nutritionally." He did and won the biggest tournament of his life!

The Era of E (or e) Has Begun

The fact that vitamin E has suddenly become such a hot and popular nutrient with the pill-popping masses may have something to do with its letter in the alphabet. According to Jamie Malanowski, writing in the April 21, 1997 issue of *Time* magazine, this is the age of the letter E. The e Cafe on Fifth Avenue in Manhattan "joins the top-rated television series *ER,* the popular magazine *Entertainment Weekly* (widely called *EW*), CBS's highly praised series *EZ Streets,* the irreverent E! Entertainment Television, the resurgent *E. coli* bacteria and the favored form of communication of the cognoscenti, E-mail, plus its multifarious electronic spin-offs, e-cash, e-commerce, et al."

Just about everybody seems to know something about E these days (*vitamin* E, that is):

Angina. Leading cardiologists now recognize that it can prevent or even slow the rate of heart disease. In a Japanese study that app eared in the medical journal *Circulation* (94(1):14-18, July 1, 1996), patients who were given 300 I.U. daily of vitamin E had fewer attacks of angina pectoris, a painful constriction around the heart caused by insufficient blood flow. A few alternative-minded cardiologists are now recommending that their patients take a *gradual* increase of vitamin E, starting out with 300 I.U. the first week and adding an extra 100 units every week thereafter until 800 I.U. per day are being taken. This enables many of their angina patients to decrease or discontinue altogether their daily intake of nitroglycerin, a standard drug for treating angina.

Burns. Word of mouth is what has kept bringing thousands of patients every year to the non-profit Shute Institute located midway between Detroit and Toronto in the Canadian city of London, Province of Ontario. The clinic has been going strong for over half a century now and has never once had to advertise for customers. It was founded by the Shute brothers, Evan and Wilfrid, whose names are virtually synonymous with vitamin E research and therapy. They believed in using this wonderful nutrient for treating heart disease, diabetes, and burns.

These doctors applied vitamin E oil externally after treating burned surface tissue with standard antimicrobial agents first in order to prevent infection by a large variety of gram-negative and gram-positive bacteria. Liquid chlorophyll was also employed in the occlusive dressings put on more serious burns.

The Shute brothers came up with a nutritional package for every burn patient treated: 400-600 I.U. vitamin E, 1,000 mg. vitamin C, 10,000 I.U. vitamin A, 100 mg. zinc, and 25 micrograms selenium every day for as long as was necessary or until there was satisfactory evidence of new skin regeneration.

Cancer. Lester Packer, Ph.D. is a big fan of vitamin E, and believes it may afford the body good protection against lung, stomach, prostate, and colon cancers. He is with the Department of Modular and Cell Biology at the University of California at Berkeley and ought to know, since he's studied this particular vitamin pretty extensively. I was in Anaheim, California for the Natural Products Expo West convention and attended his session there. He spoke to a packed house on the topic of "Vitamin E, Tocopherols, Tocotrienols, Biological Action—Health and Effects." Free radicals damage the body's DNA, which can cause malignant cell division in an uncontrolled way. But vitamin E stops this injury to our genetic blueprint for normal cell division by rendering these scavenger molecules inert. Research so far indicates that dietary or supplementary vitamin E could help reduce the risk of developing some cancers.

Chronic Fatigue Syndrome. Two naturopathic physicians, one based in Seattle, Washington and the other in Vancouver, British Columbia, have been prescribing *graduated* doses (400 to 800 I.U. over 4 weeks) of vitamin E oil for their patients suffering from chronic fatigue syndrome with outstanding success. Over 93 percent reported feeling more energy and stamina after taking vitamin E for a month.

Coronary Artery (Heart) Disease. Because of a major report that appeared in the *Journal of the American Medical Association* (273:1849-54, June 21, 1995) a few year ago and subsequently received considerable media attention, many doctors and laypeople now know that regular use of vitamin E can reduce the gradual progress of coronary artery disease (otherwise known as atherosclerosis). A total of 156 men aged 40 to 59 years old with previous coronary artery bypass graft surgery were enrolled in a special Cholesterol Lowering Atherosclerosis Study (CLAS). Supplementary and dietary antioxidant vitamins (E and C) were given to part of this cohort, while placebos were given to the remaining volunteers. A cholesterol-lowering diet was followed by all participants. Subjects with supplementary vitamin E intake of 100 I.U. per day or greater demonstrated far less occurrence of atherosclerotic lesion progression in their heart vessels than did subjects taking less than 100 I.U. per day. Evaluations of each individual were made periodically over the two-year study period at community- and university-based cardiac-catheterization laboratories in the Greater Los Angeles area.

At the end of their report, the team of seven medical researchers involved in the CLAS postulated how vitamin E might work in reducing coronary artery lesion progression. I've taken the liberty of simplifying their scientific jargon into terms the layperson can readily understand. The atherosclerotic process starts when an immune cell called a monocyte begins absorbing the oxidized "bad" cholesterol (or LDL for low-density lipoproteins). (Oxidation is the process that turns butter rancid, iron to rust, or, in this case, cholesterol into a major cause of coronary artery disease.) After the -monocyte absorbs the free-radical-damaged or oxidized LDL, it acquires a puffy quality and turns into a foam cell. It is carried through the bloodstream and soon attempts to infiltrate artery walls. While this is happening, the foam cell starts releasing free radicals and other substances that further encourage the formation of cholesterol-containing plaque. The foam cell, having stuffed itself to the hilt with LDL, grows in size and eventually gets trapped in the artery wall with many other foam cells just like itself, which leads to the cholesterol-containing plaque characteristic of coronary artery (heart) disease.

Now, the role of vitamin E in all of this is to prevent "bad" cholesterol from becoming oxidized by free radicals. In turn, there is absolutely no reason for monocytes (specifically, macrophages) to gobble up oxidatively modified "bad" cholesterol and turn into foam cells that could eventually clog heart arteries.

According to Jack Challem, writing in the December 1996 issue of *Let's Live* health magazine (p. 60), "Long-term users of vitamin E supplements [are] 60 percent less likely to die of coronary heart disease and 59 percent less likely to die of cancer than people who [do] not take the vitamin."

The "lucky number" in terms of number of vitamin E units needed each day to slow the oxidation of "bad" cholesterol seems to be 400 International Units, according to a study conducted at the University of Texas Southwestern Medical Center in Dallas. After two months, participants who took 400 I.U. of vitamin E daily had less oxidation of LDLs than those who just took 60 or 200 I.U.

Diabetes. A mounting body of medical evidence suggests that free radical damage is to blame for initiating Type 2 diabetes (the non-insulin or adult kind). Researchers think that oxidation may adversely affect sugar metabolism or damage the pancreas, the body's sole source of insulin. Now, a prospective study by Finnish researchers of 944 men provides the first epidemiological evidence that vitamin E might reduce the risk of Type 2 diabetes. Men with low blood levels of vitamin E had nearly four times the risk of developing the condition. In previous research, supplements containing as much as 1,350 International Units of alpha-tocopherol (a vitamin E factor) helped insulin work more effectively in patients with Type 2 diabetes and improved its effectiveness in elderly people with heart disease.

Muscle Pain. Vitamin E can help weekend warriors relieve their muscle pains, according to William J. Evans, Ph. D., professor of applied physiology and director of the Noll Physiological Research Center at Pennsylvania State University in State College, Pennsylvania. He found that vitamin E supplements can be of definite assistance in preventing muscle soreness in those unaccustomed to vigorous exercise.

After such strenuous workouts, muscles develop microscopic tears and show an increase in the production of oxygen-free radicals. The damage may continue for days after exercise. The body responds by trying to heal these tears.

Evans discovered that vitamin E improved the healing process by increasing the mobilization of immune cells to damaged muscle cells and reducing the production of oxygen free radicals. And while his study only focused on older, active people, he stated that younger periodic exercisers would also benefit from vitamin E. The only one who probably wouldn't benefit very much from additional antioxidants would be the endurance athlete, whose metabolism is already well-developed to begin with, according to the July 13, 1996 issue of *Internal Medicine News.*

I also recommend vitamin E in the form of wheat germ oil (see Product Appendix) as useful therapy in the management of multiple sclerosis. Take one tablespoon of this every morning with breakfast.

Neurological Disorders. It's pretty well clear by now from the evidence available that vitamin E plays a key role in normal neurologic functions in human beings, as well as in many other mammals. Various neurologic disorders arise in people deficient in vitamin E and may be slowed or even reversed with immediate vitamin E therapy. Those suffering from chronic problems of fat absorption, serious liver disease, and cystic fibrosis are believed to have the type of vitamin E deficiencies that could contribute to nerve damage.

Attention should be especially paid to those afflicted with malabsorption or maldigestion disorders. These people can be given vitamin E both as a *preventive* and protective measure in neurologic disease. Doses exceeding 1,200 I.U. may be required for some individuals and should always be administered under a doctor's supervision. Some of the malabsorptive diseases generally associated with vitamin E deficiencies include: cirrhosis of the liver, short bowel syndrome, bacterial overgrowth, sprue and non-tropical sprue, sclerodermal bowel disease, chronic pancreatitis, gluten enteropathy, and the already cited cystic fibrosis.

According to Sheldon Saul Hendler, M.D., Ph.D., author of *The Doctors' Vitamin and Mineral Encyclopedia* (New York: Simon & Schuster, 1991), vitamin E therapy may prove very useful in treating "some of the neurologic symptoms of these diseases" which he listed as including "muscle weakness, abnormal eye movements, loss of reflexes, restriction of field of vision, unsteady gait, loss of muscle mass" and "the commonest non-neurologic symptoms" of all, namely a type of "diarrhea in which one excretes a lot of fat."

Dr. Hendler also mentioned the possible benefits that vitamin E therapy might play in Parkinson's disease, epilepsy, and tardive dyskinesia. He cited a range of "400 to 1,200 I.U.s of vitamin E daily" as the potential dosages applicable for treating any of these neurological disorders.

Premenstrual Syndrome (PMS). Further along in his informative book, Dr. Hendler mentions that women suffering from the miseries of PMS have obtained relief from the symptoms with regular "supplementation of 400 I.U.s of vitamin E."

A doctor I know who specializes in women's health routinely prescribes vitamin E to all of her patients suffering from PMS, as well as taking 600 I.U. daily herself for the same problem.

Respiratory Distress Syndrome. It is estimated that about 150,000 adults in America come down with respiratory distress syndrome each year. The condition is marked by hyperventilation, increase in the work of breathing, high-pitched diffusely scattered crackles, and very low oxygen levels in the circulating blood plasma, which can lead to a gray pallor, damp skin, lethargy, and elevated agitation.

A combination of winning nutrients will reduce these and other symptoms by as much as 75 percent, if not more: vitamin E (600 I.U.), vitamin C (3,000 mg.), and selenium (200 micrograms). These supplements should be taken daily with a meal, preferably in the morning upon arising. Mucous-forming foods such as milk, ice cream, cheese, and eggs should be temporarily discontinued.

The Two Most Active Compounds of Vitamin E

Pure vitamin E was first isolated from the unsaponifiable fraction of wheat germ oil in 1936. Just two years later its chemical structure and synthesis were also reported in the scientific literature. Although alpha-tocopherol is, by far, the most widely recognized active compound in vitamin E, there is actually another one which scientists have known about for many years but only now have been looking into with intense interest. There are seven naturally occurring tocopherols that comprise this wonderful nutrient and are named after the first seven letters in the Greek alphabet: alpha-tocopherol, beta-tocopherol, gamma-tocopherol, delta-tocopherol, zeta-tocopherol, epsilon-tocopherol, and eta-tocopherol. The first four tocopherols have roughly 135, 50, 30, and 10 percent relative biological activity, respectively. Not much is known about the remaining three but their relative biological activities are quite low, ranging from 5 for epsilon-tocopherol to a mere 1 for delta-tocopherol.

Until very recently, the alpha-tocopherol had been receiving the lion's share of scientific attention and has, for some years now, been used interchangeably with vitamin E. But some of the other structurally similar tocopherols are generally packaged together by nature. In such mixtures, gamma-tocopherol usually predominates.

The April 1, 1997 *Proceedings of the National Academy of Sciences* reported that researchers from the University of California at Berkeley had discovered that gamma-tocopherol provides valuable protection from nitrogen oxides, a broad class of reactive compounds that alpha-tocopherol largely ignores. This should be of considerable interest to consumers, since all vitamin E sold in drugstores, health food stores, vitamin shops, and through multiple-level marketing schemes contains mostly alpha-tocopherol.

The California-based researchers focused on the ability of tocopherols to defuse nitrogen oxides. In the environment these compounds contribute to acid rain. But inside the human system, many serve as destructive oxidants that can alter DNA and trigger some of the damage caused by inflammation.

Working with simulated cell membranes and "bad" cholesterol (low-density lipoproteins or LDLs) taken from people who had consumed different brands of vitamin E supplements, the scientists tested the tocopherols' ability to detoxify peroxynitrite, a nitrogen oxide that is associated with inflammation. Although the alpha-tocopherol pretty much eliminates the oxidant character of the molecule, it leaves behind a reactive nitrogen component that only gamma-tocopherol is capable of handling. During a follow-up reaction, they observed this tocopherol permanently trap those remaining nitrogen compounds that were still reactive. Gamma-tocopherol exhibits a special affinity for reacting with and inactivating nitrogen oxides.

This same team, headed by Stephan Christen, induced inflammation in animals and then observed what transpired to tocopherols in the blood. Concentrations of the gamma plunged like crazy. Simultaneously, certain nitrogenous compounds increased, suggesting that the gamma-tocopherol was trapping nitrogen oxides.

Since consumption of large amounts of the alpha form tends to shove the gamma kind completely out of the body, both tocopherols should be consumed together, noted Dr. Christen. Anders G. Olsson, a physician who studied lipids and atherosclerosis at University Hospital in Linköping, Sweden, agrees with the American researchers. In the March 1st, 1997 *British Medical Journal,* he and some of his colleagues described their investigation into risk factors that could explain why Lithuanian men face four times the heart disease mortality of Swedish men the same age.

Neither conventional risk factors—such as hypertension or elevated cholesterol/triglyceride levels—nor alpha-tocopherol concentrations were radically different between the two groups. The Lithuanian men, however, did possess significantly lower gamma-tocopherol concentrations in their circulating plasma than the Swedes did. The ongoing research being done by the Americans could explain Olsson's findings.

Coronary artery disease isn't the only degenerative condition linked to low gamma-tocopherol. Robert V. Cooney's team at the Cancer Research Center of Hawaii in Honolulu has demonstrated in test-tube studies that "gamma-tocopherol pretty well blocks the formation of tumor cells at high doses. It's much more effective than alpha-tocopherol for this," he said in a telephone conversation with this author in mid-April 1997.

Sources of Vitamin E

In mentioning available sources for vitamin E, it should be kept in mind that whatever is recommended ought to include the gamma-tocopherol as well as the more plentiful alpha-form. The table below lists sources for both.

Vitamin E Sources

Alpha-Tocopherol	Gamma-Tocopherol
Sesame oil	Corn oil
Sunflower oil	Canola oil
Safflower oil	Soy milk
Salmon (broiled)	Soybean oil
Butter	Hazel nuts
Liver, beef (baked)	Walnuts/walnut oil
Peas, fresh (cooked)	Peanuts, fresh (shelled)
Tomato, fresh	Peanut butter
Beef, ground (fried)	Almond butter
Chicken breast (broiled)	Cashew butter
Apple (fresh)	Pistachios
Pork chop (fried)	Macadamias
	Avocados

Both Tocopherols
Wheat germ
Wheat germ oil (unrefined)*
Millet barley
Rye
Oats (cooked)

---

*The only vitamin E oil I've recommended for years is the one used by many veterinarians and livestock breeders. See the Product Appendix for more information on where to get it.

Vitamin F
BIOAVAILABLE NUTRITION FOR GROWTH
AND WELL-BEING

A Short-Lived History

Early in this century, G. O. Burr and M. M. Burr described some interesting experiments they conducted with white rats in the *Journal of Biological Chemistry* (82:345, 1929; and 86:587, 1930). Their research led them to conclude that in animals given a ration extremely poor in fat, a deficiency disease could result that was curable when linoleic or linolenic acids and arachidonic acids or fats containing these acids(such as lecithin from soybeans) were added to the diet. Additional support for the conception of the essential nature of these two fatty acids was contained in two reports by Evans and Lepkovsky in a later issue of the same periodical (*Journal of Biological Chemistry* 96:143; and 93:157, both 1932). They stated that growth would not take place unless unsaturated fatty acids with two or more double bonds were present in the ration.

To help the reader better understand some of the technical aspects involved in vitamin F, a brief diversion into a short discussion on fatty acids in general may be of assistance here. Fatty acids are composed entirely of carbon, hydrogen, and oxygen. They are found in all the simple and compound lipids or fats. Some of the common fatty acids are palmitic, stearic, oleic, and linoleic. There are short-chain (10 or fewer carbon atoms), long-chain (12 to 18 carbon atoms), and extra-long-chain (20 or more carbon atoms) fatty acids. Fatty acids of 10 carbon atoms or less are seldom found in animal products except for milk fat. Long-chain fatty acids occur in animal fats and most vegetable oils; the extra-long-chain ones are found in fish oils.

Scientists also classify fatty acids according to their degree of saturation or unsaturation. Certain fatty acids, such as stearic acid, contain as many hydrogen atoms as the carbon chain can hold: they are called saturated fatty acids. Others have only one double-bond linkage (two hydrogen atoms missing) in the carbon chain; they are referred to as monounsaturated fatty acids. A third group, the polyunsaturated fatty acids (which constitute, as a group, vitamin F) may have two, three, four, or more double-bond linkages in the carbon chain with four, six, eight, or more hydrogen atoms missing.

Saturated fatty acids (largely animal fats) comprise about 35 percent of the total fat in the American diet. The most common saturated fatty acids are stearic acid and palmitic acid. The fat of butter and cows' milk contains about 60 percent saturated fatty acids; those of meat vary from about 46 percent for lamb to 28 percent for chicken and beef liver.

Monounsaturated fatty acids constitute about 40 percent of the total fat in the diet of most Americans. An example of a long-chain monounsaturated fatty acid is oleic acid, which is found in appreciable amounts in many foods. It comprises nearly one-third of the fat content of chicken and about 47 percent of the fat content of margarine.

Polyunsaturated fatty acids (or the vitamin F group) are long-chain and extra-long-chain fatty acids. Most Americans consume far less of these acids than of either the saturated or monounsaturated ones. However, their intake is increasing. In 1947-1949, linoleic acid constituted 10.7 percent of the total fat consumed, and in 1973, 15.4 percent.

With this overview before the reader, we can now return to the short-lived history of the polyunsaturated fatty acids' temporary vitamin status. In 1934 a series of three papers by Evans, Lepkovsky, and Murphy appeared, in which the name vitamin F was officially given to linoleic, linolenic, and arachidonic acids. There followed a short period of comical exploitation of vitamin F by sharp businessmen seeing an opportunity for some dollars to be made.

Patients began telling their doctors about this new "miracle nutrient" they had begun taking called Vitamin F. A number of alarmed physicians wrote to the American Medical Association complaining of this new health fad and demanded an investigation into the matter. After a cursory examination of things had been made in haste, the AMA soundly denounced this nutrient as nothing better than another form of "nutritional quackery." Hence, for many years vitamin F was discredited and no longer mentioned in books on nutrition.

General Information

Fortunately, though, vitamin F has made a comeback in recent years, perhaps not by the name of vitamin F per se, but certainly in the great emphasis being placed these days on the many health benefits of the unsaturated fatty acids. There has never been an official Recommended Dietary Allowance set for them, but 10 percent of total calories consumed in one day is the usual consumption. Supporting nutrients for vitamin F are A, C, D, E, and phosphorus.

Body parts positively affected by vitamin F include cells, glands (adrenals, thyroid, and parathyroid), hair, mucous membranes, nerves, and skin. Biological functions facilitated by the presence of polyunsaturated fatty acids in the diet include the following short list, but are not limited to them:

- artery-hardening prevention
- blood coagulation
- blood pressure normalizer
- cholesterol destroyer
- glandular activity
- physical growth in early years of life
- vital organ respiration

Some of the more apparent deficiency symptoms of vitamin F might be: acne, allergies, diarrhea, dry skin, dry, brittle hair, eczema, gall stones, nail problems, underweight, and varicose veins.

The vitamin F group has certain useful therapeutic applications for a small number of health problems. These consist of:

allergies	heart disease
baldness	leg ulcers
bronchial asthma	psoriasis
cholesterol (elevated)	restless legs syndrome
eczema	rheumatoid arthritis
gall bladder problems or removal	underweight/overweight

She Grew Like a Weed

Most people won't know who Helen Foster Snow was unless the name of the famous man she became connected with in marriage is mentioned in the same breath. Still, this Utah-born native had stunted growth during a portion of her formative years. Born in 1908, she grew fairly well as was expected of girls her age then, until about the time of her eighth birthday. Then it seemed that her growth mysteriously stopped for no apparent reason.

Naturally, her parents were quite alarmed over this most unusual predicament. This was when medical science was still in its Stone Age evolution and quite primitive. It was in a time when there were no growth hormone shots or pills like there are now for such things. A number of learned doctors were concerned, but could give the worried parents no hopeful news.

An old woman in the city, who worked at a local fish market, told the Snows one day when they came in with their small girl with them, to start giving her cod liver oil and to feed her baked fish several times a week. This woman promised that, if her advice was followed, the girl's growth would begin to spurt upward again. She then demanded a $5 bill from them, which was a goodly sum in those times. They reluctantly paid her, bought their fish, and left.

However, there was a ring of genuineness to the old woman's statement, despite her rough ways and obvious con artist talents. The Fosters decided they had nothing to lose by trying what she had recommended on little Helen. For the next seven months, she was given tablespoons of cod liver oil morning, noon, and night with her regular meals. And her parents made sure she had plenty of fish. The results were not apparent at first, but then became readily evident. In just 1 1/2 years following this extraordinary diet and supplementation program of vitamin F foods, she grew an astonishing six inches, much to the delight of everyone who knew her. Doctors were baffled, to say the least, when her parents brought their no-longer-little girl into a few of their offices for an explanation as to why this had happened.

Suffice it to say, Helen grew to young adulthood and became a poised, charismatic woman with confidence and a sense of style that ingratiated her to everyone who had the good pleasure of meeting her. One of these was Edgar Snow, whom she met in Shanghai, China. He was an American news correspondent who wrote the worldwide bestseller, *Red Star Over China*. A year later she wrote a companion volume, *Inside Red China* under the pseudonym Nym Wales. Both books are still considered to be the definitive texts on the leaders of the Chinese Communist revolution, including Mao Tse-tung and Chou En-lai. The books detail the grueling 6,000-mile Long March the Communists made from Jiangxi to seek refuge from Chiang Kai-shek's forces in the caves of Yunnan.

The Chinese government in mainland China has always held the Snows in high esteem for the invaluable assistance they rendered their country and for the good reports they gave to the outside world, at a time when nobody would help them. Edgar Snow died in Switzerland in 1972 and his wife died in January, 1997 at age 89 at her home in Madison, Connecticut.

Help for Dyslexia and Crohn's Disease

Dyslexia is an impairment of the brain's ability to translate visual information into meaningful language. According to preliminary research conducted by Jacqueline Stordy at the University of Surrey in Guildford, England, it is accompanied by an impairment of the eye's ability to adapt to dark conditions. A polyunsaturated fatty acid DHA (docosahexaeonic acid) is concentrated in parts of the brain as well as in the photosensitive cells in the retina.

Stordy wondered if daily supplementation with fish oil, which contains omega-3 fatty acids identical to brain and eye DHA, could help improve dyslexics' ability to adapt to the dark. She treated five patients with 480 mg. of fish oil daily for one month. At the end of that time, all of the dyslexic patients had made significant improvement in their ability to adapt to darkness.

The findings in her studies are bolstered by other research that has shown that DHA is critical to the development of the brain and retina prenatally and in the first year of life. Adults can manufacture their own DHA from essential fatty acids in vegetable oils—even if they aren't fish lovers as such.

Crohn's disease is an inflammation of the bowel wall that causes diarrhea, flatulence, weight loss, and abdominal tenderness. It is marked by its relapse and remission periods.

Two of the polyunsatured fatty acids in the vitamin F group that are derived from fish were used in a recent study with Crohn's disease patients. These were EPA (eicosapentaenoic acid) and, of course, the now familiar DHA (docosahexaenoic acid). They were administered in enteric-coated fish oil capsules; the enteric coating protects the oils from digestive acids in the gut. Because of this, just one-third of the amount of fish oils used in previous studies were needed for this one, since the fish oils' fatty acids were more quickly absorbed by the body. Additionally, the frequency of side effects was reduced and patients were more willing to stick to their supplement regimen.

In the placebo-controlled, double-blind study, researchers gave 39 Crohn's disease patients with high risk of relapse enteric-coated fish oil capsules daily for one year. At the end of the study, 59 percent (23 patients) experienced total remission of their problem, compared with 10 patients in remission in the control group. For something as painful as Crohn's disease, anything capable of easing symptoms or increasing the span of remission periods is definitely beneficial and should be given serious attention. In fact, the vitamin F contained in fatty fish is an important part of treatment protocol for all types of inflammatory diseases. [Consult the June 13, 1996 issue of *The New England Journal of Medicine* for the full report.]

How Vitamin F Has Helped the World's Oldest TV News Anchor

Wednesday, April 16, 1997 was another typically busy day for me in my office at the Anthropological Research Center. My staff was occupied with its own tasks and duties, while I hammered away on my vintage typewriter keyboard. I received a telephone call from a most interesting fellow in Los Angeles, California. He introduced himself as Hal Fishman and gave me a little background about himself.

He started out as a news anchor at KTLA Channel 5 in 1960. "I was at the Democratic Convention here in L.A. when John F. Kennedy was nominated as the candidate for President of the United States. On June 20th, 1997, I will celebrate 37 straight years as a news anchor. I'm also the station's managing director. To give you an idea of just how long that's been, let me put things in this perspective: Walter Cronkite anchored the CBS Evening News for 19 years; I've been anchoring almost twice that long! I've been told by those in the TV news business that I am, without a doubt, the world's longest-running television news anchor!"

"What a record to be proud of!" I replied. I then told him a little bit about my own background and the type of alternative health books I write for consumers.

"I am very careful of what I eat," he returned. "I always do things in moderation. I follow what my body tells me to do. If it says, 'Eat more fish,' then I have my wife fix me more fish. She usually cooks with safflower oil all the time."

When I informed him that fish and safflower oil were high in vitamin F, he asked me what that was. I explained that it was the polyunsaturated fatty acids vitamin group. He replied, "Well, I don't get into the specifics of health things. I let my wife worry about that. My business is the gathering and reporting of the news."

Mr. Fishman told me that he had been a heavy chain-smoker until 1965, at which time he quit. "My wife got me into the 'fish thing' and she started cooking with safflower oil sometime after that." He believes that both things "helped to keep my voice strong and my larynx [voicebox] healthy all these years," even though, by his own admission, "I don't know much about nutrition like others do."

Hope for Multiple Sclerosis

Multiple sclerosis (MS) is a disorder marked by destruction of the protective outer casings of the nerves within the central nervous system (the brain, optic nerve, and spinal cord). The nerve casings, known as myelin sheaths, are composed mostly of fats; they insulate the nerves and increase the speed of electrical transmissions. In MS, patchy areas of the sheaths are destroyed (demyelinated) and replaced by scar tissue (known as plaques)—a process known as sclerosis—at multiple sites throughout the central nervous system (hence the name of the disorder).

Sclerosis impairs electrical conduction, thus reducing or eliminating transmission of nerve impulses within the affected areas. Symptoms wax and wane unpredictably and vary widely from patient to patient. Some of the more common ones, though, are physical fatigue, muscle weakness and spasticity (especially in the arms and legs), eye pain and visual disturbances, double vision, "pins-and-needles" sensations, loss of coordination, vertigo, slurred speech, loss of bladder control and constipation, emotional depression and mood swings, mental confusion, facial paralysis on one side, and partial or total paralysis of the entire body.

In the early 1980s, when people from all over the U.S. and Canada started writing to me about this problem, I began to give it some serious attention. In my own research work, I discovered along the way (through some trial and error, of course), that certain vitamin F foods and herbs were especially good for this problem. The ones I favor the most are olive oil, baked and canned salmon, and borage and evening primrose oils. All are incredibly rich in certain polyunsaturated fatty acids. They help to restore myelin sheathing to the nerves that have previously been destroyed. They restore electrical conduction through the nervous system. While not every MS case may experience total recovery, these items, when eaten or consumed on a regular basis, will *definitely* minimize many of the more common MS symptoms and allow individuals thus afflicted, to have more freedom of movement than they've had. Obviously, those with the early onset of MS are going to benefit more than those who've had it for some years. Still, there is even hope for some limited recovery for long-term patients, believe it or not!

As a rule, I've recommended 1 tablespoon of extra virgin olive oil once or twice daily with meals, and 3 to 6 capsules of borage or evening primrose oils on an empty stomach. Salmon should be consumed a minimum of twice a week. These items also help to prevent stroke and to treat stroke in the first 36 hours after its initial occurrence. In this case, olive oil and borage and evening primrose oils would be the handiest to use for quickest results in helping to reduce the paralysis that customarily accompanies a major stroke.

Foods Containing Vitamin F

The following table lists the percentages of vitamin F contained in a number of different foods.

Foods	Vitamin F Content (%)
Beef, ground	2
Butter	3
Cheese	2
Chicken leg (broiled)	23
Corn oil	57
Egg yolk	10
Lamb chops (broiled)	4
Liver, beef (fried)	11
Milk, whole	3
Nuts (general mix)	34-69
Olive oil (extra virgin)	78
Peanut butter	29
Pork chop (broiled)	9
Safflower oil	73
Salmon (baked)	81
Veal cutlet	4

Incorporate as many of these into your diet as wisdom dictates or as it seems prudent to do at the time. Your body will greatly appreciate getting a nice blend of unsaturated fatty acids in foods from natural food sources.

Supplement When Necessary

A more efficient way of getting your daily intake of vitamin F is from supplemental sources. Several essential fatty acids are available in softgel capsules: cod liver oil, omega 3 and 6 marine lipids and evening primrose oil. Lecithin granules and tablets are also good supplemental sources. Follow label directions for suggested amounts. (Check the Product Appendix on page 381 for more information on where to obtain supplements containing Vitamin F.)

Vitamin H
(SEE UNDER VITAMIN B COMPLEX—CHOLINE)

Vitamin K
THE VITAMIN THAT STOPS YOU FROM BLEEDING

Nutritional Needs for Vitamin K

The daily vitamin K requirements for humans have been estimated to be around 80 micrograms (mcg) for men and a little less for women, 65 mcg. Standard recommendations, though, have usually been much higher, averaging between 300 and 500 mcg. This should come from a combination of dietary intake through vitamin-K-rich foods and microbiological biosynthesis in the gut. It appears that the microorganisms synthesizing vitamin K in the gut must reside in the ileum, where absorption of vitamin K is possible. In human subjects, the vitamin K homologues stored in the liver suggest that almost 50 percent of the daily requirement is derived from plant sources(vitamin K-1) and the remainder from microbiological biosynthesis. In fact, half of the vitamin K of human liver is vitamin K-1 and the remainder a mixture of other K homologues (designated as MK-7 through MK-11 by scientists).

Those at risk for cardiac thrombus embolus, deep vein thrombosis (DVT), stroke, or other conditions involving single or multiple blood clots, are frequently prescribed heparin or warfarin (Coumadin)—drugs that inhibit blood coagulation. Such medications are not without obvious side effects, though they've obviously saved many lives in the process. (As a side note, I have recommended safer alternatives that include cayenne pepper, ginger root, garlic, red clover, and turmeric root.)

Such anticoagulant medications deprive the body of adequate vitamin K. Lengthy use of warfarin, for instance, increases capillary fragility, leading to hemorrhages. Prolonged intake of heparin not only drives down cholesterol levels as it's intended to do, but also eliminates vitamin K from the system. When this happens, less muscle-nerve activity and brain performance are evident. In order to reverse such capillary hemorrhaging, hypoactivity, and general malaise, some vitamin K foods need to be included in the diet periodically.

Another thing that vitamin K is essential for is in the prevention of osteoporosis, especially in the necks and spines of very elderly folks. Vitamin K plays a significant role in bone calcification. Without vitamin K present, calcium cannot be fully utilized in bone- and tooth-hardening processes. According to a report by a cellular biologist in the June 1985 issue of the *Journal of Clinical Endocrinology and Metabolism* (60:1268-69), low levels of vitamin K can be attributed to a much higher risk of sustaining fractures or developing osteoporosis.

More recent evidence indicates that vitamin K increases osteocalcin, an important protein needed for bone formation. In the early part of 1996, French medical investigators reported that older women with low osteocalcin levels had lower bone density and were especially prone to hip fractures. This inspired American researchers at Tufts University in Boston and the Johns Hopkins Medical School in Baltimore to conduct their own study with regard to osteocalcin. Nine healthy male and female volunteers were given 420 micrograms of vitamin K every day; this amounted to roughly four times the RDA. They found that osteocalcin levels increased dramatically, and various tests suggested that bone density increased as well. This definitely shows the benefit of vitamin K when it comes to building strong bones.

Things That Interfere with Vitamin K Utilization

Certain diseases are known to interfere with the absorption of vitamin K into the body. These include various liver disturbances (hepatitis and cirrhosis), cystic fibrosis and gastrointestinal problems such as celiac disease, Crohn's disease, and short bowel syndrome.

Certain drugs and nutrients can also block the absorption of vitamin K. These would include the two anticoagulants previously mentioned, large doses of aspirin or aspirin-like medications, broad-spectrum cephalsoporin antibiotics (moxalactam and cefamandole), and high doses of vitamins A or E.

Common sense suggests that in the event any of these other drugs or nutrients are necessary for some reason, then the diet should include adequate amounts of K-rich foods. By consuming such *occasionally* instead of frequently, you will allow the drugs or other nutrients to do their jobs without putting too much vitamin K back into the system, only what is necessary to prevent serious depletion.

A word or two should be said in passing with regard to newborn infants receiving the standard vitamin K injections that doctors and hospitals routinely administer following birth. This is done in order to reduce the risk of death from bleeding. While once laudable, the validity of this practice is now being brought into serious question. Two recent studies have determined that infants receiving the *injected* form of vitamin K are about twice as likely to experience childhood cancer as those who are given the same dose *orally.*

Since 1993, American hospitals have required that their doctors on staff give an intramuscular injection, rather than an oral dose, of vitamin K to newborns. Many scientists believe that this injection could very well be linked with phenol, a carcinogenic substance used in preparing synthetic vitamin K. The newborn is able to detoxify this substance when receiving it orally, but not when it is injected. While the drawback to oral vitamin K is that it requires repeated doses—especially for breast-fed babies (since breast milk is notably deficient in this vitamin)—it appears worth the trouble.

Plant Sources

The very best source for vitamin K happens to be leafy green plants. Some obviously contain more of this important nutrient than others do. With one plant in particular—green tea—exceptionally high amounts of vitamin K also seem bound together with large amounts of naturally-occurring fluoride (which makes this a handy beverage for stronger gums and healthier teeth). The accompanying table lists a variety of field grasses, seaweeds, garden vegetables, and other foods with adequate to abundant amounts of both fat-soluble and water-soluble vitamin K homologues.

Plant Source	Vitamin K (mcg/per 100 grams)
Alfalfa	167
Arame	201
Asparagus	57
Pines' barley grass*	87
Beans, green	14
Beet greens	473
Broccoli	200
Cabbage	125
Carageenan	42
Coffee	38
Kelp	109
Kombu	89
Lettuce	129
Pines' Mighty Greens*	over 600
Mustard greens	591
Nori	88
Peas, green	19
Spinach	89
Tea, green	712
Turnip greens	650
Wakame	111
Watercress	57
Pines' wheat grass*	92

*Consult the Product Appendix for more information on how to obtain these products.

Surgeon Turned Chef Stops Nosebleed with Spinach Leaf

Probably only in a book like mine would you find something as incredible and different as the following true narrative I'm about to relate.

For 15 years, Alan Resnik, M.D. deftly wielded his scalpel several thousand times as an intestinal surgeon at two Philadelphia hospitals. But then, in his own words, "I couldn't stomach the job anymore," so he quit, having become a millionaire in the process. His wife Mary Ann, who herself is still an anesthesiologist, thought her hubby had taken leave of his senses at first, and briefly considered enrolling him in some serious couch therapy with a psychoanalyst she knew. But "once she tasted the gourmet meals I cooked for her and our 14-year-old son, Andrew, she changed her mind," he laughed.

After leaving his medical practice for good, Dr. Resnik became hooked on TV cooking shows, especially those airing on "The TV Food Network" (the same cable network I've appeared as a guest on several times). This induced him to enroll at the prestigious French Culinary Institute in New York. For almost half a year he learned how to operate on hearts of lettuce, suture legs of lamb, and examine chicken livers (for their palatability, of course). He graduated in March 1997 and was promptly hired as a humble preparation chef at Philly's great five-star Le Bec-Fin restaurant. "As a prominent surgeon," he recalled with some obvious nostalgia, "I was treated like a king in the operating room. But now I'm just one of the guys in the back kitchen wearing a tall, funny white hat and white apron. But I wouldn't trade this [chef work] for anything else in the world. I mean, I *love* what I'm doing now!"

While going through the demanding rigors of chef school, though, he had an occasion to replay his role as Dr. Resnik, be it ever so briefly. "One of the other guys had a nosebleed that wouldn't stop. He tried using some ice wrapped in a bar towel and sitting down with his head tilted backwards to stop it, but the blood flow continued. Realizing how serious it had become, I looked around for something else that might work. I remembered in my early years of medical school, a long time ago, that vitamin K stops hemorrhaging immediately."

Chef Resnik saw some fresh spinach leaves lying on a table where some other chefs-in-training were working. He grabbed a leaf, tore part of it off, and pounded it to a pulp with a wooden meat mallet. He then gathered up this green mass and carefully applied it inside the other man's left nostril. Within moments it seemed, *the bleeding totally ceased*!

Everyone was amazed by this, including Resnik himself. "I knew it would work, but was astonished at just how *quicky* it did!" Resnik went from making $430,000 a year to a mere $40,000, but is happy, nonetheless. "I've made my million, so why should I have to worry anymore?" he asked. "I've got the best of both worlds right now—I get to work with food and cook for the family, as well as spend more time with our son. Who could ask for more?"

Vitamin "L"
THE LACTATING NUTRIENT

One of the Merck Vitamins

The Merck Index (Rahway, NJ: Merck & Co., Inc., 1976) is world-renowned as being the most comprehensive interdisciplinary encyclopedia of chemicals, drugs, and biological substances ever published. Chemists, biochemists, pharmacists, biologists, pharmacologists, and health practitioners the world over have come to rely upon this volume for the succinct data it offers on the use, principal pharmacological action, and toxicity of many hundreds of wide-ranging compounds.

In Merck's ninth edition vitamin "L" was briefly mentioned as representing a group of factors with vitamin-like actions to them that are necessary for lactation in nursing mothers with newborn infants. Besides brewer's yeast, the following herbs are also believed to contain this vitamin L complex: angelica, anise, basil, borage, caraway, dill, fennel, hops, Iceland moss, lavender, parsley, raspberry, stinging nettle, vervain, and walnut. The best way for childbearing women to get their daily intake of vitamin "L" is from these sources.

Vitamin M

(SEE UNDER VITAMIN B COMPLEX—B-9/FOLIC ACID)

Vitamin P

THE OTHER SIDE OF ASCORBIC ACID: BIOFLAVONOIDS
AS POTENT NUTRITIONAL AGENTS

The Rest of the Vitamin C-Complex

In the very beginning of this book, I covered Vitamin B-complex and pointed out to the reader that there were some 16 members belonging to this particular vitamin group. Not all of them, of course, might still be recognized as being valid B vitamins today, but at one time or another they were. I emphasized that while individual members of the B group were sometimes necessary to take by themselves, yet the better way was to consume them all together in one high-potency B-complex supplement.

A similar comparison of sorts can be made for vitamin C. There was a time, many years ago, when scientists viewed vitamin C as one *whole* vitamin and nothing else. But then Dr. Albert Szent-Gyorgyi, a Nobel Laureate (1937, for his discovery of ascorbic acid) turned up the first evidence of other factors associated with it that clearly showed the evidence of a vitamin C *complex* rather than just one nutrient alone.

Dr. Szent-Gyorgyi used what he later called some "intuitive guesswork" to identify these other factors as flavonoids. "I felt very strongly that this substance had to be a vitamin," he stated in a 1977 interview, "so I decided to call it 'vitamin P' for want of something better." Later, in 1950, the biochemist B. L. Oser coined the term *bioflavonoid,* which expanded the classification considerably. Szent-Gyorgyi's original understanding of his newly discovered flavonoids had been limited to numerous plant pigments known as the flavonols and flavones. Eventually both words were synthesized down into just one, flavonoids. But when Oser came along, he felt there was a pressing need for a more specific term that would

define those flavonoids that exhibited biological activities of some
kind; hence was born in his fertile mind the word *bio*flavonoids.

In the same year this word came into being, the Joint
Committee on Biochemical Nomenclature of the American Society of
Biological Chemists and the American Institute of Nutrition adopted
a firm resolution recommending that Szent-Gyorgyi's "vitamin P" no
longer be used. They claimed, in effect, that "studies have failed to
substantiate these claims" of its being a vitamin. Furthermore, they
insisted that "the identity of a substance of a vitamin nature had not
been fully established" by the man. The *New York Times* even ran a
front page story describing "vitamin P" as being "perfectly useless."
However, just because American scientists pooh-poohed Szent-
Gyorgyi's claims, the same didn't necessarily hold true for many
other countries, especially those in Europe and Scandinavia, where
even today the term "vitamin P" still remains very much alive within the medical and nutritional communities.

Bioflavonoid Types

What replaced vitamin P in the U.S. was the fancier term, bioflavonoid, of which there are a great many in nature. But, as it turns
out, relatively few of them show any clinically useful activity in
human beings. Such activity, we now know, depends on whether a
particular bioflavonoid contains certain chemical constituents known
as hydroxy or methoxy groups. A hydroxy group is made up of one
atom of oxygen and one of hydrogen. On the other hand, a methoxy
group contains one atom of oxygen, one of carbon, and three of
hydrogen. Most consumers don't realize it but there are sharp differences in activity between hydroxylated (hydroxy-containing)
bioflavonoids and methoxylated (methoxy-containing) bioflavonoids.

Knowing how they differ from each other, helps us to better
appreciate what we should be taking into our bodies for specific
health needs. The most common bioflavonoids in food plants are
hydroxylated. Some of these, which are helpful in preventing
cataract formation in the eyes, are quercetin, myricetin and
kaempferol. Hydroxylated bioflavonoids also have an antioxidant
activity helpful in preserving foods.

Methoxylated bioflavonoids occur almost exclusively in citrus. In his early research, Szent-Gyorgyi and his associates isolated two, hesperidin and eriodictyol, from lemon extract. Interestingly enough, such citrus-derived bioflavonoids are more active in the body than the hydroxylated ones coming from ordinary food plants. Besides this, the citrus kinds are more resistant to degradation in the intestinal tract, which means they are more readily absorbed from the gut.

One other thing has become more apparent in recent years is that it usually takes *twice* as much of the hydroxylated bioflavonoids to do the same jobs that the methoxylated ones can do better. A case in point is the common bioflavonoid quercetin, which readily occurs in spices like cloves, dill, onion, and pepper, in medicinal herbs such as boneset, elder flowers, and hawthorn berries, and in natural beverages like black and green tea. Quercetin exhibits antibacterial properties in spite of being hydroxylated. But so does nobiletin, a methoxylated bioflavonoid that is always present in the inner white part of the peels of grapefruit, lemon, lime, oranges, and tangerines. But you have to use at least *twice* as much of the herbs, spices, and tea to get rid of a bacterial infection within or on the outside of the body, whereas just half of the same amount of citrus materials would be required to do the same task!

This is why it's important to do some *careful label reading* before you ever purchase any brand-name vitamin C product or a bioflavonoid formula of any kind. Because regular food plant bioflavonoids that are hydroxylated are cheaper to obtain, many vitamin manufacturers like to use them over the citrus or methoxylated bioflavonoids, which are more costly to extract. If the label doesn't specify citrus bioflavonoids, then *don't* buy it. (See Product Appendix, p. 381, for more information.)

Rediscovering Vitamin P

Citrus fruits are a major source of those bioflavonoids that do the body the most good, namely the methoxylated kind. Their highest concentrations are always in the inner peel or white portion, with far lesser amounts in the juices and edible parts of the fruits themselves. Below is an arrangement showing which ones appear in each of the different citrus fruits.

Citrus Fruits	*Bioflavonoids*
Citrange (cross between an inedible trifoliate orange and a sweet orange)	Rhoifolin Lonicerin Hesperidin Sinensetin Auranetin
Citron (a creamy white citrus cultivated in Mediterranean countries and Puerto Rico)	Nobiletin Naringin Rutin Citraurin Citrantin
Grapefruit	Naringin Poncirin
Kumquat (an orange-yellow fruit indigenous to China)	Rutin Quercetin Kaempferol Iosrhamnetin
Lemon	Hesperidin Eriocitrin Citropten
Lime	Limettin Diosmin Quercitrin
Mandarin orange (a small type of sweet orange indigenous to the Orient; believed to be several thousand years old and parent to all other oranges)	Tangeretin Nobiletin Hesperidin Neohesperidin Naringin Auranetin
Orange (bitter)	Neohesperidin (up to 14%) Naringin (up to 4%) Rhoifolin Lonicerin Hesperidin

Orange (Sweet)	Neohesperidin
	Hesperidin
	Naringin
	Tangeretin
	Auranetin
	Nobiletin
Pomelo	Naringin
(believed to be the	Poncirin
progenitor of the	Marmin
grapefruit; native	Osthol
to and long a popular	Limettin
fruit in India and	Citroptene
other parts of Asia)	Bergapten
Satsumelo	Rutin (up to 3% in unripe fruit)
(a hardy hybrid	Tangeretin
of grapefruit and	Naringin
tangerine)	Poncirin
Tangelo	Tangeretin
(a cross between a	Naringin
tangerine and a	Poncirin
grapefruit)	Auranetin
Tangerine	Tangeretin
(a variety of mandarin	Nobiletin
orange with a deep	Neohesperidin
reddish-orange peel)	Hesperidin

Preferably these methoxylated components of the vitamin C complex group should be obtained from the aforementioned *fresh* citrus fruits instead of in tablet or capsule form. But because the inside white portion of the peel usually holds a slightly unpleasant taste, it is best to consume it another way.

I'm indebted to Lillian Grant, who in mid-1981 shared with others her own clever rendition of what she referred to as "my Sassy Super Citrus Bio-Applesauce." To make this terrific-tasting and very nutritious food, lightly peel two types of citrus fruit—always one sweet and the other with a slightly bitter taste. She emphasized that the peeling should be done with great care so as to retain as much of the white pulp as possible without its adhering to the discarded skins. Cut the fruits into small pieces and put into a food blender, along with a chopped apple and small cut pieces of one ripe papaya. Next add 1/2 cup of vanilla yogurt, put on the lid, and blend everything into a sauce for about 1 1/2 minutes. Then remove the lid and add a tablespoon of liquid lecithin and a little honey for taste. Replace the container cover and run the unit again for an additional minute. The "Sassy Super Citrus Bio-Applesauce" is then ready and can be eaten out of a dish with a spoon or slurped through a straw from a large glass or paper cup, as you would do with a milkshake.

Lillian told me then: "Doing this a couple of times every week will give the body more than enough of the citrus bioflavonoids it requires for optimal health." She claimed it took her a few years of "some kitchen experimentation" to finally figure out a way to make it in "a tasty form that a person won't mind eating or drinking."

While the two citrus ingredients may change with every batch made, the apple and papaya remain the same. Lillian felt that the inclusion of some hydroxylated bioflavonoids helped to balance out the large amount of methoxylated kinds found in the citrus fruits used.

Bioflavonoid Contributions to Good Health

Before giving a rundown on some of the more important bioflavonoids (hydroxy- and methoxy-containing types), it may be helpful at this point to mention in passing some of the health contributions generated by them within the human body.

Reduce Heart Disease Risk. Two foreign studies of late confirm that vitamin P factors can reduce a person's risk of developing heart disease later in life. Bioflavonoids in general seem to protect "bad" (low-density lipoproteins or LDL) cholesterol particles from oxidation (this is a chemical process that makes cholesterol's effect more deadly on blood vessel walls). Vitamin P helps reduce the tendency of blood platelets to clot. Likewise, it strengthens arteries and capillaries in the heart; this, in turn, helps avert the disease process.

Protect Against Cataract Development. Body enzyme systems occasionally go awry. One example may be seen in the activity of aldose reductase, an enzyme involved in the formation of cataracts in diabetics and in those with the metabolic disorder galactosemia.

Some years ago researchers working out of the National Eye Institute's Laboratory of Vision Research in Bethesda, Maryland tested bioflavonoids on partially purified rat lens aldose reductase. They also tested them on intact rat lenses, culturing the lenses in a medium rich in cataract-producing sugar. In both tests, they discovered the bioflavonoids to be exceptionally potent inhibitors of the enzyme, capable of as much as 80 percent inactivation of the enzyme. This phenomenal action was evidenced even in the lenses that should have been highly cataract-prone because of the culture medium. In an old issue of *Science* journal (188:1215) they suggested that bioflavonoids could be very "useful in preventing the onset of diabetic or galactosemia cataracts."

Better Stress Management. Scientists know that a certain amount of vitamin C is always stored in the adrenal cortex for immediate use when stress activity within the system rises. But ascorbic acid isn't alone there since its many accompanying bioflavonoids are added to this reserve as well. Without a full and active complement of the *entire* vitamin C complex, the adrenal cortex is less able to cope with stress.

Avert Capillary Bleeding. Bioflavonoids protect blood vessels against fragility and permeability (leakage). They increase the strength of tiny capillaries. When this happens, easy bruising, surface blood vessel damage, varicose veins, and bleeding gums are averted for the most part.

People who bruise easily or have pinpoint-size red blotches under the skin, those subject to periodic nosebleeds, women experiencing heavy menstrual bleeding or recurrent miscarriages, and individuals afflicted with hemorrhoids will all benefit from ample citrus bioflavonoids like rutin and hesperidin.

Curb Heart Attacks and Strokes. The May 1997 issue of *Harvard Men's Health Watch,* a monthly newsletter published by Harvard Medical School, included highlights of several medical reports that are part of a growing body of evidence that shows the value of bioflavonoids in helping to curb the risk of heart attacks and strokes in men. The article opened by noting that "eating apples and other foods high in bioflavonoids may indeed reduce a man's risk of heart attack and stroke."

The following four recent studies were then cited as evidence for this:

- A 1993 report mentioned 805 men between 65 and 84 years of age being examined for their intake of bioflavonoid foods. Those who ate the most enjoyed the lowest incidence of coronary artery disease, as well as having a 58 percent lower risk of cardiac death than those consuming only minimal amounts of bioflavonoids.

- An investigation printed in 1995 reviewed the link between bioflavonoids and heart disease in 16 different population groups of middle-aged men in seven nations. Where bioflavonoid intakes were high, coronary artery disease was extremely low.

- Two separately published studies in 1996 followed the health benefits of bioflavonoids in some 5,500 people. The first investigation tracked the effects of dietary vitamin P in 2,748 men and 2,385 women for 26 years. People of both genders who consumed the most bioflavonoids invariably had the fewest heart attacks and deaths from heart disease. In men especially, a high intake of dietary vitamin P correlated with a 22 percent reduction in mortality rate. The other study involved 552 male participants only, who entered the 15-year-long evaluation program when they were between 50 and 69 years of age. Results were astonishing to medical investigators: Men with a high intake of bioflavonoids had a 73 percent lower risk of stroke and heart attack!

The Harvard Medical School newsletter article concluded by naming those vitamin-P-rich foods that best corresponded to each type of health problem. The simple table below helps to illustrate this better.

Heart Attacks/Heart Disease	Strokes
Apples	Tea
Onions	Onions
Tea	

Interestingly enough, the hydroxylated bioflavonoid, quercetin, emerged as the primary winner of particular potency for these problems. Missing from these reports, however, was red wine, the fermented beverage responsible for the so-called "French paradox."

Medical investigators became attracted to red wine after discovering that the French, who love to indulge in foods rich in fats and sugars, still somehow manage to have one of the world's *lowest* rates of heart disease, heart attacks, and strokes.

Help for Varicose Veins. Varicose veins afflict about 25 percent of the populations of industrialized nations; the ratio of women over men suffering from this disorder usually runs around 5 to 1. Those who are middle-aged or older are most often at highest risk for developing this disease of the venous system.

Varicose veins are twisted, swollen veins near the surface of the skin. Vein varicosity usually occurs when weak or defective valves distributed along the walls of the veins permit blood to flow backward instead of in a normal forward pattern; the accumulation of stagnate blood within a vein can also make this happen. Sometimes chronic obstruction of the veins may produce varicosity. Varicose veins generally appear in the legs, though they also occur within the anus, where they're known as hemorrhoids.

Typical symptoms include the usual enlarged, swollen, knotted clusters of purple veins. Sometimes swelling in the legs due to fluid accumulation in muscle tissue takes place. There may also be an aching or a sensation of heaviness in the legs. Sometimes the skin may itch directly over the affected veins. In more advanced cases, skin discoloration and ulcers on the inner aspect of the ankles may occur. Periodic fatigue isn't unusual. Symptoms in women always seem to be worse during their menstrual periods.

For several decades now, a number of German doctors have routinely treated tens of thousands of cases of varicose veins with herbs rich in bioflavonoids. One of those who helped to pioneer this beneficial therapy was the late Rudolf Fritz Weiss, M.D. His medical training was highly unusual: He studied medicine *and botany* together at the University of Berlin and began his practice of internal medicine in 1922. In 1961 he retired from clinical practice and focused his efforts entirely on bringing folk herbal remedies into a more scientific and medical setting.

Two of his more notable accomplishments in this direction were the founding of a still-published medical journal, *Zeitschrift für Phytoherapie* and a wonderful medical text, *Lehrbuch der*

Phytotherapie (Stuttgart: Hippokrates Verlag GmbH, 1974). For the more severe cases, Dr. Weiss preferred using intravenous injections of certain herbal extract preparations. But he wasn't hesitant to recommend these same items used in tea or capsule form for less serious cases. The herbs he utilized are all rich in vitamin P factors and help to, as he put it, "tone up the vascular walls" of each vein so as to reduce most of the varicosity.

His three favorite herbs for treatment of venous system diseases like varicose veins were horse chestnut (not to be confused with edible sweet chestnut), yellow sweet clover, and (in the closing years of his medical practice) ginkgo biloba. I've summarized what he wrote about each of their uses in the following table.

Phytotherapie für Krampfadern [Plant Therapy for Varicose Veins]

Aesculus hippocastanum. In his excellent medical reference work, *Lehrbuch der Phytotherapie,* Dr. Weiss made clear that the chestnut he had in mind was the *in*edible kind and *not* the sweet chestnuts people commonly roast at Christmastime. But he did advise that once the shiny, brown seeds were removed from their prickly, green, globular capsules, they should be placed in a pan and roasted in the oven for about 45 minutes in order to *remove their toxicity.* Once this has been done, then they are safe to make a tea from.

Boil 1/2 pint of water. Add to it 2 level teaspoons of powder, obtained by crushing some of the roasted seeds. This can be done in a mortar with a stone pestle or by putting the seeds between two layers of waxed paper and rolling them with a rolling pin or hitting them with a wooden mallet. Stir well with a spoon, cover with a lid, and set aside to steep for 20 minutes. Strain and drink 1/2 cup on an empty stomach twice daily, in the morning and evening. *Caution:* Due to the potent nature of horse chestnut seeds, this therapy should be conducted intermittently rather than regularly, with occasional breaks in between of a week or more.

Horse chestnuts, Dr. Weiss noted, are rich in two important bioflavonoids: aesculin and aescin. These are what help to "tone up vascular walls."

*Melilotus officinalis.*Yellow sweet clover is widely distributed throughout Europe, Weiss observed, "though not native to Britain." It is also common to North America, except in the far northern states and provinces of the U. S. and Canada. The flowering yellow herb yields "a pleasant, sweetish, honey-like scent," which bees find irresistible. Honey made from such blossoms has a very delightful taste and aroma to it.

Boil 1 pint of water. Lay a clean, white cotton handkerchief (or cloth of similar size) on a flat surface. In the center, place 1-1/2 tablespoons of dried plant parts. Then draw the ends together and tie with string or thread. Set in the boiling water very briefly, no more than 2 minutes, and cover with a lid. Then set the pot aside and let its contents steep for 10 more minutes with the lid intact.

Remove the cloth bag, squeeze out excess liquid, and apply the cloth bag directly over the varicose vein site. Cover with a *dry* hand-towel or wash cloth to retain the heat as long as possible. Afterward, you can discard the bag and drink one cup of the warm tea on an empty stomach. *Caution:* Don't overdo a good thing! Give the system periodic rests from this tea at various intervals: two weeks on, one week off.

Ginkgo biloba. This tree has been around for a couple of hundred *million* years, or since the time dinosaurs roamed the earth. They disappeared, but the ginkgo remained. Considerable research on the leaves of this highly important deciduous conifer has been conducted by numerous medical investigators throughout Europe, especially in France and Germany. Dr. Weiss developed several methods of application for it in the treatment of varicose veins.

Tea	Fluid Extract	Capsules
2 tbsps. leaves in 1 1/2 pints hot water. Cover and steep for 20 mins. Drink 1 cup on empty stomach twice daily. Soak a	Combine 2 tsps. powdered leaves with 1 pint of vodka, rum, gin, or brandy. Shake every day, in the a.m. and p.m. Let set in a cool, dark place for 12 days. Remove powder by straining	Place some powdered leaves in a small saucer. Separate the two halves of a gelatin capsule (00 size) and

clean wash cloth in some of the hot tea and apply directly over varicose veins.

through layered cheesecloth or coffee filter. Store in amber glass bottles with tight-fitting lids away from heat or light. Use as needed. Take 1 teaspoonful every morning before breakfast and again at night before retiring.

slide only one of them through the powder, scooping powder into the capsule. Fit the two halves of the capsule together by sliding the empty one over the filled one. Take 3 capsules A.M. and P.M. with 8 oz. water.

The Vitamin C-Complex: Key Bioflavonoids

At present count, there are an estimated 5,000 bioflavonoids, which belong to a more diverse group of chemical compounds known as polyphenols. They are present in just about all plants in the pigments that give food plants and herbs their notable colors. Colored fruits and vegetables are particularly high in bioflavonoids, especially those that are emerald green, golden yellow, vivid orange, brilliant red, or royal purple.

Of this vast number, however, a mere handful or few hundred are believed to possess biological characteristics that may be useful to the human body in various ways. In citrus species alone, well over 70 different methoxylated bioflavonoids are known to reside, yet just a few are known to have therapeutic significance. The same holds true with the more common, hydroxylated kind so abundant in nature.

I've drawn from this large pool of compounds what I believe to be the most useful bioflavonoids, and have listed them in alphabetical order with brief explanations of what they can do for us and the plant food and herb sources that they're most readily available in. I'm firmly convinced that the very best way to obtain the majority of them is by consuming the plants they appear in. The only notable exceptions to this would be the supplementary use of rutin (50 mg.), hesperidin (100 mg.), and quercetin (25 mg.) or any of these together with citrus bioflavonoids in a mixed formula product (400 mg.) of some kind. (See Product Appendix p. 381, for more information.)

Bioflavonoids	*Biological Activities*	*Plant Sources*
Apigenin	Temporarily stops cells partway through the dividing process, which helps prevent cancer by giving cells a chance to fix genetic errors that creep in when their DNA is copied.	Apple Chamomile Milk thistle Onion Oregano Passion flower Rosemary
Betanin	Prevents cell mutations along similar lines that apigenin does; has been used by Hungarian doctors to treat many forms of cancer.	Red beet Purple eggplant Dark bell pepper Red and purple grapes
Biochanin A	Lowers serum cholesterol by decreasing intestinal absorption of it and binding it to neutral steroids and bile acids in fecal matter for later excretion.	Alfalfa Bengal gram chickpea Red clover Sweet vernal grass Timothy grass Wheat grass Woodruff Yellow sweet clover
Delphinidin	In company with vitamin E tocopherols, improves the mental and physical performance of *early*-stage Alzheimer's and Parkinson's disease patients, as well as delaying by several months severe dementia; also makes blood platelets less sticky so they don't form into clots as easily.	Blueberries Bordeaux wine Purple grape juice Red currants
Diosmin	Increases vascular tone of capillaries and promotes better circulation even more strongly than rutin does; manifests antimicrobial	Bergamot oil Hyssop (3-6%) Lemon oil Lemon petitgrain oil Rosemary

	(bacteria and fungi) properties.	Spearmint
Ellagic acid	Scavenges carcinogenic chemicals from tobacco smoke, auto exhaust, and food nitrosamines by competing for the same DNA receptors that are also used by these carcinogens; also produces sedation and prevents death from electrical shock in lab mice.	Almonds Black currant Black walnut Brazil nut Geranium Grape Oak bark Purple eggplant Radish *Raspberry (highest content) Red apple peel Red cabbage Red cherry Red currant Strawberry
Hesperidin	Exhibits strong antiviral activities against herpes simplex and influenza viruses; manifests antibacterial properties against the common cold; reduces serum cholesterol and triglyceride levels; and repairs capillary fragility.	Citrus fruits Hyssop (5-6%)
Hyperin	An MAO inhibitor and, therefore, good for mild depression or nervous disorders; halts infection by interfering with virus assembly at the cell membrane; concentrated in body near skin surface, too, for cell regeneration of damaged tissue.	St. Johnswort
Kaempferol	Has increased bile secretion in experimental animals; and exhibited unusual antimicrobial properties	Arnica Asparagus Boneset Cloves

	in vitro against *Staphylococcus aureus, E. coli,* and *Candida albicans.*	Dill Elder flowers Hydrangea Passion flower Pepper Podophyllum Senna Witch hazel
Lycopene	At the March 1997 annual meeting of the American Assoc. for Cancer Research, it was reported that people with the lowest lycopene levels had three times the risk of cancer as those with high level intake; it was even worse for blacks: those with the lowest lycopene levels had eight times the cancer risk of those with the highest levels of consumption.	Calendula/marigold Dandelion flower Sunflower Tomato and most tomato-based products (gazpacho, salsa, soup, spaghetti sauce, etc.)
Nobiletin	Prevents red cell aggregation and platelet aggregation better than anticoagulant drugs like heparin; reduces platelet adhesiveness as well as aspirin does.	Bitter orange Grapefruit Mandarin orange Sweet orange Tangerine
Nordihydroguaiaretic acid	Strong antigrowth activity brought on by inhibiting energy and nutrition transfers to and withholding critical enzyme functions within mutating cancer cells.	Chaparral (a desert shrub common to the American West and Southwest)
Podophyllotoxin deoxypodophyllotoxin	Extremely cytotoxic to tumor cells; antiviral activity against chickenpox, measles, and herpes simplex I; frequently used in Europe for treatment of testicular	Podophyllum (also known as mayapple or American mandrake)

cancer, lung cancer, leukemia, psoriasis and rheumatoid arthritis.

Quercetin	Strongly antiinflammatory; achieves this by inhibiting IgE mediated allergic mediator release from mast cells or, in simpler language, acts as an antihistamine would; also exhibits strong "blocking" action in the further production of pro-inflammatory compounds like prostaglandins and leukotrienes; and scavenges free radicals to protect against possible cell damage; also profoundly antibacterial (destroys the organism, *Clostridium botulinum,* that causes food poisoning); modifies liver transformation of cooked food mutagens to bacterial genotoxins that could lead to some forms of cancer; inactivates herpes virus; prevents dental caries.	Black walnut bark Black walnut hull Boneset Cloves Dill Elder flowers Fenugreek seed Hawthorn berry Hydrangea Juniper berry Mayapple/podophyllum Nuts Oak bark Onion Pepper Root vegetables Tea (black/green)
Quercitrin	Demonstrates capillary-strengthening activity in various small circulatory diseases; eliminates influenza type A viral infection; increases bile secretions; expedites detoxifying function of the liver; and manifests antiinflammatory activity; prevents cataract formation in diabetic animal models; has beneficial effects on hyperthyroidism.	Bilberry Epimedium/xian ling pi Eucalyptus Hops Immortelle/immortal/ everlasting Oatmeal Rye Tea (green) White oak bark Wintergreen
Rhamnazin	Exerts a mild sedative	Lemon balm/balm

action on the CNS (central
nervous system) in cases of
insomnia; its sedative
activity also plays a vital
role in treating nervous
stomach disorders and excited
hearts; relaxes muscle
spasms and nerve pains
frequently associated with
neuralgia and migraines.

Rutin	Acts mainly on the inner vascular walls of blood vessels by decreasing their capillary fragility by inhibiting production of hyaluronidase in the body; also displays a calming effect upon the heart, nerves, and brain.	Boneset Buckwheat (up to 3%) Calendula Chamomile Chaparral Elder flowers (up to 1.9%) Eucalyptus Fennel Hawthorn Hops Hydrangea Juniper berry Lemon Mandarin orange Onion Orange Passion flower Rhubarb Rue (up to 9%) Tea (up to 4%) Tobacco
Secoisolariciresinol diglycoside	This lignan precursor and vitamin P component was found to have strong antitumor effect when fed to rats at the early stage of tumor growth; its estrogen-blocking and enzyme-inhibiting actions are mostly responsible for decreasing cancer development.	Flaxseed Flaxseed oil
Silymarin	Protects the liver against	Milk thistle seed

damage from infectious
hepatitis and toxic chemicals;
hinders uptake of toxins by
liver enzyme system and
effectively blocks their
potential binding sites;
accelerates liver regeneration
through cell development.

Tangeretin	Its notable fragrance demonstrated significant immunological enhancement and psychoneurological benefit in 20 depressed male patients, aged 26 to 53, who were institutionalized in the psychiatric ward of a large university hospital in Tsu, Japan.	Mandarin orange Orange Tangerine

References:

BOOKS

James A. Duke, *CRC Handbook of Medicinal Herbs* (Boca Raton, FL: GRC Press, Inc., 1985)

Hans Flück, *Unsere Heilpflanzen* (Thun, Switzerland: Ott Verlag, 1971)

Albert Y. Leung and Steven Foster, *Encyclopedia of Common Natural Ingredients Used in Food, Drugs, and Cosmetics*, 2nd edition (New York: John Wiley & Sons, Inc., 1996)

Paul Schauenberg and Ferdinand Paris, *Le Guide des Plantes Mèdicinales* (Paris: Delachaux & Niestle S. A. Neuchatel, 1974)

Rudolf Fritz Weiss, M.D., *Lehrbuch der Phytotherapie* (Stuttgart: Hippokrates Verlag GmbH, 1985)

JOURNALS

Alternative Therapies in Health and Medicine (Vols. 1-3, 1995-1997)

Journal of Herbs, Spices & Medicinal Plants (Vols. 1-5, 1992-1997)

Renaissance of the Bioflavonoids

In the beginning of this section, I mentioned that in 1950 a group of orthodox scientists effectively quashed the matter of bioflavonoids gaining any legitimacy for a vitamin P status. Then, in 1968, the Food and Drug Administration (FDA) withdrew the rights of pharmaceutical companies to distribute and doctors to prescribe bioflavonoid preparations. In effect, the FDA declared that these were utterly worthless and totally ineffective in people "for any condition" whatsoever.

However, this didn't stop consumers from purchasing bioflavonoid products at their favorite health food stores or nutrition centers. Consumers mainly took them because of scientific evidence indicating that these vitamin P factors help to sustain ascorbic acid's own antioxidant activity within the system. Moreover, it was later determined that vitamin C is able to protect at least one of these bioflavonoids from oxidation, namely quercetin. Recent research is showing more of a "hand-and-glove" relationship between the bioflavonoids and vitamin C in much the same way that all of the B vitamins are interrelated. Hence, there is now a pretty strong case to be made for a vitamin C-complex, just as there has been for many years for the vitamin B-complex.

Beginning in the early 1980s, the popularity and acceptance of the bioflavonoids by consumers *and* scientists alike really took off in a big way. Consider this excerpt, for example, taken from an abstract of a review article in a 1984 edition of the journal *Trends in Pharmacological Sciences:* "Naturally occurring [bio]flavonoids have potent anti-allergy, anti-inflammatory, and anti-viral activity. Since they are common dietary constituents the question arises: are they natural biological response modifiers?" Given the rather bizarre history of vitamin P, this about-face statement from the scientific community really shouldn't surprise us all that much. In spite of the opposition against them for many years, there were still some scientists dedicated enough and willing to spend their research time and dollars to continue investigating the bioflavonoids. It was the gradual outpouring of their *combined* findings presented to consumers by an eager media that finally resulted in their gaining their much-deserved and prominent place in modern medicine and nutrition.

Vitamin "T"

THE STRANGE GROWTH VITAMIN THAT ONLY CHINESE DOCTORS AND HOMEOPATHIC PHYSICIANS COULD APPRECIATE

This Merck Vitamin Originates from Rather Murky Sources

I include this particular nutrient, which—believe it or not—*does* have some official status as a vitamin—at least, so far as the prestigious *Merck Index* (9th edition) goes. As was mentioned earlier under Vitamin "L," this voluminous work on chemicals and drugs, faithfully published since 1889 by the Merck Pharmaceutical Co., makes brief references to several very obscure nutrients, which by broad definition actually qualify for vitamin status in certain ways.

But before you get all fired up about this particular nutrient, you'd better read on a little more. First, the good news: It is a complex of growth-promoting substances that will probably come as welcome news to little people or size-challenged folks. Now for the *really* bad news: It is obtainable *only* from *termites, cockroaches,* and *earwigs!* A small fact that may bring a measure of relief to disgusted minds and upset stomachs is that tiny amounts of vitamin "T" can also be obtained from various unspecified yeasts and fungi that fall in the mildew category.

Homeopathic Possibilities

Not everyone would shy away from these vitamin-"T"-rich "creepy crawlies." In fact, I sincerely believe that Oriental doctors and European homeopaths might find them intriguing enough to investigate for their medical possibilities! Think I'm joking? Let me briefly introduce you to "The *Far* Side" of Chinese and homeopathic materia medica. While everything in both is definitely from *natural* sources, not everything therein is—how shall I say it?—normal and conventional.

Let's start with Chinese medicine. I went to mainland China in 1980 with a small group of medical students and a few doctors; our trip was arranged under the auspices of the American Medical Students' Association. We spent a couple of weeks there getting a real eyeful of the more hidden intricacies behind Chinese medicine. To this day, I still remember the donkey-hide gelatin, rich in many amino acids, being dutifully administered to expectant women who had previously miscarried. But as goofy as the remedy sounds, the irony of it all is that this *ejiao* stuff really works to prevent further spontaneous abortions. I'll spare the reader the agony of having to read about *rat spit* being dropped into the eyeballs of patients immediately following surgery for cataract removal in order to help heal the eye lenses more quickly.

One of my medical colleagues from the Shanghai Second Medical College in Shanghai, China sent me a book that he helped to edit (along with nine colleagues). His name is Dr. Shun Qingsheng and the gift was a beautiful, coffee-table edition of *Colour Atlas of Chinese Traditional Drugs* (volume I), published by Science Press in Beijing in 1987.

As I carefully perused its pages, I became somewhat enamored with item #58 that I found on page 110. There in vivid colors were three close-up, in-your-face snapshots of live *scorpions*! Here such horrible little creatures would be considered part of Frankensteinian medicine; but in China, it's really no big deal. You see, the Chinese use *quanxie* all the time for treatment of nervous tics, convulsions in kids, facial paralysis, muscle spasms, and tetany. What makes this weird and wacky drug work so well is its richness in lecithin, certain essential fatty acids, and cholesterol, all of which are important to healthy nerves and muscles! Many pages later the drug preparations became less extreme, as in the case of sea horse or *haima* on pages 228-229 for male sexual impotency and impaired kidney/bladder/prostate functions.

Join me now as we pay a visit to the homeopathic doctors of London, England. One of their members even treats Queen Elizabeth! It has always been said of the British that they are properly refined and highly cultured. That may be true of their social behavior, but not necessarily of their materia medica. I had open before me as I typed these words a rather handsome and very definitive work entitled *The Complete Guide to Homeopathy* (London:

Dorling Kindersley Ltd., 1995) by Drs. Andrew Lockie and Nicola Geddes.

On page 106, I discovered a full treatise on the several benefits to be expected from Tarentula, a standard homeopathic remedy for "edginess, restless legs syndrome, face twitching, and sensitive genitalia in women." Featured smack dab in the very center of the page was a six-inch-long by four-inch-wide actual size color photo of a *wolf spider!* This is a mild remedy, though, when compared with Aranea Diad. on page 117 or Lactrodectus Mac. on pages 132-133. They are, respectively, the papal cross and black widow, both *deadly* spiders! The first is used for severe facial neuralgia and the second to treat heart attacks and angina.

Of course, it's a tossup between these poisonous arachnids and *extremely* venomous snakes: yellow pit viper or fer de lance (page 120) for treating paralytic stroke, thrombosis, and hemorrhaging; rattlesnake (page 126) for right-brain strokes, cancer, and severe heart problems; coral snake (page 128) for heavy nosebleeds and profuse uterine hemorrhaging as well as strokes; and, last but not least, king cobra for intense angina pains and chronic asthma.

And you thought vitamin "T" from wood ants, roaches, and ear bugs was bad! *Tens* of millions of people in China and elsewhere throughout the Orient, as well as millions of others in Europe, India, Mexico, and the Philippines, where homeopathy thrives, let their respective doctors administer such nauseating and noxious nostrums to them on a regular basis when they're sick, without the least bit of objection. That's probably why this queer growth vitamin that was originally obtained from termites would find better appeal with Oriental and homeopathic health care providers than it would with American doctors. Aspirin anyone?

Vitamin "U"
THE ANTI-ULCER ANTIDOTE

Merck Supports Its Vitamin Status

It seems fitting to close out the biggest section in this book with
another of the *Merck Index*-sanctioned vitamins. This one, of
course, has been around quite awhile and is appropriately called
vitamin U. Serious medical research on it has been reported in
California Medicine (77:248-52, 1952) by Dr. G. Cheney, and by
Szabo and Vargha in the German medical periodical *Arzneimittel-
Forschung* (10:23, 1960). *Merck Index* lists as the vitamin's "THER-
AP[EUTIC] CAT[EGORY]: Treatment of gastric disorders."

A Great Greek Discovery

I recently interviewed Peter George Cordas, who turned 91 in 1997.
He is a retired shepherd, miner, and businessman. This small, port-
ly man with a face that has almost as many cracks as the parched
desert floor of Death Valley told me just how bad it was for Greek
immigrants like himself who came to the Beehive State in 1917 to
work in the copper mines at Bingham, located on the extreme west
end of the Salt Lake Valley.

"There were no women around in those times," he recalled
with some obvious pain to his expression. "And the job was so bad,
so dangerous, only Greeks, Mexicans, and Japanese would work in
the mines. Others didn't want the job. There were times they killed
two or three people in twenty-four hours because there was no protection. The banks were 145 feet high; and when the steam shovels
loaded the dirt, rocks came tumbling down on men working at the
bottom—just knocked them plumb down. If you got killed, the
mine carpenter built a box in a hurry, put your corpse in, and
hauled you down to Bingham cemetery, and threw you in the lot.
That's all there was to it. No one mourned anybody's passing in
those days!

"They didn't pay nothing to nobody back then. There were no unions like now. There was only a company-run carpenters' union, which spied for the mines—told the bosses what working people thought about their jobs. So the working man didn't have *nothing*. And if you didn't like it, there were always 300 or 400 other men outside just itching to get your job, and hoping you'd get riled enough to quit. That's where you were. It was rough in them days. Life was very cheap!"

Because of such mistreatment at the hands of greedy mine owners and their tyrannical foremen, young men like Peter, who started working in the copper mines while he was still a teenager, eventually developed bad cases of stomach ulcers. By the time he was in his early twenties, this Greek youth had his own digestive problems to contend with. "It was all that damned worrying I did," he muttered softly." "Always worrying whether I'd get my skull bashed in from some big rock falling down on me from above. This and just trying to stay alive gave me ulcers good."

But Peter was one of the lucky ones who managed to find a remedy for his problems. "An old German miner I knew there took me to his home once, and his wife dished me up a big helping of her homemade sauerkraut. I must have been very hungry then," he said with a laugh, "because I can still remember shoveling it all down in a hurry. The man's wife looked at me in astonishment and chuckled aloud, 'Du *frisst* wie ein Vieh!' Her husband, who was sitting nearby, slapped his thigh and roared with laughter after she said this to me." (The more correct verb for *eating* in German is *essen*, which applies only to human beings. But the other word she used, *fressen*, only applies to the way in which animals eat. Hence, she was telling him that he ate like a beast!)

George continued his narrative: "The next day when I went back to the mine again, I noticed that my stomach no longer bothered me as it usually did. There was no evidence of pain like before. It wasn't until the following morning that my ulcer symptoms returned in full force." George quickly made the connection between the sauerkraut and his stomach feeling better.

He made special arrangements with the German woman to buy some of her sauerkraut every week. He would eat small portions of it every morning before going to work. He found that when he did this, his stomach no longer bothered him. After a few months of this daily regimen, his ulcer disappeared for good. "Look at me now," he declared with some pride, "I'm gonna be 91 pretty soon, and I can eat just about anything I want. It's been 67 years I reckon and I've never had any more ulcers to hold me back from enjoying one of life's little pleasures—eating anything I set my mind to!"

Food Sources

The Merck Index states that "cabbage leaves and other green vegetables" are excellent sources for obtaining vitamin "U." Those "other green vegetables" include mustard greens, turnip greens, watercress, and spinach.

One herb that also holds possibilities for having vitamin "U" is black cohosh. Though intended primarily for women's health needs, a small amount (1/2 cup) of the *cool* tea a couple of times daily in between meals will help alleviate gastric distress due to ulcers.

Minerals

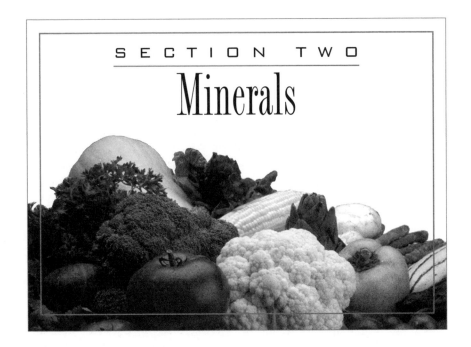

Boron

A Trace Element That Mimics Estrogen

In 1987, Forrest H. Nielsen, then director of the United States Department of Agriculture's Grand Forks Human Nutrition Research Center in North Dakota, published research to the effect that boron lessened postmenopausal women's risk of developing osteoporosis. This trace element is one of a small group considered to be *micro*minerals, in that only very tiny amounts of them are *periodically* required for the body's overall health needs. They are just the opposite of *macro*minerals, such as calcium, which the human system requires a lot of every day in order to maintain certain normal biological functions.

Dr. Nielsen's work demonstrated that boron has the uncanny ability to frequently mimic the effects of estrogen within the body.

217

A number of different estrogenic hormones, such as estradiol, are formed by the ovary and placenta in women, the testicles in men, and the adrenal cortex in both genders. Some plants, like alfalfa, black cohosh, clover, and sarsaparilla, also make them. These estrogenic hormones stimulate secondary sexual characteristics and exert systemic effects, such as growth and maturation of long bones. Synthetic versions of them are routinely used by doctors for any disorder directly attributable to estrogen deficiency or amenable to estrogen therapy.

In May 1997 I took seven boys to the Utah State Fairpark for the annual Scout-O-Rama. Some 20,000 Cub Scouts, Boy Scouts, Varsity Scouts, and Explorers gathered there for this grand two-day event. This particular Scout-O-Rama provided an amazing variety of exhibits and demonstrations. Almost 85,000 Utahns showed up to see Scouts explain such traditional Scouting topics as woodworking, beekeeping, backpacking, and knot-tying, and more exotic ones like oceanography, space exploration, and time machines. There I met a registered dietitian named Joan Flores, whose Cub Scout den had prepared an exhibit focusing on the health importance of key vitamins and minerals, including boron.

Role in Hardening Bones

A portion of the exhibit's large mineral poster was devoted to boron. A clever heading said it all: "Boron isn't boring but good for your bones!" The text mentioned that this trace element has long been used as a water softener and mouthwash. It cited a six-month study hinting at a new role for this micromineral: preventing osteoporosis. The study was said to be the first to ever examine the nutritional effects of boron in humans.

The poster text was obviously geared toward children and simply read: "Boron helped a group of older ladies lose less calcium and magnesium when they added it to their diet every day for a few weeks. The result was that their bones became harder," quite the opposite of osteoporosis. For my own benefit, Ms. Flores showed me the article from which she had adapted the text for the poster.

Chemical Marketing Reporter for November 9, 1987 told about a dozen postmenopausal women consuming a very low boron diet of 0.25 milligrams per day for 17 weeks. They were then given a daily 3 mg. supplement that represented the boron intake from a well-balanced diet. They stayed on this boron supplement for seven additional weeks.

Within a week's time the group lost 40 percent *less* calcium, one-third *less* magnesium, and about 30 percent *less* phosphorus through the urine. Their calcium and magnesium losses were lower than prestudy levels, when they were eating normally.

Ms. Flores added her own comments on the subject after I finished reading the material she had just handed me. "I've noticed that boron is vital in maintaining bone integrity. It has a remarkable effect on indicators that tell how well the body is conserving calcium or preventing bone demineralization." She told me of an article from an agricultural journal devoted to poultry raising. that made mention of boron helping chickens overcome low vitamin D levels that stunted their bone growth.

An Alternative Steroid for Body Building

In the boron research that Ms. Flores had read through, another fact kept emerging: its value in helping to build muscle mass in athletes. We discussed the role it could play in assisting body builders to gain the physical chest, arm, and thigh sizes they desired, but without having to resort to harmful drugs or synthetic steroids to do so.

The fact that one study showing a twofold increase in testosterone levels in postmenopausal women after just eight days of taking a boron supplement indicated to both of us that this was something worth exploring further in terms of athletic nutrition. We were of the decided opinion that boron might just be able to do the same thing for men's testosterone levels. However, anything beyond this, such as enhanced sexual performance, would definitely be on the scientific fringes, and something neither of us would feel comfortable endorsing.

Potential Cancer Therapy

I shared with Ms. Flores what I'd read about boron's possible role in cancer treatment in the October 1990 issue of *Scientific American*. Rolf F. Barth, M.D., a professor of pathology at Ohio State University in Columbus, and two colleagues suggested that by irradiating a non-radioactive isotope called boron 10 with low-energy neutrons (called thermal or slow neutrons), entirely new and very potent radiation therapy was possible. But unlike more conventional forms of cancer radiation that utilize protons, gamma rays, and fast neutrons and cause greater tissue damage, this boron neutron capture therapy (BNCT) would be much more *specific* and limit its destructive effects to the tumor itself.

When an atom of boron 10 captures a neutron, an unstable isotope called boron 11 is born. The boron 11 instantly fissions, yielding lithium 7 nuclei and energetic alpha particles. It takes only a very few alpha particles releasing their highly potent energy within a cancer cell to destroy it. Contrast this with the other forms of radiation which have more of a shotgun or "spread approach" and seriously damage normal tissue surrounding the tumor site.

Ms. Flores became so absorbed in what I was telling her that she almost ignored passersby stopping to read her Cub Scout pack's information posters. I mentioned another thing the article brought out. The boron-generated alpha particles don't need oxygen to enhance their biological effectiveness as the other types of radiation do. A rapidly expanding malignancy often outgrows its blood supply, so that some legions get less oxygen than normal tissues do. As a result of this oxygen depletion, the cancer can become more resistant to the effects of conventional radiation therapy. Tumor sensitivity to alpha particles is retained, though, because the particles, not requiring oxygen, can attack all parts of a tumor with equal vigor.

A third advantage of BNCT is that the lethal alpha particles it generates can kill dividing and nondividing cancer cells alike—tumors are known to have a large number of viable but inactive cells. Other forms of radiation treatment and even chemotherapy tend to work best only on the cells that are dividing.

New boron compounds are now available that show increased affinity for tumors as well as marked effectiveness in treating animal tumors. In fact, epithermal neutron beams have now been developed that permit the treatment of deep-seated tumors in such difficult to treat regions of the body as the brain, liver, and bone marrow.

I told Ms. Flores about the work of Yukata Mishima and his associates at Kobe University School of Medicine in Japan. Working with Duroc pigs, which develop human-like melanomas spontaneously, the researchers injected a boron compound around a skin-level melanoma. They followed the injection with a single exposure to thermal neutrons. Within two months the melanomas began to shrink, and eventually they disappeared.

These results soon led to clinical trials in which patients who had skin-level melanomas and who for various reasons were not candidates for surgery were treated with BNCT. A 60 to 80 percent success rate has been achieved with this highly unique boron-neutrons combination. But as with anything relatively new, it will take some time before modern medicine totally embraces it.

Food Sources for Boron

While Ms. Flores had some food sources listed on her exhibit poster for this trace element, there were others that she provided to me a few days later to make my own list in this book more complete. I've arranged them alphabetically and put asterisks next to those that yield the highest amounts of dietary boron.

Boron-Containing Foods/Herbs
(ppm=parts per million)

Alfalfa

Almond

Apple

Apricot

Avocado* (7-10 ppm)

Banana

Bladderwrack

Broccoli

Carrot

Date

Dulse

Hazelnut* (6-8 ppm)

Honey

Kelp

Oatstraw

Parsnip

Peanut

Pear

Pistachio*

Plum

Prune

Radish

Raisin

Rose hips

Soy meal* (8-11 ppm)

Turnip

Watercress

Alexander G. Schauss, Ph.D., an expert in ionic trace minerals, made the observation in his paper on all health aspects of boron that "humans eating a diet rich in foods of plant origin are able to consume between 7 and 20 milligrams of boron a day." And while American consumption of boron-rich foods is way down, European intake is quite high: "In some regions of France, the average daily intake of boron is 7 mg/day, probably owing to the high intake of fruits, vegetables, nuts, and wines in those regions."

Dr. Schauss mentioned that "dietary supplements containing boron" usually have "between 0.25 and 3.0 mg. of boron," which are levels "well within the range available by diet." (See Product Appendix, pages 382–383, for more information.)

CALCIUM
THE WONDER MINERAL THAT HELPS BUILD STRONG BONES AND TEETH AND MUCH MORE

An American Deficiency Syndrome

Believe it or not, many Americans, especially women, are getting less than the RDA (Recommended Dietary Allowance) for calcium. Ample calcium is essential for maximizing the development of peak bone mass. The mineral also reduces bone resorption in later adult life.

Nutritionists estimate that about 90 percent of the total body bone mass in females is achieved by age sixteen; 95 percent by age nineteen; and 99 percent by age 26. Unfortunately, the average American teenage girl gets a measly 300 to 600 mg. per day of calcium, when the RDG clearly states it should be between 1,200 and 1,500 mg. each day.

An irony, though, comes into play here with regard to the calcium intake of college students. Meals served to students were collected for 7 consecutive days at 50 colleges in 31 states and analyzed for various nutrients. The calcium content of the meals averaged 1,216 mg. per person per day with a range of 899 to 1,531 mg. All colleges surveyed served meals with calcium content *above* the recommended allowance for young adults.

A unique clinical test of volunteer students from each of these campuses turned up something surprising. The clinical test used to assess students' calcium status and detect deficiency was Chvostek's sign. This was accomplished by tapping the cheekbone of each student and looking for any contraction of the perioral muscles surrounding the mouth. Such contractions indicate a hyperirritability of the neuromuscular system due to calcium deficiency or, more often, a calcium-phosphorus imbalance. Students between the ages of 19 and 25 had the highest prevalence of positive Chvostek's sign: African Americans at 18.9 percent and whites at 14.8 percent. Women tested higher than men for this.

So, what's going on here anyway? If college meals average *higher* calcium content even than what the RDA suggests, then why did so many show apparent calcium deficiencies? The answer may astonish you: It was their *excessive* intake of phosphoric-acid-containing soda, hamburgers, French fries, and pizza that did it! Too much phosphorus and saturated fat in the diet drives calcium out of the system like crazy.

Body Calcium

The body contains more calcium than any other mineral around. Roughly 2 percent (0.9 to 1.4 kilograms) of the body weight of an adult is calcium, about 99 percent of which is in the bones and teeth. A newborn infant's skeleton is only partly mineralized; the calcium content is around 0.8 percent of the total body weight. Using values for the calcium content of the body at birth and adulthood and at several states of growth during childhood, values for calcium content of the body at different age levels during the formative years were estimated in the following table.

Age (Year)	Weight (Lbs)	Ca Content (oz)
1	23.4	3.5
5	41.9	7.7
10	73.4	13.9
15	121.3	28.2
20	147.8	37.7

The extent of calcium absorption varies widely among individuals; the greatest absorption always occurs in childhood when the need is greatest. Infants fed human milk were found to absorb 50 to 70 percent of the calcium ingested. On the other hand, though, adults absorb just 10 to 40 percent of the calcium in a mixed diet. As the amount in the diet increases, the percent of the intake absorbed actually *decreases*. Since calcium salts are more soluble in an acid medium, most calcium absorption takes place in the upper part of the small intestine where the contents are slightly acid following gastric digestion. The process of absorption is mostly by active transport, with a little bit taking place by passive diffusion.

Vitamin D (see the entry in the previous section) is the most important vitamin (particularly D-3 or cholecalciferol) for assisting in the absorption of calcium into the system. The antioxidant vitamins A, C, and E follow after this. Magnesium and phosphorus are the two significant minerals needed to help calcium get through the body as it should. Iron, manganese, and zinc are distant seconds in this regard.

Only small amounts (400 I.U. daily) of vitamin D from sunshine and food or herb sources is needed. The standard ratio for dietary calcium-magnesium intake has always been two parts of calcium for every part of magnesium. Under the prevailing theory that most nutritionists hold to dearly, for every 600 mg. of calcium taken a day, there should only be 300 mg. of magnesium taken. But my own work in anthropology has led me to strongly disagree with this assumption. Research into the bones and diets of early prehistoric human beings clearly demonstrates *just the reverse*—there was a 2:1 magnesium over calcium ratio in skeletal remains and consumed foods (gauged by scientifically examining human coprolites or ancient feces).This intriguing discovery some years ago prompted me to investigate the matter further by recommending 600 mg. magnesium and *only* 300 mg. calcium. In doing so, I eventually found that those who followed my suggestion had far *less* osteoporosis (brittle bones) and osteomalachia (rickets or soft bones with severe pain accompanying it). In other words, by taking *more* magnesium and *less* calcium, they were able to retain stronger bones as they became older. As I told a skeptical nutritionist once following a public lecture at a national health conference in Chicago, "It's amazing what the bones, skulls, and jaws of prehistoric peoples and their deposited feces can tell you about mineral needs a long time ago." No wonder ancient Neanderthals were a massive-framed race and strong as an ox!

Fiber interferes with the absorption of calcium, as do soft drinks, colas, coffee, and saturated fats. In a balanced study, when two adults were changed from a diet low in fiber content, with white bread at each meal, to one of high fiber content, with whole-wheat bread at each meal, negative calcium (and magnesium, zinc, and phosphorus) balances ensued. The increased loss of each mineral was by way of the feces. This loss correlated closely with increased fecal dry matter weight, which in turn was directly proportional to fecal fiber excretion, as reported in the *Journal of Nutrition* (106:403, 1976)

Calcium absorbed from the intestine is transported by the blood to all parts of the body. The normal blood calcium level of 9 to 11 milligrams per 100 milliliters is remarkably constant and maintained so by the action of the parathyroid hormone (PTH), vitamin D, and calcitonin (a hormone secreted by the thyroid gland).If the blood level falls, PTH provides more calcium by stimulating its release from storage in the bone, decreasing calcium excretion from the kidney, and, with the cooperative action of vitamin D, increasing its absorption. Calcitonin inhibits calcium release from bone and thereby lowers the blood calcium when it is higher than normal.

Bone serves as an unstable storage place for calcium. The trabeculae of spongy (cancellous) bone is the place of retention. The trabeculae are fine interlacing partitions enclosing cavities that contain marrow. At the exterior of the spongy bone is the compact bone. The unsteady stores are utilized any time that calcium may be required by the blood serum or muscle and organ tissues. Teeth, on the other hand, retain all of their calcium and don't release any of it.

The urinary excretion of calcium is relatively constant in each of us but varies widely from person to person. Calcium intake exerts a variable influence on this excretion rate. Nighttime sleep increases in a very pronounced way the urinary loss of calcium as does sitting and quietly meditating or reading; however, standing without doing anything doesn't result in a great calcium loss for some reason. It is believed by some scientists that weight-bearing on the long bones is critical in conserving body calcium.

The level of dietary protein has a notable influence on urinary calcium; increasing the protein consumed from 47 to 142 grams daily on a constant calcium intake (500 mg. or 800 mg. or 1,400 mg. daily) caused the amount of urinary calcium to just about double, in a study conducted with college-age men. In another series of clinical investigations with adults, when the protein intake was around 560 grams a day, the urinary calcium excretion was 800 percent more than when the subjects were consuming a protein-free diet, irrespective of the calcium intake (from 100 to 2,300 mg. daily), according to the *American Journal of Clinical Nutrition* (27:584, 1974). It appears that the uric acid resulting from meat consumption has a definite negative impact on calcium retention.

Calcium Content of Selected Foods and Herbs

Ordinarily, I've kept the food sources for each nutrient mentioned in this book toward the end of the entry. I've made an exception in this case, since *usable* calcium levels are so low in many Americans in spite of the inordinate amounts of *un*usable calcium consumed (such as the frequent drinking of milk or eating of cheese, ice cream, or yogurt). The following table gives an array of foods (and their assigned portions) together with their respective calcium contents. The reader is encouraged to eat as many of them as possible, with the exception of the dairy items listed (since milk and milk byproducts are poorly absorbed). *The sole exception is whey:* A milk substitute recently introduced has loads of assimilable calcium that will do the body a lot of good but *without* the allergic reactions that real milk typically produces. (See Product Appendix p. 382, for more information on this product.)

Selected Foods and Their Calcium Contents

Almonds, 1/2 cup, 160 mg

Apricots, dried, 1 cup, 100 mg

Beans (cooked, kidney, navy, etc.), 1/2 cup, 45 mg

Beef, chicken, fish, 6 oz., 30-80 mg

Blackstrap molasses, 1 tbsp., 140 mg

Bok choy, cooked, 1/2 cup, 79 mg

Bread (white, enriched), 1 slice, 24 mg

Bread (whole wheat), 1 slice, 24 mg

Broccoli (cooked), 1 cup, 140 mg

Buttermilk, low-fat, 8 oz.. 285 mg

Cabbage, 1/2 cup, 20-50 mg

Calcium-fortified cereal, 1 cup, 300 mg

Calcium-fortified orange juice, 8 oz. serving, 300 mg*

Cheese (cheddar, colby, etc.), 1 oz., 220 mg

Cheese (cottage, creamed), 1/4 cup, 34 mg

Corn tortilla, 1 medium, 60 mg

Cream, light, 1 tbsp., 14 mg

Dates, pitted, 1 cup, 100 mg

Egg (medium), one, 28 mg

Evaporated whole milk, 1 oz., 50-150 mg

Farina, enriched (instant, cooked), 1 cup, 190 mg

Figs, 10 dried, 270 mg

Green beans, cooked, 1/2 cup, 32 mg

Greens (turnip, collard, mustard), 1/2 cup, 170 mg

Ice cream, 1/2 cup, 88 mg

Kale (frozen), cooked, 1/2 cup, 78 mg

Lima beans (frozen), cooked, 1/2 cup, 17 mg

Low-fat yogurt (plain), 1 cup, 420 mg

Mackerel, 3 oz. canned, 200 mg

Milk, whole, 1 cup, 291 mg

Molasses, light, 1 tbsp, 33 mg

Nonfat milk, 1 cup, 300 mg*

Oatmeal, cooked, 1/2 cup, 11 mg

Orange, 1 medium, 60 mg*

Oysters, cooked, 3 oz., 38-76 mg

Peanut butter, 2 tbsp., 18 mg

Peas, green, canned, 1/2 cup, 22 mg

Potato, baked, 1 medium, 14 mg.

Rhubarb, 1 cup, 120 mg

Rice, 1 cup, 20-50 mg

Rutabaga, cooked, 1 cup, 72 mg

Salmon, 3 oz. canned, 165 mg

Sardines, 3 oz. canned, 372 mg

Sesame seeds, 1 tbsp., 300 mg

Shrimp, 1 cup, 80 mg

Skim milk, 1 cup, 300 mg

Soybeans (cooked), 1 cup, 130 mg

Spinach, 1 cup, 200 mg

Tofu (soybean curd), 4 oz., 150 mg*

Walnuts, 1/2 cup, 50 mg

Yogurt, 1 cup, 300 mg

*The dietary/food magazine *Eating Well* (January/February 1994; p. 88) noted that orange juice and oranges encourage higher calcium retention than cheese or even calcium-fortified milk. Along similar lines, the *Journal of Food Science* (January/February 1988) observed that the calcium in lime-treated tortillas and soybean-based tofu was 12 percent more bioavailable than calcium in non-fat milk. It appears that the ascorbic acid in oranges and limes and the fermentation involved in making tofu allow for much better calcium absorption in the small intestine. And to show just how much synergism there can be between certain fermented foods and calcium, consider this: In Vietnam, a high calcium broth is made by soaking the bones of chicken and pork in vinegar before boiling and straining the broth. Some German doctors have gone one step further by requiring their mineral-deficient patients to take adequate amounts of calcium supplement in *combination* with vitamin C *and* sauerkraut juice. What seems quite apparent from all this information is that calcium is most easily absorbed in an *acidic* environment. As people grow older, they tend to lose digestive acid enzymes.

We should also remember that certain medicinal herbs, spices, and sea weeds are high in calcium content. They are useful as a secondary backup source of calcium, and can be taken in capsule, tablet, powder, or tea forms whenever necessary.

Calcium-Rich Herbs, Spices, and Seaweeds

Acacia	Fenugreek
Alfalfa	Fo-ti
Barley grass	Ganoderma
Bladderwrack	Ginseng
Borage	Hawthorn
Chervil	Kava kava
Cleavers	Kelp
Comfrey	Parsley
Dandelion	Red clover tops
Dulse	Savory
Eucalyptus	Slippery elm bark
Eyebright	Stinging nettle
Fennel	Wheat grass

Calcium derived from huge inland bodies of glacial runoff water accumulated over aeons of time are easily assimilated and highly utilized in the body. An example of such a water body would be the Great Salt Lake, Utah's own version of Israel's Dead Sea. There are a number of products geared toward supplying the system with chelated and bioelectrically-charged (ionic) calcium (see pages 382–383 of the Product Appendix). The calcium in each of these formulas is augmented by a number of other important trace elements that provide nutritional balance to the body's present mineral reserves.

Calcium at Work for You: Bodily Functions Facilitated

An interesting thing about body calcium is that while 99 percent of the slightly over two pounds of this mineral that we carry in us is primarily located in our teeth and bones, the remaining 1 percent that floats around in our systems plays a crucial role in a myriad of physiologic events. I've arranged some of the more important bodily functions dependent on calcium in the following list with brief explanations accompanying each of them.

Aging Hearts Saved. During the month of August, 1990 the American Society for Pharmacology and Experimental Therapeutics held its annual meeting in Milwaukee, Wisconsin. Evidence was presented there by scientists studying cardiac nerves to explain why aging diminishes the heart's ability to pump harder and faster under exertion. Experiments with rats demonstrated fewer calcium "gateways" in the aging heart's sympathetic nerves. That gateway shortage diminishes the flow of calcium into those nerves, thereby impeding the transmission of signals that ordinarily would tell the heart muscle to speed and strengthen contractions as the body works harder.

As long as older hearts aren't subjected to stress, they operate just fine. But when they are put under any kind of stress, then they begin to show immediate signs of function failure. It was noted by the pharmacologist presenting this team's report that the elderly would greatly benefit from increased intake of calcium if stress of any kind becomes evident in their lives.

Blood Clot Formation. Calcium is essential to blood clotting. This process is complex, but generally occurs in three steps:

Step One: A substance called prothrombin activator is formed in response to the rupture of a blood vessel.

Step Two: The prothrombin activator catalyzes the conversion of prothrombin to thrombin.

Step Three: The thrombin acts as an enzyme to convert fibrinogen into fibrin threads that enmesh red blood cells and plasma to form the clot itself.

Calcium takes part in all of this during Step Two. Without this mineral being present there is simply no conversion of prothrombin to thrombin. Those who hemorrhage easily would do well to increase their calcium intake.

Bone Loss Averted. A few years ago I went to a local chiropractor for some simple neck and spine adjustments. While there I informed him of a slight hip pain I was then experiencing. He took x-rays of my trunk and legs before giving me some adjustments in that region of my body, which brought prompt relief. When I returned a week later, he showed me the x-rays and, at the same time, pronounced my bones as "looking really good, really healthy," with the statement afterward that "you must do a lot of walking to keep your bones so well exercised."

My purpose for recounting this little episode here is to acquaint the reader with something that very few people are aware of: While bones may appear rigid and fixed, they are actually more like muscles, capable of growing or shrinking with use. Each time a bone is moved, it bends ever so slightly, just enough to trigger electrical and biochemical changes that stimulate bone formation. The more force, the greater the bending, and the greater the stimulus for new bone formation. A normal amount of movement keeps the calcium density of bone constant, while additional bending—say, from a brisk walking routine—can cause this calcium bone mass to increase. Believe it or not, the threat of osteoporosis doesn't just come from low mineral intake. It is also primarily due to a sedentary lifestyle. Less-frequent bending translates to: "I don't need so much bone." As a result, the body reduces the storage of dietary calcium in the bones and excretes the unused excess.

The point is, if you want to avert potential bone loss later in life, then you'd better *walk a lot*, besides taking 800 mg. of calcium daily. Another thing is to stop drinking coffee and cola beverages. Caffeine is known to cause bone loss that can eventually lead to osteoporosis. Those who don't have the strength or willpower to kick their caffeine addictions should at least consider drinking a glass of milk every day or eating some of those calcium-rich foods mentioned earlier.

Building Better Bones and Healthier Teeth. Calcium, like certain other minerals, gives rigidity and permanence to our bones and teeth. Bone forms protective cavities for the heart, lungs, and brain to rest in. Although bone can withstand nearly as much weight as cast iron before breaking, it is itself amazingly light in weight.

Bone is a highly specialized type of connective tissue; it is made through two separate processes: matrix formation and mineral deposition. The chief minerals in bone are calcium and phosphorus, with smaller amounts of sodium, magnesium, and fluorine. Bone minerals exist in the form of extremely small crystal and comprise 60 to 70 percent of the weight of dry bone. Bone is continually being formed and broken down. It has been calculated that roughly 20 percent of adult bone calcium is resorbed and replaced.

Those foods highest in calcium content that were previously cited should become a frequent part of the diet. The intake of capsulated herbs or reconstituted cereal grasses is also part of this regimen. An ideal nutritional scenario for better bones would be something like this: 1 tbsp. of wheat, barley grass, or beet root powder (see Product Appendix) mixed with 8 oz. of calcium-fortified orange juice. That winning combination would deliver over 650 mg. of *usable* calcium into the system at once. Doing it often and walking every day would guarantee strong bones.

Teeth are composed of three highly calcified tissues: enamel, the outermost covering; dentin, the portion beneath the enamel and surrounding the tooth pulp; and cementum, the calcified portion covering the root of the tooth. In the center of the tooth, enclosed in these calcified tissues, is the pulp—the soft connective tissue that contains the blood vessels, lymphatics, and nerves. The pulp extends into the periodontal membrane.

Enamel, the hardest tissue in the body, is about 97 percent mineral, being comprised of calcium, phosphorus, magnesium, and carbonate. Dentin, which forms the largest portion of the tooth, is similar to bone in its composition, containing about 60 percent mineral. The chemical composition of cementum is similar to bone and dentin, but little else is known about it.

Teeth, like bones, require a certain amount of daily exercise in order to remain healthy. Your dentist may never have told you that but it's true, nevertheless. Chewing sugarless gum, a few carrot or celery sticks, or some sprigs of parsley accomplishes two things: your teeth get plenty of exercise from lots of chewing; and they get properly nourished when the vegetable matter is thoroughly masticated.

Cancer Prevention. Medical statisticians estimate that close to 70,000 Americans die annually from colorectal cancer; it is the second most common cancer appearing in men and the third leading one in women. Doctors are still pretty much at a loss to explain how this particular disease gets started in the colon and rectum. But mounting evidence appears to implicate diet, climate, and mineral deficiency.

For some time now it's been known that eating a high-fat, low-fiber diet almost surely guarantees that colon cancer will develop. The reason is believed to be that high-fat diets result in larger amounts of cholesterol and bile acids accumulating in the colon. These are converted by colonic bacteria into cancer-causing byproducts. Fiber, though, as found in whole grains, fruits, and vegetables, reduces the concentration of these by-products because it moves fecal matter, and any carcinogens it may contain, out of the intestine more rapidly. Fiber also seems to bind or inactivate carcinogens.

That's the dietary factor. Now let's examine the involvement of climate in colorectal cancer development. Epidemiologists (scientists who study disease patterns and behavior) know that people who get the least amount of sunlight (those who lived in big cities or in rural northern areas) are more susceptible to colorectal cancer. Vitamin D, the sunshine nutrient, is necessary for the complete absorption of calcium in the intestines. Without adequate amounts of sunlight, whatever calcium we ingest isn't going to be fully utilized as it should be.

This, of course, leads us right into the third reason, mineral deficiency. The calcium connection to colorectal cancer has been suspected by doctors and scientists for a couple of decades now. Colorectal cancer incidence is invariably higher than normal among those drinking soft water, which is low in calcium anyway. But people eating diets high in calcium and vitamin D always have a much lower than normal incidence of this cancer.

In a 19-year study of middle-aged white males in Chicago, the risk of developing colorectal cancer was found to be related to the amount of just two nutrients working in close harmony with each other—calcium and vitamin D—which these men got in their diets. The lower the amounts of both, the greater the incidence of this cancer. Epidemiologic studies in Norway, Denmark, Sweden, and Finland pretty much reached the same conclusion. Men who have the lowest intake of calcium are at three times greater risk of developing colorectal cancer than are those men (in the American study) who were taking in the most calcium daily. (Lowest versus highest calcium intake was gauged at 1 1/2 to 4 1/2 glasses of milk consumed daily.)

Martin Lipkin and Harold Newmark, two cancer researchers with Memorial Sloan-Kettering Cancer Center in New York City, pioneered some of the research in this important health area, which was eventually published in the mid-1980s. They studied colon cells removed by biopsy from ten people at high risk of colorectal cancer because of a positive family history. They found that the cells were dividing more rapidly than normal. But within two to three months of starting daily calcium supplementation at 1,250 mg., new biopsies showed the cells looking more like cells from people at low risk of developing such cancer. This study suggests that daily calcium intake at one and a half times the recommended daily allowance is quite useful for preventing the occurrence of this type of cancer.

Drug Metabolism. You may not realize it, but the amount of calcium you have in your system at any given time can determine the metabolic outcome of drugs, medicinal herbs, or other nutrients that you might be taking. The role of the calcium ion is central to many homeostatic processes, according to the pharmacological textbook, *The Role of Calcium in Drug Action* (New York: Pergamon Press, 1987) by Australian researcher M. Denborough. But any disturbance in the mineral concentration can cause profound metabolic effects.

Disorders of red blood cells, platelets, the heart or bones, hypertension, and asthma are all linked to this one important factor. Many drugs, some herbs, and a few vitamins and minerals can *deplete* calcium levels in the circulating blood plasma. This can lead to the problems just described. Therefore, *extra* calcium intake is highly recommended to avoid such serious breakdowns. Without adequate calcium, certain drugs, herbs, and nutrients cannot be properly metabolized as they ought to be. They would, therefore, most likely perform to less than full capacity and leave the system more quickly than anticipated.

The book underscores the need for daily calcium intake *above* 800 mg. when taking drugs, herbs, vitamins, or minerals.

Hypertension Lowered. Doctors are often prone to tell their hypertensive patients that they need medication, a low-salt diet, exercise, weight reduction, and reduction of alcohol consumption in order to control their elevated blood pressures. But recent studies have suggested that increasing calcium intake—either through mineral-rich foods or by supplementation—might just help to reduce blood pressure. Women of all ages are already being encouraged to consume more calcium to prevent fractures due to osteoporosis from occurring later in life. Now it seems that men as well as women would benefit from more calcium in their diet to control hypertension.

Gender, age, and race all play a role here: Women, the elderly, and African Americans are at greatest risk for hypertension. Some scientists believe that calcium influences the way the body responds to salt. In other words, insufficient calcium could make someone more likely to retain salt and develop high blood pressure if that individual partakes of salty food.

Hypertension has often been alluded to as the "silent disease," because many people have the problem without ever realizing it. High blood pressure can lead to heart disease, stroke, and several types of kidney disease.

So, just to be on the safe side, figure on taking a *minimum* of 600 mg. of calcium daily; most of this should come through food sources but don't rule out supplementation either, if necessary.

Intoxication Explained. It is interesting to consider that all of the ancient religious writings—scriptural, apocryphal, pseudepigraphal, and historical—that deal with matters *before* the Great Flood, never once speak of intoxication. It is only *after* this watery cataclysm that we find the first mention ever being made of someone getting drunk. Both *The Septuagint Version of the Old Testament and Apocryphia* (Genesis 9:18-27, and translated from the original Greek into English by Clondon, Samuel Bagster & Sons, 1851) and *The Works of Flavius Josephus Containing the Antiquities of the Jews* (Book, Chapter VI, Philadelphia: David McKay) tell what happened to Noah a little while after he planted a vineyard.

After gathering the ripe grapes and pressing them into juice, Noah let the liquid remain in a container as he had always done before the Flood, never once imagining the material would become subject to bacterial fermentation. For him this would become a new experience, something unknown to the destroyed Antediluvians.

He offered up a burnt animal sacrifice to God on an altar of stones and then drank what he still thought to be ordinary grape juice as part of this religious observance. However, he wasn't quite prepared for what followed next. According to both accounts, he became unintentionally "drunk, fell asleep, and lay naked in his house in an unseemly manner."

His youngest son Ham just happened to come by for a short visit and found his father in this embarrassing situation. Thinking it was funny to see a distinguished man of God in such a position, "he came laughing, and showed his brethren," Shem and Japheth, their father's unwitting circumstance. Ham hoped to incite them to the same ridicule and mockery that he was at that time heaping upon an unconscious and very naked Noah. But the other two, having far greater respect for the old man, held an article of clothing between them, "and went backwards, and covered the nakedness of their father . . . and saw not [his] nakedness . . ." After "Noah recovered from the wine and knew all that his younger son had done to him," he cursed his grandson Canaan (Ham's boy) to become a slave to all mankind.

Some 4,000 years later, we now know how the alcohol from that unexpected wine impaired Noah's brain functioning for a short period of time. According to a report published in the December 20, 1996 *Journal of Biological Chemistry,* when a person starts drinking plain alcohol, the body quickly breaks it down. Among the resulting byproducts are fatty-acid esters, believed now to be the direct agents of intoxication.

These ethyl esters speed up the movement of potassium ions, which are positively charged, from brain cells through channels in their outer membranes. This flow of ions increases the negative electric potential inside the cells, impairing the action of the voltage-dependent calcium channels.

The cells rely on calcium for responding to messages from other cells. When such alcohol esters depress calcium concentrations, communications between these cells can become uncoordinated. And when their timing is off, then typical symptoms of drunkenness are likely to occur, not to mention a breakdown in the inhibitory pathways that would normally curb slurred speech and drunken stupor. This report is the first to demonstrate such profound changes in the electrical functions of a brain cell at concentrations of alcohol that are present after people drink.

What this intriguing data suggests is that an intake of several thousand milligrams of dietary (milk or green vegetable juice) or supplemental calcium might very well *reduce* an intoxicated state far better than hot coffee would. Had Shem and Japheth known about these things, they could have persuaded their father to drink some warm animal milk. The calcium in it would have substantially *decreased* the negative electrical energy inside the affected brain cells and restored normal communication between them.

Leg Cramping Alleviated. A number of obstetricians sometimes prescribe extra calcium to pregnant women and older folks who complain of leg cramps. The dosage varies from 600 to 1,600 mg. This is usually recommended in supplement form instead of from food sources rich in this important mineral.

Muscle Contraction and Relaxation. Where would we be without the muscles continually contracting and relaxing? Quite simply, we wouldn't be able to move at all. Muscle contraction is a complicated process requiring muscle proteins, enzymes, and minerals. Scientists themselves don't even know all that goes on when muscles contract and what chemical changes take place. Actin, myosin, and troponin are the proteins in the skeletal muscle most directly involved in muscle contraction and mechanical work. The stimulus that produces muscle contraction is an electrical impulse delivered by the motor nerve to the muscle cell. It travels along the membrane of the muscle fiber. The electrical activity increases the permeability of the membranes of the sarcoplasmic reticulum to calcium ions. The ions pour into the cell cytoplasm, activating the troponin-inhibited contractile mechanism. Troponin inhibits muscle contraction by blocking the interaction of the proteins actin and myosin, unless it is combined with calcium. Following contraction, calcium is promptly evacuated and returned to the storage sacs in the sarcoplasmic reticulum, and the muscle once again eases into a temporary relaxed state.

Daily calcium intake from food and supplemental sources makes for good muscle contractions and relaxations in work and play. But sporadic intake can lead to reduced levels of this mineral, which result in poor mechanical actions due to electrical interference between motor nerves and muscle cells.

Nuclear Detoxification. When above-ground testing of nuclear devices was being done a few decades ago, considerable strontium-90 was lofted into the atmosphere as a result of the fallout from each of these mighty explosions. This is a very radioactive and extremely long-lived isotope of the element strontium. Nuclear scientists have calculated that it will probably be several more *centuries* or longer before most of these isotopes disappear from our atmosphere (assuming, of course, that no further above-ground testing is done).

Strontium and calcium are both very similar in their metabolic behavior and distribution throughout the human body. More than 95 percent of both minerals is deposited in the bones and teeth. The body preferentially absorbs calcium and preferentially excretes strontium by way of the kidney. This discrimination, however, depends on ample amounts of calcium being in the blood supply and muscle and organ tissues at all times. The mineral helps safeguard the system against the accumulation of radioactive strontium.

While I'm on the subject and since there isn't a separate strontium entry in the mineral section, it may be worthwhile to say a thing or two about the *non*radioactive form of this interesting trace element. Anthropologists like myself who've studied the skulls and bones of very early human creatures always notice how much *more* strontium they contain compared with values for the same mineral in modern men and women. The increased strontium levels help to account for greater bone density and hardness in prehistoric subjects. This isn't totally surprising considering the close affinity both minerals have for each other, and strontium's own ability to replace calcium to a limited extent.

For years I puzzled over the source of so much nonradioactive strontium in primitive peoples. I suspected it came through the diet, but wasn't quite sure if it was through consumed foods or via swallowed water drunk from the runoff of melting glaciers. Finally, the matter was pretty well settled in my mind after I read *The Analysis of Prehistoric Diets* (Orlando: Academic Press, 1985; p. 347) edited by archaeologist Robert I. Gilbert, Jr. and anthropologist James H. Mielke. They presented evidence showing that wild game, wild root vegetables, grains, and especially nuts and seeds were good sources of strontium. While the former three ranked below five parts per million (ppm) in the mean elemental concentrations of this particular trace element, nuts and seeds ranked a whopping *60 ppm*. So eating more almonds, cashews, hazel nuts, pecans, pine nuts, pistachios, and walnuts, not to mention sunflower seeds, is going to give you more than enough strontium for stronger bones and teeth.

Premenstrual Symptoms Reduced. In April 1997, 98 percent of the city of Grand Forks, North Dakota (population 50,000+) was destroyed by floodwaters spilling over the banks of a very swollen and turbulent Red River. But just a few years preceding this unhappy chaos, in the drier times of 1991, researchers at the USDA's Agricultural Research Service studied ten healthy women who experienced mild behavioral and physical symptoms the week before and during their menstrual periods. The researchers randomly assigned the women to either high (1,300 mg.) or low (600 mg.) daily doses of calcium, added to their food in liquid form. Halfway through the six-month study, the two groups switched dosages.

Nine out of the ten women reported a reduction in premenstrual mood problems—such as crying, irritability, and depression—while on the high-calcium regimen. The extra calcium also seemed to allay the physical discomforts accompanying menstruation itself. For example, seven out of the ten women reported a reduction in cramps and backaches while on the high-calcium diet.

Another study briefly reported in *Science News* for October 27,1990 (vol 148:263) mentioned that women with premenstrual syndrome (PMS) could have low blood levels of zinc. This suggests that trace amounts of zinc may help regulate key hormones like progesterone that could play a role in menstrual difficulties. It seems, then, that if calcium (1,300 mg.) and zinc (75 mg.) are taken together daily or every other day, they just might bring relief of PMS symptoms.

Buying Guide to Calcium Supplements

Guidelines issued by the National Institutes of Health some years ago indicate that adults need from 1,000 to 1,500 milligrams of calcium each day. But surveys show that they consume, on average, only about half of this. Over time, this calcium deficit is a significant risk factor for thinning bones and other metabolic disorders.

My own recommended intake of this mineral is just the opposite of what conventional nutrition has been suggesting for many years now. As stated earlier in this section, paleolithic (Stone Age) diets had a 2:1 magnesium-over-calcium ratio. The *correct* intake, therefore, based on research done by physical anthropologists like myself with ancient human remains and fecal matter (called coprolites) should be 1,200 mg. of magnesium, but only 600 mg. of calcium.

A dizzying array of calcium supplements are available to choose from. One large New York City health food emporium that I did a book-signing in recently had *42* different brands of calcium by my count. You should know right off the bat that supplemental calcium *never* comes by itself, but is always partnered with another substance. Available forms include calcium carbonate, calcium citrate, calcium phosphate, calcium lactate, and calcium gluconate.

Calcium carbonate is by far the most common form on the market today. It's found in most calcium pills, including popular antacids like Rolaids and Tums. Common sources of calcium carbonate include ground limestone or oyster shells. I don't favor either one for several very good reasons. Crushed and heated limestone is widely used for a number of industrial purposes: making porcelain and glass; in purifying sugar; in preparing laundry bleach; in softening hard water; and in mortars and cements. And so far as oyster shells go, considering just how polluted the oceans are now it is very likely to contain heavy metal and bacterial contaminants.

For older people, calcium carbonate is difficult to properly break down inside the gut for absorption. That's because many elderly people have a condition known as atrophic gastritis, which is a deficiency of stomach acid. Only when they have just eaten and the stomach has secreted acidic juices will sufficient acid be present to break down a calcium carbonate tablet.

That's why I always recommend calcium hydroxyapatite or calcium citrate instead. Both are from much safer sources in nature and easily absorbed by the body. They are found in many calcium-containing products. Readers are advised to consult the Product Appendix, pages 382–83, for more information on how to obtain any of these calcium products.

Before closing, I probably should say a thing or two about a few of the calcium medications available in homeopathy. This is a system of medicine developed several centuries ago by itinerant practitioners who believed in creating like symptoms to match those of any given disease in order to effect a cure. The following calcium-based items are a part of this distinctive but very debatable medicine:

CALC. CARB. (Calcarea Carbonica). This remedy is made from oyster shell-derived calcium carbonate and is intended for backache, joint pain, fractured bones that are slow in healing, and painful teething in very young children.

CALC. FLUOR. (Calcarea Fluorica). This is one of a dozen vital tissue salts introduced to the world by a German homeopathic doctor, Wilhelm Schussler, between 1872 and 1898. He believed that many diseases were due to mineral deficiencies, and that adequately replacing them with minute doses of mineral salts might effect a cure of some kind. This particular tissue salt is used for maintaining tissue elasticity.

CALC. PHOS. (Calcarea Phosphorica). This is another Schussler tissue salt prepared chemically from dilute phosphoric acid and calcium hydroxide. Primarily employed for bone and tooth pain, growth problems in children and adolescents, mental weariness, physical fatigue, digestive discomforts, and feelings of discontentment.

CALC. SULF. (Calcarea Sulfurica). Yet another Schussler tissue salt believed to be useful in treating open sores and flesh wounds, as well as any skin eruptions (abscesses, boils, carbuncles, cysts, or infected eczema).

For those wishing to venture into this realm of healing who want to obtain any of the above homeopathic remedies, write to: Standard Homeopathic Co., 210 W. 131 St., Los Angeles, CA 90061.

Chlorine

THE NUTRITIONAL MARRIAGE WITH SODIUM THAT MAINTAINS THE BODY'S ACID-BASE BALANCE

The Chlorine-Sodium Marriage

In spite of the adverse effects sometimes experienced from the chlorination of public water, chlorine itself is a fairly useful trace element, especially when joined in minute quantities with sodium to form sodium chloride. That's the form in which these two minerals almost always appear in human and animal bodies. The tissue of the average adult human being contains roughly 60 grams of sodium and somewhat less chlorine.

Sodium chloride has several vital functions. It helps maintain the acid-base balance of the body and is largely responsible for the total osmotic pressure of the extracellular fluids. It also facilitates the formation and free flow of saliva, gastric juices, and intestinal secretions. Although sodium can't be replaced by any other ion, it's thought that chlorine could be replaced in part by bicarbonate ions from calcium dioxide.

Man and beast alike have always craved salt, otherwise known chemically as sodium chloride. Ordinary table salt usually contains tiny amounts of calcium and magnesium chlorides, too, which absorb moisture and make it cake. Human intake of salt is typically in excess of our needs, since the food we eat contains adequate amounts to ever prevent the occurrence of any deficiency of chlorine or sodium. Salt intake can be highly variable in animals. Herbivores require salt in the diet, but carnivores do not because a sufficient amount is obtained from the flesh and blood of their prey.

Under experimental conditions it's possible to demonstrate with animal models in the laboratory that life is unable to continue with sodium and chlorine missing in the diet. But the amount is less than one would expect at first glance because when the intake of salt is at a minimum, the body makes an adjustment whereby the output of sodium and chlorine in the urine nearly ceases. The kidney is the regulatory organ which, through its secretory activity, controls the concentration of electrolytes in the blood.

Both chlorine and sodium are critical for human and animal perspiration needs. The liquid secreted by the sweat glands (glandulae sudoriferae) of humans has a distinctive salty taste and a pH that can vary from 4.5 to 7.5. Sweat produced by the eccrine sweat glands is clear with a faint characteristic odor, which is evident of chlorine. It contains water, sodium chloride, and traces of albumin, urea, and other compounds. Its composition varies with many factors, e.g., fluid intake, external temperature and humidity, and some hormonal activity. Sweat produced by the larger, deeper, apocrine sweat glands of the axillae (armpits) contains, in addition to the others, organic material which on bacterial decomposition produces an offensive odor.

Here's how these two trace elements work synergistically to evoke the sweating phenomena. Sodium does the "pushing" of waste materials from the body, while chlorine "opens" the skin pores to let them out. A similar "pushing" and "opening" action is evident in the way the kidneys work, too.

The Good and Bad Sides

A few more remarks on chlorine in particular are in order. It stimulates the production of hydrochloric acid in the gut, keeps joints and tendons agile, and assists in the distribution of hormones throughout the body. When coupled with sodium, it can serve as an electrolyte replenisher, an emetic, and a topical antiinflammatory. In veterinary medicine sodium chloride is frequently administered to animals orally as an emetic, stomachic, or laxative or to stimulate thirst for the prevention of kidney stones. When given intravenously as an isotonic solution, it helps elevate blood volume and combat dehydration. Veterinarians like to use sodium chloride to help irrigate wounds and sores and as a rectal douche in smaller animals.

The downside to chlorinated water, beside possible skin rash, is elevation of "bad" lipoproteins that carry cholesterol into the bloodstream, but without any changes in the "good," high-density lipoproteins that remove cholesterol from the blood. Additionally, excessive consumption of chlorinated water has been known to trigger liver cancers. (See *Science News,* 135:342.)

Those who swim a lot are at high risk for acid erosion of their dental enamel, according to the *American Journal of Epidemiology* (123:641-47, 1986) An epidemiologic survey of 747 swimming club members in a Charlottesville, Virginia private pool showed that over 54 percent of them had experienced some kind of dental enamel erosion in the course of time.

To help curb some of this tooth enamel erosion, a fairly regular swimmer should take daily doses of calcium (600 mg.), magnesium (1200 mg.), phosphorus (800 mg.), and silicon (in the form of the herb horsetail shavegrass—1 capsule daily with a meal).

Natural Sources

The following land-grown plants contain measurable amounts of chlorine in them: borage and comfrey (the highest), elm leaves, pennyroyal, horehound, catnip, lobelia, tansy, wormwood, sassafras, spikenard, wood sage, prickly ash leaves, catnip, and bitterroot and bittersweet. All of the various seaweeds cited under Fluorine, such as kelp and carrageen (Irish moss), are also exceptionally rich in chlorine.

Chromium
THE SUGAR REGULATOR

A Critical Nutrient That Is Hard to Come by in the Food Supply

Chromium deficiency is very common in America. Poor soil, food refining, and high dietary sugar intake (which requires extra insulin that diminishes chromium reserves) are responsible for the shortage. Tissue levels of chromium also decline with age and too much exercise.

Eating a varied diet won't help that much to meet your body's chromium requirements. Unless you're fond of eating nasty-tasting and horrid-smelling brewer's yeast—considered to be the premier source of absorbable chromium—you won't find that much in other foods known to contain small amounts of this important trace element: beef liver, beets, blackstrap molasses, grapes, honey, raisins, mushrooms, whole grain cereals, and whole wheat bread.

Supplements Necessary

Chromium is available in different supplement forms. Besides the obvious brewer's yeast, there are several chelated kinds: chromium nicotinate, chromium gluconate, and the more famous chromium picolinate. However, this last form of the trace element *cannot* be used for long durations, since it has been found to cause chromosomal damage. Modest intake of chromium picolinate should never exceed 100 micrograms per day or be taken for longer than a month at a time without several weeks rest in between before resuming consumption.

Chromium picolinate tablets are available, but since one tablet contains 200 mcg. of chromium, it's only necessary to take it every *other* day. There are also products using two kinds of chelated chromium surrounded by six other minerals and one of the B-complex vitamins. Both are good, each in its own way. (See Product Appendix for more information on pages 381–383.)

Regulates Blood Sugar Efficiently

Chromium influences the performance of insulin within the body. Insulin is a hormone produced by the islets of Langerhans within the pancreas that assists in regulating blood glucose (sugar) levels. Chromium enables insulin to bind to appropriate cell receptors so glucose can enter cells (glucose tolerance). Lack of this trace element results in impaired glucose tolerance. Chromium insufficiency is also implicated in elevated blood glucose levels, high blood cholesterol, and aortic plaques.

Consequently, chromium is of considerable therapeutic value in treating sugar diabetes, elevated cholesterol, and arteriosclerosis. It has become very popular recently in treating obesity. It has proven itself to be quite effective in weight management because of the mineral's ability to regulate blood sugar levels, thereby reducing sugar cravings.

We all need to be careful about what we eat. Watching personal sugar intake is very important if you want to have good health. Often it isn't so much staying away from white sugar per se, but rather scrutinizing package labels of what you intend to eat. There are many forms of "hidden" sugars made from cane, beet, corn, or high-fructose syrups that are listed under more oblique terms. If you find ingredients that end in "-ose," assume they are sugars of some kind. Such simple carbohydrates are abundant in the American food supply. They tend to create a relaxed state at first because, like all carbohydrates, they stimulate serotonin, a chemical in the brain that has a calming effect. However, if these sugared foods are consumed frequently enough, the mellow state turns into unexplained exhaustion. A person's effort to counteract this fatigue creates stress that in turn encourages an individual to indulge in more stimulants such as caffeine or alcohol.

High-sugar foods also displace more nutrient-rich staples from the diet, causing a junk-food-induced form of malnutrition. Even when not all that obvious in the form of gauntness or wasting, such malnutrition can trigger tiredness, lowered work capacity, and ultimately stress. Adding chromium to the diet will help ameliorate this situation somewhat, but practicing healthier food habits is even more important if you want to stay well for longer periods of time.

Capsules are available to help regulate blood sugar more efficiently that bring together Japanese aged garlic extract and the trace element chromium. Usually two capsules daily are adequate for most people's needs. (See Product Appendix, pages 383–84.)

Staying Young

Chromium is of value in promoting dehydroandrosterone (DHEA), a vital anti-aging hormone in the news a lot these days. High insulin levels suppress body production of DHEA. But frequent supplementation with chromium picolinate can boost DHEA production *dramatically!* Since DHEA dwindles with age, older people should periodically supplement their diets with "biologically active" chromium to improve brain function, immune system activity, and muscle strength.

Cobalt
The Mineral Twin to Vitamin B-12

Role in Human Health

Cobalt's chief function is to be the biological twin of vitamin B-12 (also known as cyanocobalamin). Much of its behavior and purpose have already been discussed in the first section of this book under Vitamin B Complex in connection with B-12. Hence, I will only concern myself here with some of the mineral's other biochemical and nutritional roles in relation to human health.

Cobalt is widely distributed in nature in minute quantities. It activates a number of body enzyme functions, including many of those ordinarily triggered by zinc.

In pharmacologic doses cobalt can stimulate production of red blood cells. It also has a positive impact on bone marrow and lymph tissues, helping them produce more antibacterial and antiviral substances with which the immune system can successfully ward off encroaching infection.

Very tiny amounts of cobalt are necessary for the synthesis of vitamin B-12. In cud-chewing animals (sheep, cattle, deer, camels, and giraffes) this always takes place in the proximal portion of the intestine from which the vitamin is then absorbed. In other animals and humans, though, in whom bacterial formation of B-12 happens only in the colon, absorption is quite limited. Therefore, to be of nutritional value for humans, cobalt must be ingested or else injected as vitamin B-12.

Animal glandulars, which are very popular with naturopathic and homeopathic doctors, are rich sources of cobalt. Usually those derived from beef are prescribed for patients suffering from pernicious anemia, poor circulation, and stunted growth. Eating cooked beef liver or heart will also supply the body with some cobalt.

Copper
A MINERAL PROTECTANT FOR AUTOIMMUNE DISORDERS

Helps Arthritis

I remember seeing a couple of John Wayne Westerns years ago in which the Duke wore a copper bracelet on one wrist. It was occasionally conspicuous when the actor raised that particular hand or the camera focused on it momentarily as he was in the act of reaching for his holster during an impending gunfight with the bad guys.

It was not a charm bracelet or something for good luck that he wore. Rather, it was intended to help alleviate some of the pain he suffered in that particular wrist due to osteoarthritis. There was a time when doctors used to debunk such a treatment as nothing more than harmless quackery. But not any longer, since a mounting body of evidence now indicates that millions of victims suffering from some form of arthritis have elevated blood levels not only of copper but also of the protein ceruloplasm, which acts as sort of a fire extinguisher or emergency antioxidant in the terrific inflammation caused by several different autoimmune disorders.

Arthritis sufferers have a great deal *more* copper content in their synovial joint fluids than nonarthritic people have. As it turns out, copper acts as something of a protectant and the higher levels indicate the body's efforts to collect as much of it as possible in an attempt to fight off the disease. Copper apparently plays an important role in the body's response to inflammatory disease. Ceruloplasm, to which copper is bound, is a scavenger of free radicals that are invariably liberated in various autoimmune disorders such as arthritis or lupus erythematosus.

Associated with Cancer

For a number of years researchers were puzzled by the elevated copper levels they discovered in the blood of those suffering from breast cancer, Hodgkin's disease, leukemia, lung cancer, lymphoma, multiple myeloma, and stomach cancer. In the beginning it led them to erroneously postulate that copper was involved in carcinogenesis. But later on, after further studies on the matter, they concluded that the increased copper was a consequence and not the actual cause of the disease process.

Copper's role in the development of cancer is an indirect one—it antagonizes selenium. Selenium affects the enzymatic processes that inhibit the activation of some carcinogens, as well as increasing the efficiency of DNA repair mechanisms in the wake of carcinogenic damage. Copper is pulled from various parts of the body by cancer cells for protection against these helpful benefits from selenium. The obvious solution is to drastically reduce intake of copper-containing foods and instead greatly increase the intake of selenium-bearing foods and a selenium supplement.

Zen Master Finds Protection against Cardiovascular Disease

A renowned Zen master, who asked that I only identify him by his first name of Stephen, saw his father, uncle, and one brother go to early graves before their 50th birthdays due to coronary heart disease. In every case their low-density lipoprotein (LDL) or "bad" cholesterol levels were extremely high. At age 32, he decided to have a thorough physical examination to learn if the disease might be genetically inherited (it was) and if he might have it (he did).

"That's when I decided to do a *complete* makeover on my life," he confessed in an interview. First he began by putting out of his life as much materialism as possible and retaining only the necessary parts that would help him to earn a modest income to live on. Next, he committed himself to a Zen Buddhist belief which entails allying oneself to the three pure precepts where one promises to do no evil, to do good, and to do good for others or free all beings. I asked him what distinguished Zen from other forms of Buddhism and was told that emphasis is placed more on what he termed "sudden enlightenment," rather than the more traditional step-by-step awareness growth fostered by other schools of Buddhist practice and thought. "At any moment you can have realization," he said. "You need to cultivate the mind through practice and by developing concentration. But the enlightened moment is always a sudden experience."

Stephen then turned the conversation to the last change he made in his life in order to protect himself from ever suffering cardiovascular disease like members of his family had done. "I started eating foods that were high in copper values," he noted. These included nuts (especially Brazil nuts, pecans, peanuts and peanut butter, pistachios, and walnuts), legumes (especially lentils and Navy beans), avocado, raisins, black strap molasses, soybeans (especially tofu products), cocoa powder, dark chocolate, and green tea. Since he was a strict vegetarian, he avoided all forms of meat.

Another interesting thing he did along with this radical dietary change was to take a zinc supplement every day. "I had a clinical nutritionist inform me that if I kept my zinc-to-copper ratio somewhere around 8 to 1, that my copper levels would be okay and not get excessive." At the time of my interview with this very softspoken man, he had been rigorously following this very different lifestyle for close to 15 years. "My last medical checkup a year ago," he added, "showed *no* signs of coronary heart disease at all. The doctor checking me over told me that I had one of the best high-density lipoprotein (HDL or 'good' cholesterol) counts he'd ever seen in 24 years of practice."

Stay Away from Fructose

In the 1970s Sheldon Reiser of the Agriculture Department's Carbohydrate Nutrition Lab in Beltsville, Maryland conducted studies with animal models that suggested that diets high in fructose reduce the body's ability to absorb copper. He observed in his published reports that copper-deficient animals fed fructose started dying in about a month of catastrophic heart disease—such as ruptured hearts—while similarly copper-deficient animals whose sugar source was cornstarch managed to survive comfortably enough. He claimed that in the fructose groups, "every index of unfavorable metabolic effect was magnified" many times over.

Furthermore, fructose not only inhibits copper metabolism, but also greatly elevates serum cholesterol levels in the circulating plasma. So stay away from anything that has fructose in it!

She Overcame Chemical Hypersensitivity

I am indebted to Sherry A. Rogers, M.D., who was in private practice in environmental and nutritional medicine at the Northeast Center for Environmental Medicine in Syracuse, New York in the early 1990s, for the following.

"We had a 33-year-old lab technician who visited us awhile back. This poor woman was suffering from chemical hypersensitivity. She couldn't stand being in shopping malls, driving or riding in cars, and numerous other situations on account of her being quite chemically sensitive to them. She felt disoriented, fatigued, and complained of constant migraines whenever she breathed the higher levels of chemicals commonly encountered in these environments. She almost died one time when a coworker came in one morning after having had her hair permed the night before at her local hair stylist.

"We did a thorough blood workup on the woman and discovered that she was seriously deficient in copper. We corrected that immediately by giving her 4 mg. of copper daily. Within one month she was free of all her symptoms and could go just about anywhere and be around anyone without the least bit of problem."

Improve Your Immune Functions

Most people only get about 1 mg. of copper a day, compared to the recommended 1.5 to 3.0 milligrams. A study published in the August 1995 *American Journal of Clinical Nutrition* demonstrated that a diet deficient in copper affects the human immune system, reducing the activity of some cells that attack invading bacteria.

Darshan S. Kelley, Judith R. Turnlund, and their colleagues at the Western Human Nutrition Research Center in San Francisco conducted the study as part of a larger USDA project assessing the role of dietary copper in the body. They put 11 men on a liquid diet—

balanced in all nutrients except copper—for 3 months. At several points in their investigation, they measured the number and immunological activities of various immune cells in blood samples. Some cell activities decreased markedly, while others didn't change at all. One cell population, that of antibody-producing B cells, actually increased.

Clinically speaking, this combination of effects was rather difficult for them to sort out. "Immune function is a very, very complicated field," Turnlund noted in an interview. She admitted that her team didn't "really know what normal ranges for some of these immune function indices" were. Another study finished about the same time by Mark L. Failla of the University of North Carolina at Greensboro found similar changes in the immune system in moderate, yet chronic, copper depletion in rats.

When Failla was contacted by phone, he stated that "copper may have closer ties to the immune system than we ever realized." He considered it to be "a very promising mineral for better immune health" and placed it in the same league as zinc. "If you want to get lots of copper naturally," he added, "then eat more seafood (especially shellfish) and organ meats (kidney, brain, liver, heart)."

Copper Is an Effective Conductor of Our Body Electricity

Copper is a reddish metal and is an extremely good conductor of both heat and electricity. It is softer than iron but harder than zinc and can be polished to a bright finish. In the Periodic Table of the Elements, copper is put with gold and silver to form the Ib group; this trio is outstanding for electrical conductivity.

The chief commercial use of copper throughout the world is based on its wonderful conduction abilities (second only to that of silver, I might add). About 50 percent of the total annual output of copper is employed in the manufacture of electrical apparatus and wires. Copper is incorporated into the bottoms of more expensive cookware because it transfers heat more evenly. Copper tubing is used a lot in plumbing for the transfer of hot water. And, because of its high electrical conductivity, it is a standard part of heat-exchanging devices such as refrigerator and airconditioner coils.

Copper finds its greatest use, however, as a vital nutrient inside every living, breathing, moving human being. Without a *little* copper in each of us, we would be dead in a hurry. There flows through every body a continual stream of bioelectricity that, according to the authors of *The Body Electric* (New York: William Morrow, 1985), wouldn't be there were it not for copper and other essential trace elements like gold and silver. The eye-opening book by Robert O. Becker, M.D. and Gary Selden presents a dazzling array of evidence to show that copper (and other nutrients) is essential for cell life, brain activity, heartbeat, bone function, nerve transmission, and muscle movement. Very minute quantities of copper are carried by blood plasma as it continually circulates throughout the body. Everything requiring this mineral gets whatever tiny portion is necessary. Without copper present at all times the body's own self-generated bioelectrical forces would not remain constant but become faulty. In due time, a number of unfavorable pathological situations would arise to spell trouble for the individual's state of health.

Copper may not be as glamorous as calcium or as glitzy as chromium, but it is still an integral component of what keeps everything alive within our physical beings. Were it not for copper, animation as we know it would cease to exist in each of us. Therefore, we need to make sure that our copper levels always remain adequate and in balance with everything else to guarantee for us the quality of life we've come to cherish and expect.

Fluorine

THE BAD AND GOOD IN A CONTROVERSIAL MINERAL

The Roots of Fluoride

Approximately 60 percent of America's drinking water is fluoridated. How it got that way, at a concentration of 1 mg. per liter, makes for an interesting tale. In the 1930s, epidemiologist H. Trendly Dean, M.D. noticed that very-white blotches on the front teeth of children, were most common in areas where fluoride concentrations exceeded one part per million (ppm).These stains (called dental fluorosis) became more common at about 1.5 ppm. Severe mottling and tooth disfigurement were widespread at 2 ppm and more.

But the real surprise he turned up was that kids drinking water with 0.9 to 1.4 ppm had one-third *fewer* cavities than those in areas with 0.4 ppm. In a 1938 report that solidified his title as "Father of Fluoridation," he mentioned the possibility of bringing fluoride levels to a uniform 1 ppm in drinking water to reduce both cavities and fluorosis.

An experiment intended to verify fluoride's effectiveness in preventing tooth decay got underway in 1945 when Grand Rapids, Michigan; Newburgh, New York; and Brantford, Ontario (Canada), became the first cities in the entire world to fluoridate their water supplies. This trio, and eventually six other cities, would drip 1 ppm fluoride into finished drinking water. Rates of tooth decay in the fluoridated cities would be monitored for 10 to 15 years and compared with those of fluoride-free cities.

The benevolent role of fluoride in protecting children's teeth was confirmed without a doubt by the study. In Grand Rapids, for example, kids from 12 to 14 years old had 50 to 63 percent fewer cavities in 1960 than they did in 1945. Only a small handful of fluorosis cases were evident in this age bracket. Similar encouraging results came in from the other cities taking part in this lengthy and comprehensive evaluation.

But it was only five years into the experiment, in 1950, that the Public Health Service (PHS) announced that communities contemplating fluoridation should proceed. Just a year later the American Medical Association followed the PHS lead in approving fluoridation. The American Dental Association climbed on the rolling bandwagon in 1953, sending a brochure to every local and state dental society in the nation extolling the benefits of this mineral, encouraging its widespread adoption, and laying out a clever campaign to effectively deal with any public resistance on the matter.

Fluoride Facts

Fluorine is a member of the halogen family, that includes chlorine. It is a flammable, *toxic* gas. Fluorine is one of the most powerful oxidizing agents, breaking down minerals, metals, organic compounds, and water. Fluorine combines readily with other chemicals to produce *fluorides,* which are very common in the Earth's crust.

Natural fluorides, leached from the earth, can be found in groundwater (as opposed to surface water) in many parts of the country at concentrations of up to 14 parts per million—the hot states are Arizona, Arkansas, Colorado, South Dakota, Tennessee, and western Texas. Throughout the nation, some 1,300 mostly-rural community water systems (serving an estimated two million drinkers) naturally contain at least 2 ppm fluoride. The federal Environmental Protection Agency (EPA) estimates that about 10 percent of the children who drink this amount of fluoride will suffer moderate to severe fluorosis; 50 percent will be affected at 4 ppm.

Currently, 41 of the nation's 50 largest cities add about 1 ppm fluoride. The fluorides we ingest come from some strange places. *Fluosilic acid,* the most common fluoridation agent, is highly corrosive, and a byproduct of phosphate fertilizer manufacture. *Sodium fluoride,* less commonly used to fluoridate drinking water, is a salt byproduct of the process that turns bauxite ore into aluminum. *Stannous fluoride,* used in toothpaste and which we get way too much of in our bodies when brushing daily, is a byproduct of steel-can recycling operations.

Fluorides are so corrosive that they would eat through a steel tank in a matter of hours. Liquid fluorides are *always* transported in rubber-lined tanks.

The Harmful Effects

We have people like the late Martha C. Johnson to thank for the U.S. government's failing to reach its goal of having 95 percent of the public drinking water in America fluoridated by 1990. When I met this spry 87-year-old in the winter of 1992, she had been devoting the last 27 years of her life to fighting fluoridation in her home state of Michigan. She regularly lobbied the legislature in Lansing to inform them of the mineral's potential harm to human health. "I'm always armed with the facts," she said very matter-of-factly. "I'm one for *detail*. I really do a great deal of research and always go into every session [of the legislature] armed to the teeth *with facts*! Those boys [the state politicians] may not like what I bring them, but there's no denying that I'm right with what I've got."

She and hundreds of others throughout the country did it all without pay or with meager compensation at best. They depended largely upon donations from others and spent thousands of hours poring over every report that came out in regard to fluoridation. "Ours is a *health war*," I remember this woman with the gray hair telling me. "But we fight it *religiously*!"

She was extremely generous in sharing with me some of the more select pieces of research out of a mountain of photocopied paper materials she kept stored in her cluttered Lansing home. From an old rolltop desk, she pulled data that showed beyond a shadow of doubt that fluoridation is *bad* for human health. I've condensed the data below for easier and quicker perusal by the reader:

Collagen Disease. Collagen is the primary protein of the white fibers of connective tissue, cartilage, and bone. Fluoride rapidly interacts with this substance turning it into something akin to Teflon (a polyfluorocarbon). Collagen disease is on the rise in scary proportions all across the nation. The proverbial "tip of the iceberg" is manifested in diseases like AIDS and cancer. The rest of the problems that lie below the surface include sudden pneumonia, carpal tunnel syndrome, bursitis, kidney failure, neck and spine stiffness, arthritis, pyorrhea, lupus, artery disease, heart lining and valve inflammations, skin disorders, asthma, brittle bones, knee weaknesses, and Alzheimer's disease. Every one of these is clearly a manifestation of damaged connective tissue leading to fibrinoid autoimmune disorders.

Hip Fractures. Two separately published reports that appeared in the April 1, 1991 *American Journal of Epidemiology* and the August 12, 1992 *Journal of the American Medical Association* proved that men and women past the age of 65 who drank fluoridated water regularly stood a 50 percent greater chance of incurring hip bone fractures than did similarly aged individuals living in communities without fluoride in the water.

Hip fracture is a major public health problem, costing about $7 billion a year in America alone. It's the second most common cause of admission to nursing homes, accounting for almost 60,000 admissions annually. Not surprisingly, hip fractures, according to a third study, have randomly increased 20 percent or more since the widespread introduction of fluoridated public drinking water in the early 1950s.

Kidney Stones. Two reports, appearing in successive months, reported that fluoride can dramatically increase painful kidney stones. The journals in which this information appeared were *Clinical Biochemistry* (18:109-113, Mar.-Apr. 1985) and *Nutrition Reviews* (43:140-41, May 1985).

Cancer. Fluoridated and chlorinated public water supplies have been implicated in certain forms of cancer, according to the *Bulletin of Environmental Contamination and Toxicology* (34:815-23, Jun. 1985)

Foiling Fluoride

If you're feeling somewhat perturbed by now over the prolific use of fluoride in our drinking water, there are some things you can do to greatly offset the harmful effects it would eventually produce in your body. First of all, brush your teeth every night with baking soda, toothpaste containing it, or a natural toothpaste such as the brands sold in many health food stores. Just be sure it doesn't contain any fluoride.

More importantly, dose up on calcium (dairy products, sardines, salmon, and tofu), phosphorus (codfish, beef, milk, cottage cheese, yogurt, chicken, brewer's yeast), and magnesium (found in many foods). When you're deficient in any of these minerals, then your body will start using fluoride as a building block instead of them.

(*Note*: I am indebted to Steve Coffel of Florence, Montana for some of the information used in this particular entry.)

Germanium

TUMORS DON'T STAND A CHANCE WHEN THIS
MINERAL IS AROUND

The Ultimate Panacea

I remember visiting local supermarkets in the Salt Lake City area in the month of December 1987 and seeing several well-known tabloids displayed near the checkout counters. Various headlines screamed "Miracle Pill a Boon to Mankind!" or "Health Miracle on the Way!" and "New Miracle Nutrient Cures EVERYTHING!" Opening the pages of one of them, I noticed brief quotes from a couple of physicians claiming that this item was"*the* best thing that's ever happened on the planet" and calling it "a landmark development in the field of nutritional medicine."

All of this attention, of course, was being focused on the trace element germanium. As a result sales of this mineral skyrocketed and a number of supplement manufacturers became instantly wealthy almost overnight. The media furor and selling frenzy have since died away, as is common with all overly-hyped substances. But germanium is still with us, only dispensed now in a more quiet and dignified way as it should have been from the very beginning.

Antitumor Protection Substantiated

Credit the Japanese for having been the first ones to really put germanium on the map so far as its protection against cancer goes. Microbiologists such as Nobuo Tanaka, M.D. of the University of Tokyo and Fujio Suzuki, M.D. of Kumamoto University Medical School carefully evaluated this trace element and reported in the scientific literature that it exerted "direct cytotoxic activity" on tumor growth and "displayed host-mediated anticancer activity" as well.

Germanium seems to directly impact the immune system in a positive way in order to bring about this inhibition of malignant growth. According to Tanaka's observations in the *Journal of Biological Response Modifiers* (4:159-68, 1985), this trace element "induces interferon and activates natural killer cells and macrophages," all immune-system-generated substances that play major roles in the defeat of cancer within the body.

Suzuki has defined what he meant by germanium displaying "host-mediated" anticancer activity. The trace element is able to help "modify the relationship between the tumor and its host by modifying the host's (human or animal model) biological response to the tumor cells, with resultant therapeutic effects. In other words, germanium not only destroys the tumor itself, but can also alter the body's own ability to cope with this malignancy by slowing down its rate of growth, denying the tumor access to important nutrients it may require, and compelling the immune system to deal with the matter more aggressively than it otherwise would." One of his articles, published in the *British Journal of Cancer* (52:757-63, 1985), explained it in more detail.

Natural Sources

Besides coal, germanium appears in a number of different plants, some of which are quite common and others less so, but all of which are widely utilized in Oriental folk medicine. It is present only in *very minute* quantities, though, say just a few parts per *billion* (ppb). The data in the accompanying table were prepared by Yoshiki Mino and associates at the Osaka College of Pharmacy and the Department of Pharmaceutical Sciences at Tokushima University in Japan and were published in *Chemical and Pharmaceutical Bulletin* (28:2687-91, 1980). I've adapted one of the tables from their report for easier reading in this text.

Analytical Results for Germanium in Various Medicinal Plants

PLANT MATERIAL	GERMANIUM CONTENT (ppb)
Garlic bulb (Allium sativum)	1
Seeds of Job's Tears (Coicis lachryma-jobi L.)	6
Ginseng root (Panax ginseng)	5-6
Wild American ginseng root (Panacis quinquefolium L.)	1

Gromwell root (Lithospermum erythrorhizon)	1
Mountain bean root (Sophora subprostrata)	4
Tea leaves (Thea folium)	9
Fomitopsis rosea	1
Chinese matrimony vine fruit (Lycium chinense)	1
Comfrey leaf (Symphytum officinale)	1
Comfrey root (Symphytum officinale)	2
Reishi mushroom* (Ganoderma lucidum)	5

*Leung and Foster, *Encyclopedia of Common Natural Ingredients*
(New York: John Wiley & Sons, Inc., 1996; p. 256).

The handiest sources, of course, are green tea made from the boiled leaves and commercially produced formulas (see Product Appendix, pages 381–384). In the case of something as biologically potent as germanium, always remember that a little bit goes a *long* way!

Iodine

Radiation All Around Us

There was a period in the 1950s, 60s, and 70s when above-ground nuclear testing was a common occurrence. Not only were there regular, almost monthly, explosions, but occasionally there were weekly or even biweekly tests. Our planet's atmosphere became heavily polluted with radioactive isotopes, which could then be inhaled and accumulated within the body over an extended period of time, eventually causing cancer. Several thousand people living in Southern Utah, "downwind" from clouds of nuclear fallout that routinely passed over from the Nevada testing grounds next door, developed all kinds of cancers many years later. At first the cause wasn't known, but mounting research soon proved it came from the many atomic blasts and that the federal government was to blame. Most of the "Downwinders" died before they could realize the settlement of a massive class-action lawsuit against the United States, but at least their families finally received some federal compensation for the damage that had been done.

Today there isn't much of this type of testing anymore, except for periodic reports coming out of China, Russia, or France. But another form of radiation exists that in many ways is even more dangerous than the nuclear threat our parents faced. This is the widespread presence of electromagnetic radiation. Like nuclear radiation, it is invisible and very subtle in the negative impacts it makes upon the human body. But no big government agency has anything to do with this radiation. *We alone* are the makers and perpetrators of the same. Every time we turn on the television or radio, cook food in a microwave oven, dry our hair with a blowdryer, shave with an electric shaver, talk to someone on a cordless or cellular phone, sit in front of a computer screen, run copies of an original document off on a photocopy machine, or enjoy the service of *any* other electrical gadget, then we are getting bombarded with unseen radiation!

A fan of mine from "Down Under," an Aussie named Geoff Sandford, wrote me a letter about his own physical debilities due to living close to a giant TV transmission tower. He attributed his terrible chronic fatigue syndrome to the electromagnetic radiation emissions constantly coming from it. He declared in no uncertain terms: "We are living in electromagnetic *soup* . . . and guess who are the *croutons!*" Once he took the necessary steps to shield himself better from this radiation, he became well again! (For his nearly complete letter, see the entry under Sodium.)

The most definitive work I've ever read on this subject is *The Body Electric: Electromagnetism and the Foundation of Life* (New York: William Morrow, 1985) by Robert O. Becker, M.D. and Gary Selden. It describes in concise detail our own bioelectric interactions with the much larger electromagnetic environment that our wonderful(?) technology has created and, in the process, enveloped us with.

Your Nutritional Insurance Policy against Radioactive-Induced Cancer

Not much can be done to clean up the atmosphere of all the nuclear fallout and debris of decades past. What's done is done! But there are some things we *can* and *should* be doing to shield ourselves against electromagnetic radiation. The most common-sense approach is to evaluate each and every electrical item we use on a regular basis and honestly ask ourselves, "Do I *really* need this?"

I'm going to be truthful here and admit that I use some electrical items, and that I think about the effects the electromagnetic radiation generated from them might be having on my system. Do I worry myself sick about it? No, of course not. Do I use them only when absolutely necessary? Yes! Do I take other precautions? Absolutely! What are some of them? I regularly consume garlic and ginseng root, which are medically known to remove radiative particles from the system. (See Product Appendix, pages 383–84 for more information.)

But my very best nutritional insurance policy is found in the trace element, iodine. According to Sheldon Saul Hendler, M.D., Ph.D. in his book, *The Doctors' Vitamin and Mineral Encyclopedia* (New York: Simon & Schuster, 1990), this mineral is by far "the most effective blocker of radiodide uptake [from radioactive fallout] by the thyroid." Iodide (the mineral salt form of naturally occurring iodine) also protects *all* major glands and organs from the harmful effects of electromagnetic radiation bombardment.

I get my daily RDA of 150 micrograms of iodide several different ways. One is by drinking an 8 oz. mixture of Mighty Greens superfood blend and Pines organic Beet Juice Powder. I add a table-spoon of the former with one teaspoon of the latter in eight ounces of water or juice, stir thoroughly, and drink. The Mighty Greens contains different seaweeds and algaes known to be rich in iodine.

I also periodically use a product that provides my body not only with iodine, but a rich array of many other trace elements that help form a nutritional shield against invading electromagnetic radiation waves.

Last but not least, there is that wonderful seaweed called kelp. It is by far *the* richest source of natural iodine that I know of. I like to sea-son some of my food with it in preference to table salt or black pepper. You can buy powdered or granulated kelp in any supermarket or health food store.

Thus, I'm always assured that there is adequate iodide floating around in my circulating plasma to protect me from ever getting radiation-induced cancer. But it just doesn't stop with supplements, for there are a number of seafoods extremely rich in natural iodine: fish (flounder, haddock, halibut, swordfish), lobster, clams, shrimp, and oysters, to mention just a few.

Cruciferous foods such as cabbage, kale, kohlrabi, Brussels sprouts, and cauliflower are good to eat since they are high in sul-phur (see the entry for Sulphur). But, along with soybeans, they have an *antagonistic* effect toward iodine and can deplete it from the body if consumed too often.

Iodine may also prove particularly useful in "reliev[ing] [the] pain and soreness associated with fibrocystic breasts . . . in pre-menopausal women, as well as in postmenopausal women taking supplementary estrogens," according to Dr. Hendler.

Wonderful Antiseptic

On the number of occasions when I've traveled to exotic regions of the earth to do folk medicine research among primitive cultures, I've never been without tablets containing tetraglycine hydroperiodide. This is the form of iodine that world travelers and campers use to purify questionable drinking water. *Never* use elemental iodine as it can be fatal!

Had I not had the good sense to take along this iodine substance, I probably would have ingested itty bitty microorganisms with big, long-sounding Latin names that are quite capable of creating body miseries too unpleasant to write about here. I also favor packing povidone iodine in the organic form of Betadine, which is a superb topical antiseptic agent to ward off fungal infection caused by contact with plants and soil.

Preventing Mental Retardation Early in Life

For many years, doctors have recognized that extreme iodine deficiency during pregnancy nearly always induces severe mental retardation in developing infants. A recent study of boys between the ages of 9 and 15 now shows that childhood iodine deficiency not only impairs learning but also the motivation for achievement that goes with it.

Researchers at the Sanjay Gandhi Post Graduate Institute of Medical Sciences in Lucknow, India focused on 100 boys from villages in eastern India. Though very poor, each child had attended school, where he had learned to read and write. Approximately 50 percent of the youngsters had goiters of varying grades, a sure sign of little or no iodine content in their bodies.

Compared to boys their age from neighboring villages who had no overt signs of the deficiency, boys from the goiter-prone areas proved slower learners on all tests except the recall of verbally played information. This data appeared in the May 1997 *American Journal of Clinical Nutrition*. Children from the severely deficient communities also improved less after practice drills than did boys from the other villages.

Although children from the iodine-deficient villages might have suffered minor nerve damage during earlier development that continued to affect their ability to learn, it seemed the older children often performed more poorly than younger ones—suggesting a cumulative impairment.

The most dramatic difference between the two groups, the Indian scientists reported, was a strikingly lower motivation to achieve in those from the most iodine-deficient villages. "These abnormalities may prevent millions of children from achieving their full potential, even if learning opportunities are made available," the researchers concluded. Seafood, seaweed, and iodized salt could supply the iodine needed for normal function of the thyroid, whose hormones play a vital role in cognition and learning, the report concluded.

While I'm not particularly fond of homeopathy in general, yet the Iodum remedy has been prescribed with *some* good success by naturopathic and homeopathic doctors for children and youth who are mentally restless and extremely forgetful. The iodine used in this remedy is largely derived from seaweed and saltpeter deposits in Chile.

Iron

REENERGIZE YOUR LIFE WITH IRON

Health Secrets of the Mountain Men and Fur Trappers of the Old West

Very few people today are aware of the famous exploits of a number of mountain men and fur trappers who helped pave the way for the eventual settlement of the Rocky Mountains by pioneers in the mid-nineteenth century. Such rough-and-tumble characters as Jim Bridger, Etienne Provot, Miles Goodyear, Thomas Fitzpatrick, Jedediah S. Smith, Kit Carson, Robert Campbell, Peter Skene Ogden, Louis Vasquez, David E. Jackson, Milton G. Sublette, Joseph L. Meek, and a host of others braved the elements, fought Indians, and sometimes barely managed to survive in order to procure animal pelts that they sold for a living.

A number of them became, each in his own way, quite famous. Some had cities named after them: Provo and Ogden, Utah. Jim Bridger is credited with being the first white man to discover the Great Salt Lake in the late autumn or early winter of 1824. An occasional few soared into fame on the kite tails of others' much publicized accomplishments: "Kit" Carson barely made it as a mountaineer on his own, but thanks largely to explorer Colonel John C. Fremont, he acquired a second, though undeserved, reputation as a skillful frontier scout.

It took keen eyes, a sharp brain, a cunning heart, and considerable stealth to outwit the animals they were continually in pursuit of. The beaver was the trickiest of them all and certainly the hardest to catch. But with a good beaver pelt fetching anywhere from $6 to $8 in St. Louis, Missouri throughout the heyday of fur trapping, which ran from about 1819 to 1831, it was definitely worth the effort involved. As one biographer of mountain man Jim Bridger so eloquently put it: "The trapper must learn to be as wise as the beaver itself, outwitting it in its own cunning."

But it would be unfair to suggest that fur trappers and hunters were just out to pit their wits against the beaver. Active and versatile trappers laid their snares and aimed their guns at all kinds of fur and skin, making gain out of every creature that came their way. The skin of the buffalo, elk, and deer were always prepared for shipping or for clothing or camp use. Grizzly bear skins were especially prized when taken in just the right manner; and for nearly every one of them, there was some sort of thrilling narrative to accompany it. Besides these animals, otter, raccoon, foxes, and even muskrats were taken in large quantities. Both the Hudson Bay Company and the American Fur Company paid equally well to get as many of these prized skins as possible. Therefore, it behooved them to treat these mountain men like kings when they brought their booty in for cash payments.

Catching the animals involved a lot of mental work and emotional patience. But skinning them and properly preparing the pelts demanded a great deal of physical labor and considerable dexterity with a sharp knife.

Traveling sometimes alone or more often in small companies, the trappers quickly learned to adapt to the harsh wilderness life. The solitude of the great outdoors became their constant companion. When traveling together, they learned to share with and look out for each other. If they didn't play by these rules, they would soon go insane from the extreme loneliness or else perish on account of starvation, frigid cold, or hostile natives.

When resupplied and well stocked with the usual victuals of flour, sugar, coffee, tobacco, and whiskey before returning to the Rocky Mountains for another hard fall and winter, they ate pretty well when regularly supplementing their meals with different varieties of wild game. Sometimes wild nuts and berries and occasional fish from lakes, rivers, and streams provided a change of pace to their usually dulled taste buds. But in times of scarcity, they had to resort to cooked animal flesh and dug-up plant roots in order to survive. All things considered, their diet wasn't bad at all for these times.

Annual summer-fall rendezvous at designated locations in the Rocky Mountains often brought together hundreds or sometimes several thousand individuals from many scattered points on the compass. Beside the trappers, hunters, and scouts themselves, together with occasional spouses and children, there were many friendly Native Americans who joined in the weeklong festivities.

While whiskey invariably flowed like water, stories of adventure, like gossip about the weather, were bandied about. Bartering was common between the whites and Native Americans, each one exchanging things of value for something else the other had. There were also the gambling games, the personal combats, and the disgraceful brawls. But when added all together, such motley and fascinating gatherings proved to be meaningful and anticipated events for nearly everyone involved.

Now from this short overview of the colorful lifestyles of these hardy mountain men and fur trappers of long ago, we can determine some of their unreported health secrets.

Mental Activity. From all that they had to be on the lookout for, it is highly doubtful that even a single one of them suffered from laziness of the brain. Their minds were keen and their wits sharp at all times; in this way they prospered and survived. If postmortem medical examinations of their brain tissues could be done today, it would be found that the gray thinking matter in each one would definitely be thicker than that of most modern people. They had no time for anxiety, depression, or loss of self-esteem, because their focus was always outward upon the surrounding environment instead of continually being internalized on their own presumed unhappiness or misfortunes.

Physical Labor. In the early North American frontier a great deal of manual labor was always needed. Putting up camp at night and dissembling it in the morning was for starters. Then followed the daily attention and care given to their riding and pack animals—horses and mules were regularly fed, watered, and doctored as needed. After this came the gathering of suitable dry wood and the making of a good campfire. Next in order was the cooking of the food that would be eaten and shared with others that night. Following the washing of utensils, the camp perimeters would be carefully checked for marauders or prowling wild animals such as wolves and bears. This, plus the tough job of pelt preparation, combined to give every one of them the type of consistent daily workout that today's athletic wannabes can only dream about in their air-conditioned, music-filled training gyms and health spas.

Endurance and Cooperation. Mountain men of old possessed that rarest of qualities—the ability to undergo any kind of adversity without ever giving in. And they learned to stand and work together under the most trying situations, even when they may have had personality differences among themselves.

Neighborly. There was an irony of sorts attached to their periodic rendezvous. After not being close together for many months on end, yet a real sense of community spirit seemed to pervade such infrequent gatherings. A heartfelt interest was felt by one and all and genuine pleasure or sadness expressed in others' good luck or misfortunes. Assistance was seldom ever asked for, but freely given when true needs became apparent. They abided by an unwritten code of wilderness life that suggested a material respect for another man's property, honesty in all business dealings, an appreciation for someone else's skills and knowledge in a certain area, and readily acknowledged gratitude for whatever services were rendered free by another party. Contrast these behavioral characteristics with today's upwardly mobile and very busy condo, apartment, or home dwellers who reside within the same locale but hardly know or speak to each other any more.

The Real Key to Mountain Men Strength

What I'm about to unfold to you may come as nothing new on the one hand, but again will probably be something of a surprise on the other. The enduring physical strength of the mountain men can be primarily traced to the iron they ingested. The fact that iron gives muscle and blood strength is of itself nothing new. But the type of iron and the particular sources of it are really what this chapter is all about and will hopefully be received by the reader with enthusiasm and delight.

First of all, let's look at iron itself. For a number of decades now nutritionists have been saying that people who want to muscle more iron into their diets should select beef, chicken, and other animal-based items. That's because some of the iron they contain is a form of the mineral called *heme* iron, which the body is better able to assimilate than the non-heme iron that is found in beans and other plant foods.

But animal foods are not similar in their heme iron content—despite the fact that nutritionists have also said heme iron makes up about 40 percent of the iron in the animal foods we eat. The 40 percent figure is an average obtained by lumping together the amount of beef, chicken, and other flesh foods Americans are fond of heaping on their plates.

In truth, though, beef contains much more than 40 percent of its iron as heme iron, and chicken contains much less. With red meat consumption way down right now and poultry consumption climbing, the 40 percent average could be out of date for many.

That's why researchers at Utah State University in Logan believed it was important to take a second look at the proportion of heme versus non-heme iron in various foods. Their findings, obtained with more precise methods than those used in the past: 55 to 80 percent of the iron in beef is heme iron (depending on the cut, of course), but the heme variety of iron makes up no more than about 40 percent of the total iron in chicken. If you're talking light meat instead of dark, heme iron comprises only about 29 percent of the iron present.

The researchers also checked out the heme iron content of various cuts of pork, lamb chops, and ground turkey. When compared to a small 3 oz. cut of sirloin steak with 2.2 mgs. of heme iron, the same serving sizes of pork loin (0.2 mg.), lamb chop (1.1 mg.) and ground turkey (0.6) fell way below this figure.

In addition to this, the iron that is derived from traditionally iron-rich vegetables such as spinach and lettuce is always the non-heme variety and, therefore, poorly absorbed. For instance, just 1.4 percent of the iron from spinach can be taken in by the body; other vegetables yield slightly more: 1.6 percent from black beans, 4.4. percent from lettuce and 7 percent from soybeans. Vitamin C can enhance the utilization of non-heme iron, but substances like tannin from green or black tea as well as cereal fiber and plant phytates can inhibit it. So, drinking a glass of orange juice with a Caesar salad will help to convert more of the non-heme iron to the heme kind, but drinking English tea with the same salad will have just the opposite effect.

The mountain men and fur trappers who lived in the first quarter or so of the last century almost always subsisted on wild animal flesh of some kind. Venison was the most common, dark in nature, and with a gamey flavor to it. In spite of its being stringy and tough at times, it served to satisfy their hunger. But more than that, it provided sustaining strength for longer periods of time. This was due to the simple fact that virtually all wild game such as antelope, buffalo, deer, elk, and moose are exceptionally all high in heme iron—in some cases in far greater amounts than beef is known to contain. *This* was the real key to their seemingly endless reservoir of physical strength.

Iron's Diverse Biological Functions

The diversity of this mineral's many capabilities accounts for the wide-ranging impact of its deficiency. The metal is best known for its role in the transport of oxygen in blood. As a component of hemoglobin, iron helps the molecule pick up oxygen in the lungs and shuttle and release it throughout the body. About 73 percent of the body's iron is found in hemoglobin, where it is constantly recycled as more red blood cells are made.

Of the balance of the body's iron, 12 to 17 percent is stored in two molecules—ferritin and hemosidern—both of which can bind large numbers of iron atoms. (Each molecule of ferritin alone binds up to 4,500 iron atoms.) Myoglobin accounts for another 15 percent of the iron, acting as a reservoir of oxygen for muscle cells. A small but extremely important amount (0.2 percent) of body iron is bound to transferrin, a compound that shuttles iron from sites of release to sites of need. Lactoferrin—a compound usually found in breast milk, mucosal tissues, and white blood cells or leukocytes—also binds a percentage of the body's iron so that it isn't available for bacterial growth, thereby stemming infection.

The minute amount of iron not accounted for by these compounds is found in myriad enzymes crucial to metabolism. These enzymes include oxidases, catalases, reductases, peroxidases, and dehydrogenases. Each enzyme plays an important role as a reversible donor or acceptor of electrons during cellular metabolism.

Iron Deficiency

"Iron deficiency," wrote Nevin S. Scrimshaw in the October 1991 *Scientific American* (from which the foregoing and present data was obtained), "is the most prevalent nutritional problem in the world today." Anemia is, by far, the most pervasive form of this nutritional disorder. It cuts across cultures and social, economic, and religious boundaries to be found "in all societies, developing and industrial alike." Scrimshaw cited, for example, that "in the U.S., Japan, and Europe, between 10 and 20 percent of women of childbearing age are anemic."

Of all vitamin or mineral deficiencies, iron deficiency still remains the most unrecognized disorder by doctors. Due to "subtle symptoms such as pallor, listlessness, and fatigue," Scrimshaw observed, "this disorder is not regarded as life-threatening by the medical community at large. Yet iron deficiency has a host of bad effects, one of which can be death."

In recent years medical researchers have found that iron deficiency is associated with the often irreversible impairment of a child's learning ability and other behavioral abnormalities. Low levels of this mineral can have a tremendous adverse impact on brain function. Beside this, diminished levels of iron in adults can affect how they work and what is accomplished, as well as increasing their chances of getting and dying from infection because of impaired immune defenses.

Sometimes a passing health food fad may incline many toward excess consumption of a particular substance. Those who've foolishly overindulged in chromium picolinate, for example, have iron knocked out of their systems because it tightly binds with transferrin, the substance that transports iron around in the blood.

The Mystery Source of Iron for the Early Fur Trappers

Previously it was shown that *heme* iron is much better utilized by the body than the non-heme variety is, and that beef has the highest source of heme iron. It was also explained that fur trappers and hunters of the early North American frontier obtained their daily intakes of heme iron from a variety of wild animal flesh such as buffalo, deer, and elk.

But there was an even better source of iron in addition to what the wild game provided. In an exceedingly scarce and long out-of-print biography, *James Bridger: Trapper, Frontiersman, Scout and Guide* (Salt Lake City: Shepherd Book Company, 1925), historian J. Cecil Alter mentioned that when an inventory was once taken of the old mountain man's possessions, everything else except his cast iron cooking pot was valued below $4.00—it alone received a higher value!

Cast iron cookware has been around for a very long time. Before the Great Flood in Noah's time, Tubal-Cain, the eighth-generation descendant of Adam, forged instruments and utensils out of bronze and iron, as suggested by Genesis 4:22. Pieces of a very ancient cast iron cooking pot dating back to 2900 B.C. were discovered by archaeologists many years ago during their excavations around the Great Pyramid of Giza, presumably built in Abraham's day. Various Hittite cooking utensils of iron have been found, dating from 1900 to 1200 B.C. Almost 2,500 years ago, the ancient Chinese had independently invented the blast furnace and were already in the business of making cast iron cookery. In the West, the Romans inherited ironworking techniques from the Greeks, carried them to a high degree of perfection, and spread their knowledge to northern and northwestern Europe. Evidence of Roman cast iron cooking utensils has been found in the Czech Republic, France, and Great Britain.

So what the early mountain men depended upon to cook all of their food in was a form of cookware that had become established over several thousand years. According to Dick Stucki, of South Salt Lake, one of America's leading experts on iron skillet (Dutch oven) cooking: "Pioneers, frontiersmen, scouts, cavalry troops, and even the Indians regarded their cast iron pots and pans as some of their most prized possessions. Next to their rifles, knifes, and horses, their Dutch ovens were indispensable. They would sooner be willing to lose furniture, books, wagons, pack animals, blankets, bedrolls, and even personal articles of clothing, than give up their pots and skillets."

So, exactly how much extra iron is imparted to foods cooked in cast iron? The accompanying table, which I modified from one that appeared in *Modern Nutrition in Health and Disease,* 5th edi-

tion (Philadelphia: Lea & Febiger, 1976; p. 300) by Robert S.
Goodhart, M.D. and Maurice E. Shils, M.D., may surprise you.

Food items	Cooking time in minutes	IRON CONTENT, mg/100 gm	
		Glass dish	Dutch oven
Apple butter	120	3.0	52.5
Beef hash	45	1.52	5.2
Gravy	20	0.43	5.9
Potatoes, fried	30	0.45	3.8
Rice, casserole	45	1.4	5.2
Scrambled eggs	3	1.7	4.1
Spaghetti sauce	180	3.0	87.5

An additional health tip from the October 1990 issue of the
University of California, Berkeley Wellness Letter (page 1) just goes to
show how dependable a source for this mineral Dutch ovens really
are: "Cooking in cast-iron pots is a good way to increase the iron in
your diet. The more acidic the food (such as tomato sauce) and the
longer it cooks, the more iron." We may not know how acidic the
food content of the mountain men was, but available records of that
period do inform us that they boiled or fried their meat in such
cookware for longer times than we do. Hence, their intake of iron
would have been considerably higher than it is for most of us.

Eyesight As Sharp As an Eagle's

One of the many things that iron is known to do inside the body is
to transfer oxygen to tissues by way of hemoglobin and myoglobin.
Good vision depends, in part, on ample oxygen flow to the eyes.
When the amount of oxygen being transferred at any given time
suddenly drops for very long, then clarity of vision becomes diminished. Experiments conducted with monkeys in which iron deficiencies were created for several months revealed a much higher
incidence of cataract formation than in monkeys given ample iron in
their diets.

Correcting Hypothermia

Hypothermia is caused by exposure to cold air or water, especially in wind and rain. It may occur indoors as well, especially among infants or the elderly. Hyothermia is a drop in internal body temperature to a below-normal level (less than 94° F). Common symptoms include shivering, numbness, pallor, slurred speech, confusion, and stumbling.

Beside the obvious procedure of rewarming the body, there is something else that can be done to bring body temperature back to normal again. This is placing the hypothermic individual on an iron supplement and recommending the consumption of iron-rich foods for several months straight.

A group of women who were put on low-iron diets for 2 1/2 months lost almost 30 percent more body heat while sitting in a drafty room than they did after their iron stores were replenished. What's more, according to researchers at the USDA's Human Nutrition Research Center in Grand Forks, North Dakota, they were able to tolerate the cold for slightly longer periods of time when they were given adequate amounts of iron. In a separate study at Pennsylvania State University, women with low levels of iron in the blood were found to have sharper falls in body temperature following submersion in cold water than those with normal blood levels of the mineral.

You do not have to be suffering from out-and-out iron-deficiency anemia to respond poorly to the cold, though. Even a relatively mild deficiency can increase the likelihood of experiencing chills and shivers, which is reason enough for everyone to make an effort to follow a diet that supplies adequate amounts of iron. And by eating an accompanying food rich in vitamin C, such as citrus fruits or juices, or tomato sauce, tomato soup, salsa, or tomato juice, your body will be able to better absorb the non-heme iron found in enriched breakfast cereals and grain products, wheat germ, eggs, and poultry. But when consuming those foods high in heme iron content—beef liver, organ meats, wild game, and fish—it isn't necessary to eat something else containing ascorbic acid.

Body Iron Requirements

Women need more iron every day than men do. Women between the ages of 25 and 50 require on average 15 mg. of this mineral every day. Their need for iron increases during pregnancy and lactation, but returns to normal after birth and breast-feeding are done with. Women over 50 and men over the age of 24 only need 10 mg. of iron daily.

Lead

A Popular Remedy in Ancient Times

Lead is one of the metals that was known to the ancient world. The Egyptians were using it almost 4,000 years ago. Later on the Greeks and Romans widely employed it for a variety of applications. Lead has a lustrous silver-blue appearance when freshly cut. But it quickly darkens upon exposure to moist air due to the rapid formation of an oxide film. This film, by the way, protects the metal from further oxidation or corrosion.

All lead compounds known to man are inherently poisonous! This is because the human body, in effect, always mistakes it for calcium, and stores the majority of it in the bones where it can literally remain for a lifetime. Lead in the bloodstream attaches to and disrupts enzymes essential to functioning of the brain and other cells. And since lead is an element, it never decomposes into another, more easily tolerated substance.

But in spite of the obvious health risks known to ancient people, they still enjoyed using this dangerous metal for many different purposes. The translation of one of the world's oldest surviving medical papyri, *The Papyrus Ebers: The Great Egyptian Medical Document* (Copenhagen: 1937) by B. Ebbell made available for the very first time valuable data on the wonderful variety of Egyptian medicines and drugs. Both plants and minerals were often compounded together in prescriptions.

One formula called for galena, the most important native ore from which the Egyptians obtained lead, and carbon—referred to euphemistically as "wall soot" and scraped from above Egyptian fireplaces. They were mixed with a generous amount of goose fat and then compounded into the eye makeup that gave Egyptian women that striking, almond-shaped expression frequently seen by archaeologists in wall drawings inside the royal tombs of long-deceased pharaohs.

Hippocrates (460-380 B.C.), the purported "father of modern medicine," borrowed many things from the Egyptians himself. He expanded the use of lead beyond mere cosmetic purposes, employing it frequently as a wound dressing. Following the actual operation, the Greek *iatros* or surgeon would take a clean pad of wool and dip it into a solution known as *enaimon* (usually anglicized as *enheme*). Some excess liquid would be gently squeezed out before the material was laid directly over the incision and tightly bound in place. The *enheme* or "drugs for fresh wounds" consisted of equal parts of *verdigris* (copper acetate), *flower of copper* (copper oxide), *molybdaina* (lead oxide), roasted Egyptian alum, myrrh, frankincense, gall nuts, vine flowers, and wool grease diluted in an unspecified amount of wine.

As a wound drug, this medicated wine was probably better than nothing at all. The four inorganic salts (including lead) probably stung a bit but also helped to kill any bacteria within reach. Myrrh and frankincense, two of the gifts brought to the baby Jesus by the Three Wise Men of the New Testament, would add a touch of perfume to the proceeding and join the fight against bacteria. No harm was likely to come of the gall nuts and vine flowers. The only dubious ingredient was the grease of wool, essentially a crude form of lanolin smelling strongly of sheep and probably not too hygienic either. But the Greeks seemed to love its texture, smell, and taste.

Sometimes the *enhemes* were in the form of dry powders intended to be sprinkled directly over the wound. They could be washed off later on with vinegar or wine. Here are four that were used to prevent suppuration: lead oxide; lead oxide powdered with zinc oxide; black-copper oxide and copper sulphate; and alum, of course. These powders were crude antiseptics, in that they killed bacteria at the price of destroying tissue cells also (not to mention the danger of inflicting lead poisoning down the road)

Lead Poisoning in History

The Romans really got carried away with lead, in a big way! Not only did they utilize it more often in their medical practices, but the stuff showed up in their food and beverages as well. For flesh wounds sustained in battle, Roman soldiers were treated with an interesting composition called barbarum. Here is the formula given in metric equivalents:

copper acetate	48 grams			
lead oxide	80 grams		oil	250 cc
alum	4 grams	*mix with*		
dried pitch	4 grams		vinegar	250 cc
dried pitch resin	4 grams			

When mixed together in a testing laboratory, these ingredients yielded a murky, brownish lotion. It was quite evident that barbarum was an effective, though highly dangerous, antiseptic.

Cornelius Celsus was one of three great Roman authors (the other two being Varro and Pliny) who wrote encyclopedias about fifty years apart. It is apparent from reading his work that Celsus was something of a doctor himself, for he appears to have known a great deal about the medicine of his day. He prescribed numerous antiseptics for treating wounds; almost all of them contained heavy doses of lead and copper salts. In many of these formulas, the doses of toxic mineral salts were quite generous, making up 1/2 to 2/3 of the mixture. An example: equal parts of lead acetate (*cerussa*), lead oxide (*litharge*), and antimony sulphide (*stibium*) combined with wax and suet.

Through the written observations of Celsus, we have recorded for the first time in ancient history some of the potential symptoms usually associated with lead poisoning. He noted that many of the wounded soldiers treated with his antiseptic formulas would afterward show signs of unexplained fatigue, mysterious muscle paralysis, unexpected abdominal cramps and pains, occasional convulsions and shakes, and sometimes sudden comas. Not knowing what these strange symptoms were due to, he called what was presumed to have been a mystery ailment *saturninus,* after Saturn, the Roman god of harvests.

For almost a week every year, beginning on December 17th, Rome would basically shut down as the equivalent of a New Orleans Mardi Gras commenced. At this festival, the Saturnalia, gifts were exchanged, schools and courts were closed, war was outlawed, and slaves and masters ate at the same table together for a change. All manner of debauchery was indulged in: drunkenness (and with it the stupor of thought and stumbling gait); excess gluttony (and the accompanying stomach spasms, nausea, and vomiting); and extreme and often violent promiscuity (leading to periodic heart attacks, great physical weakness, and incredible groin pain, in men especially). An interesting historical sidelight to the Saturnalia: The Christmas holiday celebrated by hundreds of millions of Christians around the world has its roots in this pagan celebration!

On other special holiday occasions similar to the Saturnalia (but not quite as elaborate), Celsus reported seeing the same symptoms, though in lesser numbers. If only he could have made the connection with what he wrote elsewhere in his *De medicina:* Romans drank water from lead plumbing; they definitely sipped it with their wine; a wine preservative was made with *must,* which was boiled in leaden vessels; and Roman courtesans (high-priced prostitutes) smeared lead-white on their faces and dusted it onto their hair in order to make themselves more attractive to the men. He was witnessing classic cases of lead poisoning yet never knowing exactly what to attribute the strange medical behavior to.

As weird as it may seem, the decline of the Roman Empire can be directly blamed on lead poisoning! So declared Dr. Jerome O. Nriagu, a Canadian scientist, in an interview with a newspaper reporter that was published in the *New York Times* (March 17, 1983; p. A-19). By carefully reviewing the personalities and habits of Roman emperors from 30 B.C. to 220 A.D., he discovered that fully two-thirds of them, including crazy emperors like Claudius, Caligula, and Nero, "had a predilection to lead-tainted diets and suffered from gout and other symptoms of *chronic lead poisoning.*"

"The coexistence of widespread plumbism and gout during the Roman Empire," he declared, "seems to have been an important feature of the aristocratic lifestyle that has not been previously recognized. This provides strong support . . . that lead poisoning [led] to the decline of the Roman Empire."

In the same newspaper there was published in the May 31, 1983 edition (pp. A-1; C-3) another story to support Nriagu's research. Dr. Sara C. Bisel, a classical archaeologist and physical anthropologist from Rochester, Minnesota, reported finding strong evidence of lead poisoning in Roman skeletons killed during the powerful eruption of Mount Vesuvius in 79 A.D. She told a packed lecture hall at the annual meeting of the American Association for the Advancement of Science that a chemical analysis of the bones of these once apparently healthy and well-nourished people showed that most of them had suffered *chronic* lead poisoning, and never even knew about it! She and her coworkers made the discovery of the skeletons at the Mediterranean seacoast town of Herculaneum in Italy.

Dr. Bisel examined the bones of 55 victims in all—30 adult males, 13 adult females, and 12 children. She found in her analysis that the bones contained a mean level of 84 parts of lead per million, which she concluded was "significantly high." In contrast, the bones of some prehistoric people discovered in a Greek cave contained just 3 parts per million of lead. She drew parallels between these high Roman skeletal lead counts and those measured in the bones of modern Americans and Britons, which averaged between 20 to 50 parts per million. Most of the adults she studied ranged in age from 30 to 45, with none more than 50 years old. One woman, about 24 years of age, was pregnant, carrying a 7-month-old fetus at the time the volcanic ash and terrific heat killed her.

More recent evidence, given at the First Joint Archaeological Congress held in Baltimore during the latter part of January 1989, revealed that modern Americans and Britons had *1,000 times* more lead in their bones than did people who lived a millennium ago. University of California (Irvine) anthropologist Jonathon E. Ericson and his colleagues used meticulous laboratory techniques to gauge their measurements. They collected bones after autopsies of modern-day residents of the U. S. and England and then compared lead levels with those in the bones and teeth of ancient Incans living 1,600 years ago, and with the coastal Chumash villagers near Malibu, California and the Arizona Anasazi Indians, both of whom lived around 1000 A.D. In all three examples, the lead content of these ancient remains was much lower.

Skeletal remains are always a good indicator of just how much lead individuals accumulated within their bodies. Up to 95 percent of this toxic metal is stored there and stays in place for literally many centuries.

Lead poisoning continued for a number of centuries after the fall of the Roman Empire, but e x p a n de d on a much larger scale with the advent of the Industrial Revolution. Pewter was the chief tableware in England (the pewter center from the Middle Ages onward) and in colonial North America. Pewter was made from tin, lead, antimony, copper, bismuth, and zinc. Italy, Germany, and France also favored it, but not as much as the Brits or Yankees did. Invariably, lead would leach from the pewterware into whatever food was placed on or in it. Many of the bizarre moods and strange behaviors attributed to a number of government and religious leaders during that period can definitely be linked to lead poisoning from pewter dishes and goblets.

But lead could enter the body in other ways as well. Take the lead poisoning of the great Spanish painter Francisco José de Goya y Lucientes (1746-1828), otherwise known as Goya. Art historians have always wondered about his sudden change in art style, moving from pleasant court portraitures to intensely grotesque social commentaries. His mysterious mental illness was caused by the large quantities of white paint made from lead carbonate that he preferred using in his masterpieces. Lead carbonate will seep through intact skin and also give off noxious vapors. As a result of consistent and prolonged periods of exposure to a toxic lead compound, Goya absorbed enough lead into his bloodstream to produce permanent brain damage. A New York City psychiatrist, William Niederland, M.D., who profiled Goya's illness in detail, noted that all of the artist's symptoms—vertigo, mental confusion, hallucinations, and impaired balance, hearing, and speech—are characteristic of fulminating lead encephalopathy.

Samuel Hahnemann, an itinerant German doctor and chemist, devised the system of medicine that became known as homeopathy. It caught on in the 1790s and eventually became one of the most popular alternative forms of healing in the nineteenth and twentieth centuries in Europe, Scandinavia, Asia, and the Americas. One of the most common homeopathic remedies is Plumbum metallicum, which is nothing more than lead acetate or lead carbonate. While undoubtedly proving to be somewhat useful for those suffering from arteriosclerosis, typical side effects that can be expected from this drug include a slowing down of brain activity, some memory loss, and difficulty with perception.

The invention of tinned food in the year 1810 soon became a major contributing factor of lead poisoning worldwide, but in such a subtle manner that no one really knew what to look for when bizarre actions set in. One of the most tragic instances of lead poisoning involved the fateful 1845 voyage of Sir John Franklin and his men, who were looking for the Northwest Passage. A study of the bones of all 129 of Franklin's sailors found on Canada's King William Island and of the bodies of 3 others found on Beechey Island shows that their remains contained higher than normal levels of lead. The chemical composition of lead varies according to its source. The study showed that the lead found in the skeletons came from a single source and that it matched lead in the solder used to seal food tins found in a Beechey Island cache.

Owen Beattie, an anthropologist at the University of Alberta, participated in the study and called my attention to it recently. He noted that if the lead didn't kill all those men, it surely affected their judgment, leading to poor decisions that ultimately contributed to their deaths. I speculated that similar tragedies involving large groups of individuals probably occurred within the last 175 years due to tinned food., but no one until now has made the connection. He ceded my point.

Lead Poisoning Today

Over the years the Anthropological Research Center in Salt Lake City has collected a great deal of published information regarding lead poisoning. Much of it, however, is contemporary and shows in explicit detail that the generations of our grandparents, parents, ourselves, and our children are all victims of lead poisoning to some degree. When I undertook to include this particular mineral entry, I didn't want to spend a lot of time delineating the matter in terms of the modern world we live in. Instead I opted for a very different focus that would take the reader almost back to the beginning of civilization and then bring him or her forward through time. This has been my chief purpose here.

There have been dozens of major reports on the topic of lead poisoning that have appeared in the 1980s and 1990s in a wide range of publications. Some of the better ones are referenced below for the reader's own perusal:

"Eliminating the lead in your tap water . . . and in your pottery." *University of California, Berkeley Wellness Letter* (April 1987), pp. 1-2.

"A Lead-Laden World?" *Awake* magazine (August 8, 1990), pp. 26-27.

"Lead and Your Kids." *Newsweek* magazine (July 15, 1991), pp. 42-48.

"Lead & the Issues Involved." *ECON* (March 1992), pp. 10-31;42-57.

"Water risk in 130 cities: Lead." *USA Today* (October 21, 1992), pp. A-1; A-13.

Collectively, these and similar reports discuss the `inherent dangers of lead and potential sources for it: drinking water, glazed ceramicware and pottery, painted walls, batteries for cars and trucks, flashlights, and some battery-powered toys, brass objects, gun firing ranges, clay flower pots, soldering and welding, manufacturing of steel and other metals, mining, some prescription and over-the-counter (OTC) drugs including a number of ointments, salves, and lotions, talcum and baby powder, restaurant food cooked in heavy aluminum pots and pans (that have lead mixed in with the aluminum), wine drunk from crystal goblets and brandy stored in expensive decanters, the printing on plastic bags, packaged folk medicines imported from Taiwan, Hong Kong, and Mexico, hair coloring formulas to remove grayness, stomach antacids, roll-on antiperspirants, city smog, and many others too numerous to mention. In a word, *we have become inundated with lead* to an unbelievable extent!

Little wonder then that hundreds of articles keep popping up all the time in newspapers, popular magazines, and medical and scientific journals informing us of *other* health problems connected with lead poisoning that we didn't know about before:

- sociopathic and psychotic violence
  (*Salt Lake Tribune,* July 31, 1983, p. A-2)

- hearing difficulty and maintaining physical balance
  (*Science News* 135:54, January 28, 1989)

- disturbance in the menstrual cycle, sterility, miscarriage, premature birth, and birth defects
  (*Science News* 136:373, December 9, 1989)

- lowering of mental intelligence or brain I.Q.
  (*Salt Lake Tribune,* October 30, 1992, p. A-24)

- some autoimmune disorders
  (*Environmental Health Perspectives,* December 1994)

- essential hypertension of unknown origin (which affects an estimated 48 million people in America alone)
  (*Science News* 149:382-83; June 15, 1996)

Ways to Neutralize the Lead in Your Body

It was mentioned earlier that approximately 95 percent of all lead absorbed into the body orally or through the skin is permanently stored in the bones. Only about 5 percent manages to float around in the circulating blood plasma; but this small amount can do significant damage to the brain and nervous system. Therefore, it behooves us to have it removed as soon as we can before further damage is done. By understanding these two points clearly, we can successfully tackle the twin problems of how to neutralize what we already have in our skeletal structures and getting rid of the rest that's freely moving around inside us.

Lead can virtually be sealed into bones permanently without risk of ever leaking by making absolutely sure that your body receives an adequate *daily* intake of those few minerals known to *harden* the bones: boron, calcium, and magnesium. (Consult each of these individual mineral entries for further information as to suggested supplemental dosages and likely food sources.)

Boron can be obtained in the food supply by frequently eating vegetables like celery, cauliflower, turnips, rutabagas, potatoes (with the skin intact), and beets. Beets can also be juiced with their fiber intact in a food blender, but they need to be lightly cooked first. In fact, a food blender is essential to making the following juice recipes that are very high in boron content. (See Product Appendix, p. 383.)

RED CABBAGE AND BEET BEVERAGE

1/4 cup cranberry juice

1/4 cup apple juice or cider

1/2 cup red cabbage, steamed until tender

1/2 cup canned beets, with 1 tbsp. beet juice

1/4 teaspoon tarragon vinegar

1/2 cup ice cubes

Place all ingredients in the food blender. Secure the lid in place. Run on high speed for 1 1/2 minutes or until smooth. Serve cold or else heat on the stove for a couple of minutes to make a warm drink. Makes 1 1/4 cups. (See Product Appendix, p. 383.)

BEETS WITH BERRY MEDLEY

3/4 cup cold cranberry juice

1/4 cup whole cranberry sauce or fresh cranberries

1 small beet, steamed

1/4 cup fresh or 1/3 cup frozen strawberries

2 teaspoons honey for flavor

2/3 cup ice cubes

Place all ingredients in the food blender. Secure the lid in place and run on high speed for approximately one minute or until smooth. Makes 1 2/3 cups.

You can also make a refreshing beet juice drink in an instant by placing one teaspoon of beet juice powder in an empty 8 oz. glass, filling it with warm water almost to the top, and then stirring thoroughly with a spoon. (See Product Appendix, p. 381.)

Certain medicinal herbs also have a respectable boron content. They include alfalfa, cleavers (also known as bedstraw or couch-grass), milk thistle, stinging nettle, sassafras, and wintergreen. They can be taken in capsule form or as a tea. Except for alfalfa, no more than two or three capsules or one cup of tea of the others should be taken in one day. However, since alfalfa is so nutritious and good for you, a person can take up to six capsules a day or drink two cups of the tea without any problems.

There will be sufficient boron in these different vegetables and herbs to help toughen the bones. An additional hardening agent, which I didn't mention with boron, calcium, or magnesium, is strontium. There are *no* known supplements containing enough of this trace element to do an adequate job of bone hardening. But by periodically snacking on *whole* nuts and seeds, eating fresh- or salt-water fish pretty regularly, and using granulated kelp to season your food (or else taking kelp tablets), you will take in sufficient strontium.

The importance of both boron and, to a lesser extent, strontium in the bone hardening process cannot be overstated. My own research work as an anthropologist with prehistoric bones taught me a long time ago the value of both minerals in maintaining super-strong skeletal structures, such as the Neanderthals were widely noted for. Often, though, too much emphasis is placed on more common minerals such as calcium and magnesium, thereby crowding out minor trace elements like boron and strontium which in their own way play as important a role as the others do.

The other two minerals associated with bone strength are calcium and magnesium, of course. But they are intended more for the actual composition of bones than their hardness. It is very important that older people, especially women who've entered menopause, make sure they have an adequate intake of both minerals *every day.* If they don't they run the risk of developing osteoporosis, which in turn can lead to lead poisoning.

Here's how the scenario plays itself out, according to an article, "Bone-lead climbs as old bones decline," which was published in *Science News* (135:181; March 25, 1989). When mineral depletion sets in there is some loss of phosphorus, but a much greater loss of calcium. The wrists, hips, and vertebrae in the spine are the most common sites for this to happen. The lead that has been stored in these areas of the skeletal frame for decades is suddenly released "in potentially toxic amounts," the report noted. This type of unexpected but very dramatic lead poisoning occurs three times more frequently in white women than in African American women.

The most reasonable solution, it seems, is for a woman in or past menopause to make sure she gets enough Calcium and magnesium every day. But, as I pointed out earlier under the Calcium entry, the ratio should always be 2:1—that is, for every 2 milligrams of magnesium consumed, there should be just one milligram of calcium. This is in reverse order to what nutritional science suggests and certainly contradicts everything that has been written about the higher calcium-lower magnesium intake. But I've based my conclusions on the solid science of physical anthropology: analyses of prehistoric human bones nearly always have shown a *greater* magnesium and *lower* calcium content. The way to look at magnesium is as more of a hardening agent and calcium as needed for bone composition itself. Women who've followed this counsel have noticed definite reversals of their existing osteoporosis or else strong protection from its ever occurring.

Two products that I highly recommend older women use in order to keep their bones healthy and strong are calcium and magnesium supplements (see Product Appendix, pages 382–83). Tablets of these supplements taken with a meal can provide 400 to 800 milligrams *each* of calcium and magnesium, along with 2.5 mg. of boron and 60 mg. of phosphorus (two other bone-hardening minerals). Calculate the correct number of tablets to take so that you receive twice as many milligrams of magnesium over calcium, thereby giving you that desirable 2:1 ratio I was speaking about before. Since these minerals are ionic, meaning that they are charged and in a form the body easily recognizes, they are more quickly absorbed with very minimal loss.

In addition to this, I've included some more drink recipes that mention the specific amounts of calcium and magnesium to be found in each of them. These can all be made using a food blender that retains the fiber. (See Product Appendix, p. 383.)

Before launching into the recipes, I should mention, though, that the calcium-magnesium ratios in each of them is going to be more in favor of the former and less so for the latter. This is primarily due to the fact that the recipes contain dairy products such as yogurt and buttermilk, which are high in calcium to begin with. But the small problem of getting more calcium than magnesium can be easily solved by crushing in advance six tablets of a magnesium product and adding this powder to each drink recipe before blending begins. This way a person will be sure of getting a *true* 2:1 magnesium-over-calcium ratio as I've previously recommended.

Good Morning Shake

1 nectarine, quartered and pitted

1 cup plain low-fat yogurt

1/4 cup orange juice

2 tablespoons wheat germ

1 teaspoon honey

1/2 cup ice cubes

Place everything in a food blender, secure the lid, and mix well for 1 1/2 minutes or until contents have a smooth consistency. Yields 1 3/4 cups.

CALCIUM 434 mg.   *MAGNESIUM 92 mg.*

Cereal-in-a-Glass Shake

1 cup plain low-fat yogurt

1 medium-sized banana, peeled, frozen, and cut into chunks

1/4 cup dark raisins

1/4 cup coarsely chopped unpeeled apple

1 tablespoon wheat bran

Place everything in a food blender, secure the lid, and blend thoroughly on high speed for 1 minute or until smooth. Yields approximately 1 3/4 cups. (See Product Appendix, p. 383.)

CALCIUM 445 mg.   *MAGNESIUM 109 mg.*

KUKUMBER KOOLER

1 cup buttermilk

1 two-inch cucumber section, peeled and cut into chunks

1 medium-size banana, peeled and cut into chunks

4 sprigs of peppermint

1/4 cup ice cubes

Place everything in a food blender, secure the lid in place, and mix on high speed for 45 seconds until contents are creamy. Yields 1 1/2 cups.

CALCIUM 308 mg.   MAGNESIUM 68 mg.

BUGS BUNNY SHAKE

This shake is named after the famous Warner Brothers' cartoon character, Bugs Bunny, on account of it containing carrots, which, according to Elmer Fudd, the cartoon character most annoyed by Bugs, "Dat wabbit pwobabwe stwole fwum my gwaden!"

2/3 cup carrot juice

1/2 cup low-fat vanilla yogurt

1 medium-sized banana, peeled and cut into chunks

1/4 teaspoon vanilla extract

1/4 cup ice cubes

Put everything in a food blender, secure the lid, and mix on high speed for 45 seconds until contents are creamy. Yields about 1 cup. (See Product Appendix, p. 383.)

CALCIUM 241 mg.   MAGNESIUM 75 mg.

Drinks and soups are the quickest and easiest way for someone to get calcium and magnesium in a hurry. Between such liquids foods and the two supplements previously mentioned, there will be ample amounts of both minerals to keep lead locked up in the bones for the rest of a person's life.

Getting the Lead Out (of Your Blood, That Is)

Having learned some clever ways of permanently locking up lead accumulations in your bones for an entire lifetime, we now turn our attention to the second matter mentioned in the beginning of the last subsection. While a 5 percent lead content freely moving around in your circulatory system might seem like a small amount, yet it packs a pretty big wallop in terms of the health damage it can do to your brain, nerves, and kidneys.

Over the years I've discovered some herbs—all of them taken as teas—that are very capable of *pulling* this free lead out of your bloodstream for good. Since lead is a stubborn mineral to get rid of, a two-pronged approach must be used in attacking this dilemma. Certain herbs high in calcium and magnesium need to be consumed in *capsules* an hour *before* drinking any of the designated teas that will flush this nasty mineral out of the body.

The idea here is to have adequate plant minerals introduced ahead of the tea, so that they can bind themselves to the free-floating lead particles and make it easier for them to be evacuated with the liquids later on. Making the tea is quite simple. If the plant materials are root, bark, stalk, or seed, then they need to be *simmered* for five minutes followed by steeping. On the other hand, if they're more delicate materials such as flowers or leaves, they can be immediately steeped for 20 minutes *without* simmering them first. Once the tea is lukewarm, it can be strained and drunk, always on an empty stomach.

Herbal Beverages for Removing Lead from the Bloodstream

Herb	Quantity	Boiling Water
Burdock root	11/2 tbsps.	1 1/2 pints
Celery seeds	1 tsp.	1 pint
Comfrey leaf	2 tbsps.	1 1/4 pints
Dill seed	1 1/2 tsps.	1 pint
Fennel seed	1 tsp.	1/2 pint
Flax seed	1 tbsp.	1 1/2 pints

Ginseng root*	1 tbsp.	1 1/2 pints
Horseradish root*	1 tsp. (grated)	1 pint apple cider vinegar
Lavender flower/leaf	1 1/2 tbsps.	2 pints
Lovage rootstock	1 tsp.	1 pint
Mormon/Brigham tea or Ephedra herb	2 tbsps.	1 pint
Nettle plant*	3 tbsps.	1 pint
Parsley plant*	1 1/2 tbsps.	1 pint
Peppermint leaf*	2 tbsps.	1 1/4 pints
Sarsaparilla rootstock*	2 tsps.	1 pint
Sassafras bark	2 tsps.	1 pint
Sorrel plant*	1 tsp.	1 1/2 pints
Watercress leaf/shoot	2 tsp.	1/2 pint

Encapsulated Herbs High in Calcium and Magnesium

Acerola	Fenugreek	Red clover
Alfalfa	Fo-ti	Savory
Borage	Ganoderma	Slippery elm
Chervil	Hawthorn	Stinging nettle
Dandelion	Kava kava	Watercress

This course of treatment should be consistently followed for six weeks and then discontinued for two to three weeks before recommencing for another identical period of time, but *only if necessary!*

Magnesium
THE MINERAL SURPRISE THAT'S GOING TO HELP YOU A LOT

A Deficiency of Historic Proportions

In a lengthy article devoted exclusively to magnesium in her "Personal Health" column in *The New York Times* (January 15, 1992, p. B-8), writer Jane E. Brody observed that this mineral "has been all but ignored by nutrition enthusiasts who tout an alphabet-soup of supplements to correct purported deficiencies, to counter various ailments and to enhance overall health." The chief reasons for magnesium having been such an overlooked and underutilized mineral for so long is that it "was not considered to play a role in nutritional problems nor was it regarded as a 'sexy' nutrient."

"Researchers have found that magnesium deficiencies may be far more common than doctors" ever realized. "Many doctors are unfamiliar with the effects of magnesium deficiency and few patients are ever tested for it," Brody wrote. Even when tests are run, she added, they "nearly always measure magnesium levels in blood and may not reflect the amounts found in muscle cells, bone and other tissues in which the mineral plays crucial roles."

Burton Altura, Ph.D., a professor of physiology and medicine at the State University of New York Health Science Center at Brooklyn, was quoted in the July-August 1996 edition of *Alternative & Complementary Therapies* (vol:218) as believing "that 75 percent of people in the Western world are magnesium deficient"—falling way short of the 350 mg. RDA for men and the 280 mg. RDA for women. According to Jane Brody, "National food consumption studies have shown that most Americans, with the exception of preschool children, do not consume the recommended amount[s]."

In the early 1990s, Dr. Robert Whang of the University of Oklahoma Health Sciences Center studied over 1,000 hospitalized patients who had been tested for abnormalities in their blood chemicals. He discovered, to his astonishment, that 49 percent of them had abnormally low blood levels of magnesium. More amazing still was the fact that only a mere 10 percent of these abnormalities had been detected by tests ordered by the patients' different physicians.

Brody commented in her article, "Such shortages can compromise a patient's chances for survival." A Baltimore study of 199 people with congestive heart failure, for example, showed that 1 in 5 patients who had low magnesium levels would not survive beyond 1 year, as compared with other patients with the same disease but with normal levels of this mineral. In another study, among 193 patients in the intensive care unit after surgery, a full 61 percent had low magnesium levels in the blood and the postoperative death rate was three times higher, 41 percent, among them than among patients on other floors.

A Very Delicate Role

Magnesium is responsible for many different bodily functions. But the only one I intend to cite here is probably its most important role of all. In fact, this mineral occupies a very delicate role at a cellular level, with our overall health hanging in the balance.

Magnesium's greatest function is as the *prime regulator* of calcium flow within cells. It is this delicate collaboration that is the major determinant of the rate at which each of our cellular flames burns. Put another way, magnesium enters into a special partnership with calcium in the production of the very gem of biologic energy, adenosine triphosphate (ATP). Without ATP, living cells run short of the basic "energy currency" they need to function properly.

ATP fuels *everything* we do. This vital molecule is created within mitochondria, the extremely tiny, sausage-shaped "energy factories" that exist inside living cells. Magnesium controls the gateway through which calcium must enter into cells to make sufficient ATP for a host of vital functions, such as the heartbeat, for instance.

According to geneticists from Emery University in Atlanta whom I spoke with by telephone, *magnesium deficiency is the prime culprit* in cellular energy shortages. Furthermore, they said, *this is the common link* among many different diseases affecting the brain, heart, muscles, and other organs of the body. Restore magnesium to the body in ample amounts, they declared, and "a whole host of seemingly unrelated problems suddenly begin to clear up."

Do You Have a "Hidden" Magnesium Deficiency?

Chances are that whoever is reading these words right now probably suffers from some degree of magnesium shortage. If you're a man older than 20 and haven't been getting at least 350 mg. every single day, then rest assured that your magnesium levels aren't much to brag about. If you're a woman over the age of 50 and haven't been getting 300 mg. daily or a woman who is pregnant or nursing and not taking 450 mg. during these periods, then your magnesium count is probably too low.

Another way to tell if you're deficient is to look for some of the general physical characteristics: muscle weakness, muscle twitches and tremors, irregular heart beat, insomnia, leg cramps, restless or jumpy legs, slightly shaky hands, slight, involuntary nodding of the head, eye flutters, or any other *little* body tic or twitch that is *occasional* and pretty much escapes notice.

Deficiencies are most common among people with prolonged cases of diarrhea, kidney disease, obesity, diabetes, epilepsy, or alcoholism and in those who take diuretics to lower their blood pressure. These conditions and medications put people at risk for developing magnesium deficiencies.

Beside these problems, I've arranged a short alphabetized list of some other common maladies that have been helped considerably with the addition of supplemented magnesium. I've included my reference sources as well for those wishing to investigate matters further at their leisure.

Angina. Swiss research shows six months' magnesium supplementation decreased attacks of severe chest pain in people diagnosed with coronary heart disease. (*Natural Health,* vol:26, Sep.-Oct. 1995.)

Atherosclerosis. Slightly high magnesium intake can prevent cholesterol-clogging of heart arteries. (*Science News,* 137:214, April 7, 1990.)

Asthma. Researchers from the University of Nottingham (England) found that high dietary magnesium improved lung function and greatly reduced the risk of wheezing in asthma attacks. (*Natural Health,* vol:26, Sep.-Oct. 1995.)

Autism. French psychiatrists noticed definite clinical improvement in autistic children given a nutritional combination of vitamin B-6 (30 mg/kg up to 1 gram) and magnesium (10-15 mg/kg) daily. (*Biological Psychiatry,* 20:467-78, May 1985.)

Cardiovascular Disease. Researchers concluded that 615 men of Japanese ancestry residing in Hawaii had no history of cardiovascular disease or essential hypertension because their daily intakes of dietary magnesium were extremely high. (*American Journal of Clinical Nutrition,* 45:469-75, 1987.)

Cerebral Palsy. Researchers at the Centers for Disease Control and Prevention in Atlanta concluded that giving pregnant women magnesium sulphate may significantly reduce the incidence of cerebral palsy in premature infants weighing less than 3.3 pounds. (*Journal of the American Medical Association,* 276:1805-10, Dec. 11, 1996.)

Chemical Intolerance. Individuals who suffer from chemical hypersensitivity or are unable to tolerate their surrounding environments suffer from severe magnesium deficiencies. (*Clinical Ecology,* 4:17-20, Jan.-Mar. 1986.)

Crohn's Disease. Of 25 patients hospitalized with severe inflammatory disease, 84 percent had evidence of magnesium deficiency when measured for content of this particular mineral. (*Journal of the American College of Nutrition,* 4:553-58, Sept.-Oct. 1985.)

Congestive Heart Failure. Those suffering from this disease invariably have low levels of magnesium. (Brody article in *New York Times,* previously cited.)

Diabetes. Magnesium (260 mg. daily) eases diabetic blood pressure. Administration of magnesium to patients with type-2 diabetes reduced their insulin resistance considerably. (*Science News,* 138:189, September 22, 1990; and *Therapie,* 49:1-7, 1994.)

Excitability. Those who become emotionally reactive and highly excitable over mundane matters show decreased levels of magnesium in their cerebrospinal fluids. (*Pharmacology Biochemistry & Behavior,* 5:529-34, 1976.)

Heart Attacks. At the Royal Leicester Infirmary in England, 2,316 patients admitted to the coronary care unit were given either intravenous magnesium or a placebo. Heart attacks were ultimately diagnosed in 65 percent of these patients. After a month the death rate was a mere 8 percent among those given magnesium, but much higher in those receiving only the placebo. (*Lancet,* 2:1553-58, June 27, 1992.)

Hypertension. High blood pressure was prevented in rats that had been treated to initiate salt-induced hypertension. All it took was spiking the rats' drinking water with 4 to 8 times their RDA of magnesium. (*Science News,* 133:356, June 4, 1988.)

Hyperventilation. German scientists determined that hyperventilation is the result of low magnesium and elevated calcium levels rather than being a neurosis, as many doctors are inclined to imagine. (*Magnesium,* 4:129-136, Mar.-Jun. 1985.)

Migraines. Alexander Mauskop, M.D., director of the New York Headache Center in Manhattan, made the remarkable discovery some time ago that *ionized* magnesium, the biologically active form of this mineral, was much better in treating food-allergy-induced migraine headaches than regular magnesium in patients with low magnesium concentrations. (*Alternative & Complementary Therapies,* vol:217, Jul.-Aug. 1996.)

Premenstrual Syndrome (PMS). Women afflicted with PMS received measurable relief from their symptoms of anxiety, irritability, mood swings, breast tenderness, fatigue, and headache when they increased their dietary and supplemental intakes of both magnesium and zinc, as well as taking a multipurpose vitamin formula. (Sheldon Saul Hendler, M.D., Ph.D., *The Doctors' Vitamin and Mineral Encyclopedia.* New York: Simon & Schuster, 1990; p. 160.)

Radiation. Twenty patients at the Lady Davis Carmel Hospital in Haifa, Israel received radiation treatments for three to six weeks for their cervical carcinomas. Following the treatment, all developed radiation-induced proctosigmoiditis (inflammation of the rectum and sigmoid) and were hospitalized after a couple of days of severe diarrhea. Ten patients were treated conventionally with a low-residue diet and loperamide (sold in the U.S. under the brand name of Imodium A-D); their diarrhea cleared up in two to six weeks. The other ten were given 50 mEq of magnesium in the form of magnesium sulphate daily by i.v. infusion over ten hours; their diarrhea disappeared in just three days. Radiation dramatically decreases serum magnesium; pretreatment with a slow-release magnesium supplement is highly advisable for cancer patients undergoing irradiation. (*Magnesium,* 4:16-19, Jan.-Feb. 1985.)

Restlessness. My colleague and longtime friend, Lendon Smith, M.D., made this observation on Salt Lake City's KUTV Channel 2 "Noon News " on May 18, 1979: "Magnesium deficiency in kids causes them to be itchy, restless, jumpy, nervous, sassy, temperamental—the usual to be expected in most of them. But as a pediatrician, I've always favored giving them 150 to 200 mg. of magnesium a day, which calms them down and makes them tolerable to be around again. I also prescribe 150 mg. of magnesium each night for Moms to give their young children to prevent bedwetting. You'd be surprised how much this helps."

Stress. Daily magnesium intake enables the body to cope better with physiological stress; this is especially true for women. (*Science News,* 151:279, May 3, 1997.)

Suicide. Of 41 unmedicated psychiatric patients, 11 women who attempted suicide had significantly lower cerebrospinal fluid levels of magnesium than did nonsuicidal patients and controls. Magnesium is essential to maintain normal serotonergic activity in the central nervous system. When supplemented with ample magnesium, these same 11 women reported feeling no further urge to take their lives. (*Biological Psychiatry,* 20:163-71, February 1985.)

Available Sources

Tiny amounts of magnesium are to be found in many different kinds of foods. But the greatest concentrations of this mineral occur in nuts (especially almonds, cashews, and peanuts), in dried beans like soybeans, in lentils, in seeds such as sunflower and pumpkin, in whole grains (rye, millet, and barley especially), and in seafood (canned tuna, canned salmon, canned mackerel, shrimp, and lobster). To a lesser extent, it may be found in raw, leafy green vegetables and fermented tofu.

Common over-the-counter products widely available in drugstores everywhere contain magnesium salts: milk of magnesia, the antacid magnesium hydroxide, and magnesium sulfate (Epsom salts). While helpful for relieving constipation, they are not the best way to obtain your daily magnesium but ionized magnesium products are available (see Product Appendix, pages 383–383, for more information).

Manganese
AN ELEMENTAL ENIGMA STILL BEING DEFINED

An Evolving Role

Manganese is one of the microminerals that has been with us since the 1960s. In 1966 the *Journal of Biological Chemistry* (241:3480) reported the first manganese metalloenzyme isolated from chicken liver. This was pyruvate carboxylase, a mitochondrial protein which is heavily dependent on the B-vitamin biotin and manganese for its existence.

Under the entry for Magnesium I discussed in some detail the role of the vital molecule, adenosine triphosphate or ATP, without which nothing in our bodies at a cellular level could run. In addition to magnesium, the trace element manganese is essential to complete a series of enzymatic reactions in bacteria that convert glucose to pyruvate by way of an intermediate agent, forming ATP. The binding of manganese with biotin to form pyruvate carboxylase is a part of this complex process.

The energy that fuels our bodies comes in two different ways: *respiration,* which is the exchange of molecular oxygen and carbon dioxide between the atmosphere and body cells to release free energy; and *glycolysis,* which involves the conversion of glucose to the simpler compounds lactate or pyruvate (that result in ATP) with the assistance of friendly bacterial organisms that survive without molecular oxygen.

The manganese-biotin-dependent enzyme pyruvate kinase is a crucial link in the enzymatic-driven process of glycolysis, the end products of which are ATP and pyruvate. Consequently, without adequate daily intake of dietary manganese, estimated to be between 5 and 7 milligrams, there will be disruptions in the smooth delivery of bacterial energy from the intestinal tract and liver.

A few years later scientists discovered yet another manganese enzyme produce by nonpathogenic (harmless) *E. coli* in the intestinal tract. This particular superoxide dismutase protects the cells against dangerous levels of the highly toxic free radical superoxide, which is generated by the reduction of molecular oxygen in many biological oxidative situations, Hence, another puzzling feature of manganese was unraveled, that of being a heretofore unknown antioxidant.

In the course of time and further research, other manganese-dependent enzymes have been discovered in the intestines, liver, pancreas, and spleen. These are involved in ATP production, in the metabolism of fatty acids, and in the synthesis of cholesterol. It can be said with definite certainty that manganese is an activator of enzymes (in which it serves as an enzyme cofactor) in numerous reactions but a constituent of an enzyme (or metalloenzyme) in only a few. More recently, manganese was found to be functioning in protein synthesis by stimulating RNA (ribonucleic acid) polymerase activity. (The synthesis of protein is directed by DNA, or deoxyribonucleic acid, located within the nucleus of the cell. From this "information center," specific genetic data is transcribed for protein synthesis, and carried forth by messenger RNAs.)

A group of doctors from Montreal Children's Hospital reported at a meeting of the American Chemical Society in August 1977 that epileptic children had only half as much manganese in their blood as was essential for good health. Their studies showed, in general, that children with convulsions had less manganese in their blood than did healthy children. They believed that by adding manganese-rich foods to the diets of these youngsters, epileptic seizures could be prevented.

Foods to Improve Your Mood

Nature has known all along what 's good for our bodies to consume and has judiciously placed within different foods that balanced mix of manganese, magnesium, and vitamin B-6 that can keep us happy, energetic, and anxiety-free. It should, therefore, come as no surprise that magnesium-rich foods are also manganese-containing foods, with appreciable amounts of pyridoxine thrown in for good measure.

Complex carbohydrates from whole grains and vegetables are the keys to improving your mood. Not only do such foods help with problems like schizophrenia and other personality disorders, but they also have a definite positive impact on hypoglycemia. Those afflicted with low blood sugar often are plagued with milder forms of mental illness, which can be easily corrected once their blood sugar levels are raised and their overzealous insulin productions are cut in half. They begin to feel and think better from emotional and mental perspectives. It's as if they've been suddenly freed from a dungeon of malnourishment in which they've been imprisoned for a long time due to low levels of manganese, magnesium, and vitamin B-6.

Breakfast is the single most important meal of the day for those wishing to regain their mental health and physical energy again. Cooked oatmeal with milk or a short stack of buckwheat pancakes with maple syrup or two whole wheat muffins spread with a tiny bit of sesame butter and blueberry jam are just a few of the complex carbohydrate meal possibilities for the morning.

Lunch is the second most important meal of the day for mentally ill patients, hypoglycemics, and yeast-infected people (particularly women) who wish to get well. A grilled ham and cheese sandwich on rye bread, a toasted tuna fish sandwich made on pumpernickel bread, a BLT (bacon-lettuce-tomato) minus the mayo on whole wheat or multigrained bread, a baked potato with its jacket, or a dish of pasta are some likely noontime scenarios.

Dinner should include some kind of tossed green salad and a cooked vegetable accompanied by a meat dish of your choice (preferably fish, game, beef, or some kind of poultry but not chicken or turkey since they cause cancer more readily). Desserts should be used very sparingly on account of their simple carbohydrates, which greatly disturb the manganese levels in the system.

Beverages high in manganese are green tea, instant coffee crystals, cocoa powder, and canned pineapple juice. These can be rotated, with the possible exception of the last one on account of its high natural sugar content.

Snacks are an absolute must and should be periodically munched or chewed on throughout the day in between the three regular meals. Peanuts (and peanut butter), pecans, walnuts (and other nuts), carrots, bran flakes (eaten straight out of the cereal box without milk), and, my favorite, shredded wheat (but with milk) are some possibilities.

Manganese supplements (40 mg. per capsule) are available, and some other supplements contain measurable amounts of this trace element as well. When soil is fertilized with a little manganese sulfate (1 gram to 15,000 grams of soil), the vitamin C content of vegetables like tomatoes practically doubles, as does their beta-carotene content!

Molybdenum
MINERAL DETOXIFIER EXTRAORDINAIRE

A Medical Mystery Unraveled

In the summer of 1980, I spent the months of July and August in the People's Republic of China in company with 29 medical students and 3 other faculty advisors. We were there on behalf of the American Medical Students' Association and as special guests of the Chinese government. Our purpose was to investigate their peculiar systems of healing utilizing herbal medicine, acupuncture, moxibustion, and simple diet, among other things. Aside from these, I had my own personal religious reason for going there as the following short narrative reveals.

After considerable bureaucratic hassling, I finally managed to obtain special permission (to everyone's astonishment) from the Minister of Culture, Office of Artifacts in Beijing, to depart from the rest of the medical group temporarily, and journey with a guide by train to the province of Shandong, located halfway between Beijing and Shanghai. We left Tianjin a little before midnight and arrived in Tai'an the next morning. This "City of Peace" sets at the foot of Mount T'ai Shan.

Early in the morning, my local guide Chou Yu-tsen and I climbed ancient China's most sacred mountain in a drenching downpour. For thousands of years Chinese writers have eulogized T'ai Shan as "the supreme mountain," surpassing all others in spiritual height and significance. This is where the legendary T'ai Shan, the son of the Emperor of Heaven, held court with China's mortal rulers and acted as a divinely appointed liaison between them and the god he served.

The ancient Chinese believed that the souls of those who died went to a hill at the foot of the peak. There T'ai Shan himself passed judgment on the good and evil a person had done in his or her life, in behalf of his father, the much-feared Emperor of Heaven. The expression "going to T'ai Shan" became a common euphemism for dying. As the peak of the east endowed with the power of dawn, the mountain was also regarded as the source and shaper of life. Through underlings occupying the maze of offices that made up his massive heavenly bureaucracy, T'ai Shan determined everything that would happen to a person—birth, position, honors, fortune, and death—according to the will of his father.

I came from this blissful experience back to the world of medical reality when I rejoined my group in Suzhou, which lays directly west of Shanghai some four hours by train ride. We visited the Chinese Traditional Medicine Hospital and spent the entire day there. Ding Huai-ren, the medical director of the acupuncture ward, and other hospital staff members drew our attention to a great nutritional discovery that is little known or seldom mentioned in the West.

For over 2,000 years the inhabitants of the Lin Xian region in Honan Province in northern China have suffered from the highest incidence of esophageal cancer anywhere in the world. In fact, we were told this is a common problem throughout much of China and responsible for nearly 20 percent of all cancer deaths. Now the esophagus is a muscular tube extending from the pharynx to the stomach which serves to transport ingested materials. The lining within the esophagus is scaly or plate-like except for the final portion of abdominal esophagus, which is lined with a columnar covering. Roughly 65 percent of esophageal cancers are of the squamous cell variety in that they attack this scaly lining.

For a long time the origin of the cancer problem of Lin Xian had baffled Chinese doctors. Not until soil scientists took samples of dirt in the area and had them analyzed in a laboratory was the cause finally determined—*an extreme lack of molybdenum*! In order for nitrates present in the soil to be reduced to nitrogenous substances (amines) necessary for plant nutrition, a molybdenum-activated enzyme called nitrate reductase (found in nitrogen-fixing bacteria) is needed. Molybdenum deficiency decreases the activity of this enzyme, and, instead of being converted to amines, the nitrates got transformed to nitrosamines, known as potent cancer-inducing agents.

The doctors at the hospital facility in Suzhou informed our group that the people of Lin Xian were also lacking in ascorbic acid, which has been demonstrated to convert deadly nitrosamines to more harmless forms, thereby offering some protection against them. Once the problem was fully comprehended, the Chinese government undertook to enrich the soils in Lin Xian with molybdenum and provide the residents there with supplemental vitamin C supplied from Europe. Consequently, the incidence of esophageal cancer in the entire region virtually disappeared for the first time in two millenniums!

An Incredible Asthma Recovery Story

I am indebted to Jonathan V. Wright, M.D. of the Tahoma Clinic in Kent, Washington for the following true case study. Dr. Wright has been in private practice there for a number of years and specializes in food and environmental allergies and sensitivities. He works entirely along natural lines and fully utilizes vitamins, minerals, trace elements, amino acids, enzymes, and medicinal herbs to help heal his patients.

In 1983 Dave Berger lived in the Deep South and encountered his first episodes of asthmatic wheezing. Believing that it had a lot to do with the extreme humidity and heat, he relocated to an environment that was drier and cooler. But in 1986 his asthma returned. By then he had to resort to two different types of inhalers—one for dilating his bronchial tubes and the other for blocking allergic reactions. In addition, he had to use cortisone (prednisone) frequently (5 mg. four times daily).

He came to Dr. Wright's clinic where an oral health history and complete medical checkup were done. Dave was also given a urinalysis and sulfite test in the clinic laboratory; both tests came back abnormal. His urinary sulfite was 4 to 7 parts per million (ppm), whereas normal is zero. His conjugated sulfate was zero; normal is 10 to 15 percent or above.

Dr. Wright put him immediately on a series of intravenous treatments with molybdenum and associated nutrients. Within two months, the man's asthmatic wheezing and attendant symptoms had disappeared.

Dave was discharged and given oral molybdenum to take thereafter. Within a year's time, he contacted the clinic and reported that his wheezing was "just beginning to return" in spite of faithfully taking his oral molybdenum every day without fail. Urine tests were repeated and showed that the patient's sulfite had risen from

4 to 7 ppm again and his conjugated sulfate had dropped to just 3 percent. Repeated intravenous treatment eliminated the wheezing once more and improved his test results again. Some changes were made to improve his oral supplement assimilation and, thereafter, no further wheezing occurred.

Molybdenum Detoxifies Food Preservatives

Dr. Wright and I have met at a number of National Health Federation conventions held in different locales around the country. In a visit at one of those gatherings, I remember him telling me about the great success he's had with molybdenum in helping flush certain types of allergic food preservatives out of the body.

A group known as sulfites (sulphur dioxide, sodium bisulfite, etc.) is commonly used to preserve foods such as dried fruits (to prevent them from going stiff), packaged luncheon meats (to keep them from spoiling so quickly), shrimp and frozen potatoes (to keep them from darkening), and fine wines (to keep them from turning to vinegar).

These sulfites accumulate within the system, and can induce allergic reactions such as asthma and hay fever. But with the administration of supplemental molybdenum the symptoms of difficult breathing, frequent sneezing, and eye itching quickly disappeared as these offensive food additives were bound up by molybdenum molecules and rapidly excreted in the urine.

Molybdenum Sources

This trace element occurs in certain organ meats such as beef heart, liver, kidneys, brain, and sweetbreads, as well as whole grains (wheat, barley, rye, millet), legumes (lentils and beans), leafy vegetables (spinach, bib lettuce, watercress, mustard and turnip greens), and milk (cow and goat).

Molybdenum also may be found in the ionic waters of the Great Salt Lake. There are products available that are made with this water and provide molybdenum in drop form. (See Product Appendix pages 382–83 for more information.)

Phosphorus
GIVING ATHLETES THAT COMPETITIVE EDGE

Improving Personal Performance

As part of my civic duties as a citizen of the community in which I reside, I am active in several different service clubs; I served as President of the Salt Lake Lions Club (1996-97). Every Thursday afternoon we meet from noon to about 1:30 p.m. in the historic Lion House located in the heart of the downtown business district.

During one of these weekly meetings a while ago, one of our members told us about his son, who is a high school senior and track runner. He lamented the fact that " my kid keeps coming in third or fourth in his track competitions, when he feels he should be coming in first. Heaven only knows how much practice he has put into perfecting his running, but things just don't seem to be clicking very well for him."

Someone pointed his finger at me and said, "There's the man you want to ask. Hey, Mr. President, what should he give his kid to make him run faster?" I told the father to go to any health food store and purchase two products: a phosphorus and potassium supplement in tablet form and a high-phosphorus juice (see Product Appendix, pages 382–83). I mentioned that the phosphorus and potassium supplement was to be taken *with tomato juice* an hour or two before his running event began. I suggested having the boy pack some small cans with lift-off tops along with both products in his backpack when he went to school; then he'd have the juice when he needed it. After the event was over, the boy was to take some of the high-phosphorus drink to help get back his wind and energy more quickly. Furthermore, I encouraged the father to buy some lecithin granules and have his son take one tablespoon of them in orange juice or milk every morning at breakfast.

A couple of weeks later at another club luncheon, the member who had inquired for the other one asked him, "How did your son do in his last two track meets? Did that stuff that Mr. President here recommended do him any good?" The other gentleman smiled and said, "John may be crazy as a hoot owl when it comes to his brand of politics but he *definitely* knows his stuff when it comes to nutrition. My kid won his last two meets, finished second in regionals, and almost tied with another boy for first in the state finals. He told me, quite excitedly, after coming that close to taking first in the state meet, 'Dad, I've never had so much energy in my life. I feel as if I could run forever with the stuff you've been having me take.'"

Foods for Bone Hardening

Earlier in this section under another entry (Boron), I spoke about the roles that certain minerals played in the hardening of bones. To that short list of boron, calcium, and magnesium, I would like to add phosphorus. In the form of phosphate, it is critical for the process of bone mineralization and helps make up the structure of bone.

Suggested daily intake ranges between 800 and 1200 milligrams. It is best to obtain as much of it from dietary sources as possible. The accompanying table mentions the phosphorus content of different foods by serving size.

Foods	Serving Size	Phosphorus (milligrams)
Liver (fried)	3 oz.	456
Cheese (cheddar)	1 oz.	145
Shredded wheat	1 biscuit	97
Bread (whole wheat)	1 slice	71
Haddock (fried)	3 oz.	210
Beef, lean round (braised)	3 oz.	182
Egg (medium, fried)	1 oz.	80
Ice cream (regular)	1/2 cup	67
Bread (white, enriched)	1 slice	27
Milk (whole)	1 cup	228
Baked beans (with pork and tomato)	1/2 cup	118
Corn (cooked kernels)	1/2 cup	60

Oatmeal (cooked)	1/2 cup	68
Broccoli (frozen, cooked)	2/3 cup	69
Green beans (cooked)	1/2 cup	23
Orange (peeled)	1 medium	26
Grapefruit (peeled)	1/2 medium	19

Putting Passion Back into Your Love Life with Phosphorus

Besides the obvious sex hormone, testosterone, there are other hormones produced by the pancreas, thyroid, and adrenal glands that affect human sexual functioning and response. These glands depend to a certain extent on small amounts of phosphorus to help them do their jobs effectively. But when chronic stress of any kind adversely affects them, their production of these other sex hormones drops dramatically. As a result physical, mental, and emotional fatigue set in and the flames of passion are fairly well burned out, as they say.

But working more foods into the dietary scheme that are relatively high in phosphorus can reignite those special sparks for some very meaningful and intense moments. There are certain foods, in particular, that can accomplish this in a nifty way: curry, chutney, hot sauces, brewer's yeast, wheat bran and wheat germ, and seeds of pumpkin, squash, and sunflower.

To shift one's sex drive from neutral or low to a higher and faster gear, an individual would do well to start taking more lecithin (two tablespoons of granules every *evening* in juice or yogurt), Vitamin E, and Vitamin B-6 (one 500 mg. tablet at night). (See Product Appendix, p. 381.)

Phosphorus is present in lecithin in the form of phospholipids, which are a unique mixture of nitrogen, fatty acids, and glycerol. These phospholipids help different organs of the body secrete greater amounts of the hormones that are involved in sexual response.

Potassium
PROTECTING YOUR BODY AGAINST HYPERTENSION AND STROKES

Potassium Saves Lives, No Doubt about It

Recently I had the opportunity to talk with a young musician who performed at the University of Utah. He proceeded to tell me about his father, aged 47, who suffered a very mild stroke two years earlier. "The doctors kept telling Pop that he'd probably have another one sometime soon that would be worse than the first and maybe even leave him partially paralyzed," he said in almost one breath. "But Momma and me, we figured there was something Pop could take to keep this from ever happening. So Momma asked around and someone told her about potassium." He paused and asked in earnestness: "You know what potassium is, don't you?" I nodded and he continued with his narrative.

"Well, anyhow, Momma went to a health food store and bought a jar of potassium tablets and had Dad start taking them every morning with his breakfast. He's been doing this now for awhile. He went back to the doctor for another checkup at Momma's insistence. And the doctor was as surprised as could be. He checked Dad over from top to bottom, and swore it wasn't the same guy who had come in after his first stroke. He said Pop's blood pressure was normal and there didn't seem to be a `chance of him ever getting another stroke, so long as he kept on doing whatever he was doing. And that's the honest-to-gosh truth!"

Over the years I've heard dozens of other tales told about how this mineral has saved the lives of many from serious high blood pressure, stroke, muscle weakness, heart failure, soft bones, and even cancer. But nothing I've heard was quite as telling or original as this. His genuineness was all too apparent and the excited way in which the story tumbled from his lips made it all the more convincing to me.

The following table gives the potassium content of various foods, per serving size. Because the recommended range of daily intake fluctuates between 2,000 and 4,000 mg., and considering just how much of a mineral lifesaver it's been proven to be, I advise eating as many of these foods as possible.

Where Does Our Potassium Come From?

Milligrams	Food Servings
1,200	Butternut squash, 1 cup baked
1,200	Lima beans, dry, 1 cup cooked
1,160	Spinach, 1 cup cooked
1,000	Black beans, 1 cup cooked
970	Soybeans, 1 cup cooked
940	Pinto beans, 1 cup cooked
790	Navy beans, 1 cup cooked
750	Acorn squash, t baked
720	Green lima beans, 1 cup cooked
710	Papaya, medium
680	Cantaloupe, 1/2 melon
650	Avocado, 1/2 medium
650	Raisins, 1/2 cup
630	Kidney beans, 1 cup cooked
600	Chard, 1 cup cooked
600	Prune juice, 1 cup
590	Parsnips, 1 cup cooked
590	Split peas, 1 cup cooked*
580	Blackstrap molasses, 1 tbsp.*
520	Dates, 10 medium
500	Potato, cooked
500	Orange juice, 1 cup
490	Skim milk powder, 1/4 cup
480	Beet greens, 1 cup
440	Banana, medium
430	Low-fat milk, 1 cup
430	Kohlrabi, 1 cup cooked

420	Peas, fresh, 1 cup
420	Brussels sprouts, 1 cup cooked
420	Nectarine, medium

*Ingredients used in accompanying recipe.

POTASSIUM SOUP

1 clove

1 medium yellow onion, peeled

8 cups beef stock

1 bay leaf

1 lb. split peas, rinsed

1 tbsp. blackstrap molasses

2 cloves garlic, peeled and minced

1 tsp. finely chopped fresh thyme

2 tbsp. butter

2 tsp. chopped fresh mint

Press the clove into the center of the onion. Then set the onion into a large stainless steel saucepan. Add the stock, bay leaves, and split peas. Bring to a boil over high heat, then reduce that to medium and simmer, skimming periodically, until the split peas are tender, about half an hour.

Discard the onion and bay leaf, and stir in the garlic, thyme, butter, and blackstrap molasses. Reduce heat to a medium-low setting and cook, just below simmer, for 12 minutes, allowing the flavors to integrate. Ladle into bowls and garnish with mint before serving. If desired, this soup can also be pureed in a food blender. This serves about 6 people. (See Product Appendix, p. 383, for a juicer/blender that retains produce fiber.)

Selenium

BEATING CANCER AND SUPER GERMS AT EVERY TURN

Lessons Learned from China

Since the 1970s a voluminous accumulation of ongoing published research in medical journals throughout the world has shown that the trace element selenium can prevent many forms of cancer as well as shrink existing tumors in a number of instances. Public acceptance of such findings has been well received and many individuals started taking selenium supplements on their own without any encouragement from their medical doctors.

Governments, being the big bureaucratic dinosaurs that they are, have been much slower to act. No political body on earth, with the exception of one, has even dared to issue a public proclamation in support of this mineral as an outstanding nutritional cancer preventive. The leaders of mainland China, however, had the courage to take the necessary steps to see that many of their citizens had access to this trace element in order to prevent the spread of cancer in that country. The story unfolded in the *Journal of Orthomolecular Medicine* (4:124-25; 1989).

Cancer had always been a major health problem in China, with close to three-quarters of a million Chinese dying annually from the disease. Shanghai alone has the highest cancer rate anywhere on the globe: 25 percent of the city's population is expected to eventually die of cancer.

Government leaders with the Ministry of Health in Beijing worked in concert with politicians, scientists, and doctors at the provincial, regional, and metropolitan levels in areas where cancer rates have been extraordinarily high, to find natural ways to reduce the incredible death rates from this terrible disease.

China's traditional or folk medicine hearkens back to several millenniums of origin and use. It is an extremely diverse materia medica that includes a vast array of medicinal plants as well as a number of other useful drugs compounded from some rather "interesting" sources that include rocks, reptiles, mammals, insects, and animal excrement. Mineral drugs derived from stones have been standard medicine in China for a very long time.

Government leaders were intrigued by a particular set of drugs collectively known as "jiang-shi." These are selenium-enriched calcium carbonate nodules taken from yellowish-brown, windblown deposits (*loess*), which have been repeatedly mentioned throughout traditional Chinese medical literature as being useful in the prevention and treatment of cancer. So, the Ministry of Health in Beijing commissioned researchers from the Chinese National Corporation of Traditional Medicine and from Jiangshui Hospital in Xingtai to do some field tests in order to determine if such claims were valid or not.

In 1974, large numbers of "jiang-shi" concretions were dropped into the drinking water wells of an area of Xingtai in Hebei province, having a population then of about 90,000. The result was that in the next 15 years cancer mortality rates plunged dramatically. More surprising, though, was what happened in five separate villages in Bainan. There, five new wells were constructed, either using calcium carbonate nodules as building material, or else containing large numbers of these "jiang-shi" concretions. Prior to 1974, cancer deaths were being reported annually from each of these villages. But in the next 15 years, there were *no more cancer deaths recorded*!

As a consequence of these and other findings elsewhere in China, the government in Beijing began a massive campaign in areas with high cancer mortality rates to dispense powdered "jiang-shi" and selenium to several million barefoot doctors (called so because of their walking from village to village without the benefit of shoes or sandals). These rural health care providers started giving the stone powders to people they knew ran a great risk of developing cancer.

In fact, the Chinese government became so convinced that selenium can beat cancer that they granted rare permission to the Zhou Kou Area's First Pharmaceutical Factory of Henan Province to start selling supplements containing selenium and other trace elements. Delegates from the world over were there at the time attending the International Symposium on Environmental Life Elements and Health. The government allowed this company to advertise its selenium products on the back cover of the Conference *Abstracts,* a publication that was sponsored wholly by the Chinese Academy of

Sciences and the National Natural Science Foundation of China. Nothing like this had ever been permitted before. Selenium was well on its way to becoming Communist China's number one government-backed trace mineral supplement! The President, Congress, FDA (Food and Drug Administration), and CDC (Centers for Disease Control) should take note—there are some valuable lessons to be learned here for the benefit of the American public!

The Arizona Study

A large number of studies involving both animal and human models have been conducted since the 1970s to show that selenium is one of the greatest anticancer nutrients around, second only in importance, perhaps, to vitamin C. Interestingly enough, according to a Finnish nutritionist from the University of Helsinki, ascorbic acid improves the bioavailability of dietary selenium. What the report in the *Human Nutrition & Clinical Nutrition* journal (39C:221-26, May-Jun. 1985) suggested was that if you want your body to utilize most of the selenium obtained from foods, then eat or take something with them that is high in vitamin C content. In other words, if you're about to consume 3 oz. of cooked red snapper for lunch or dinner and want to make absolutely sure you're getting nearly all of the 150 micrograms of selenium it contains, then drink with it *one cup* of the following juice selections that contain vitamin C: cranberry (40 mg.), grapefruit (93 mg.), orange (124 mg.), papaya (137 mg.), or tomato (39 mg.)

Of the many fairly recent studies that have reported on selenium's wonderful antioxidant properties in connection with cancer reduction and prevention, none has made as major an impact as the one headed up by epidemiologist Larry C. Clark, Ph.D. of the University of Arizona Cancer Center in Tucson. It included a total of 16 coauthors, was entitled, "Effects of Selenium Supplementation for Cancer Prevention in Patients with Carcinoma of the Skin," and appeared in the *Journal of the American Medical Association* (276:1957-83; 1984-85; December 25, 1996) with a follow-up editorial directly behind it ("Selenium and Cancer Prevention"). One idea strongly advocated by the journal editorial was the possible inclusion of supplemental selenium into a number of manufactured food products in much the same way as is currently being done with folic acid.

This decade-long study covering health data on 1,312 patients turned up some unexpected surprises. For one thing, selenium *did not* reduce skin cancers as researchers had hoped it would. Yet, on the other hand, there was an astonishing 40 percent decrease in *overall* cancer risk. Interestingly enough, the biggest reductions came in three of the major cancers: prostate (63 percent decrease); colorectal (58 percent decrease), and lung (45 percent decrease). Unfortunately, no changes were noticed in head-neck, breast, or bladder cancers, as had been hoped.

Clark and his research team speculated that selenium prevents cancer by inhibiting tumor growth and inducing a form of chemical "suicide" within malignant cells. Half of those enrolled in the study were given 200 micrograms of selenium (from high-selenium yeast) every day for 4.5 years, while the other half received only a placebo. The average age of the subjects was 63.

Halting the Spread of Dangerously Mutating Viruses

Selenium functions as an antioxiant and a component of another antioxidant, glutathione peroxidase. Deficiencies of either substance impair the body's immune system and ability to fight infections. E. Will Taylor, Ph.D., a viral researcher at the University of Georgia in Athens, told a reporter, "It is intriguing that a number of viruses have emerged from [those] regions in Africa, which appear to be *selenium deficient*."

The more research one does into this matter, the more sense it seems to make. Consider two reports that were separately published in the *Journal of Medical Virology* (43:66-70, 1994) and *Journal of Nutrition* (124:345-58, 1994) having to do with a benign coxsackievirus. Coxsackieviruses infect more than 20 million people annually in America and can cause illnesses ranging from a common cold to heart inflammation. But since most of them are relatively harmless, only about 10,000 infected people ever become ill at any given time. The articles explained how one of these run-of-the-mill coxsackieviruses quickly mutated into a deadly, rapidly reproducing strain when an infected person or animal was deficient in selenium or vitamin E. This new form didn't mutate, though, in animals eating a selenium-rich diet. Yet, once fully mutated, the virus could infect and be deadly to a human or animal despite the person or beast eating adequate selenium. A third study published later in *Nature Medicine* (1:433-36, May 1995) identified six specific changes in the genetic structure of the virulent coxsackievirus strain when selenium levels were minimal in animal models.

The coxsackievirus infection is made worse because selenium deficiency weakens the host's immunity, preventing the virus from being effectively challenged by T-cell lymphocytes or antibodies. As a result, the mutated virus can reproduce faster than it would in a relatively healthy person. In addition, the lack of selenium prevents the quenching of mutation-causing free radicals, so when the virus reproduces, it also mutates at a much faster rate.

There has been a growing concern among many doctors about the alarming spread of antibiotic-resistant bacteria. A report presented to the annual meeting of the American Lung Association and American Thoracic Society in the latter part of May 1997 noted that drug-resistant *streptococcus pneumoniae* has been on "a steadily increasing curve" since 1994. Where once ordinary penicillin would have been sufficient to treat bronchitis, pneumonia, and middle-ear infections, now it has virtually no effect on such a strain of "super bacteria."

The most interesting part of this report had to do with the *regional differences* in America concerning this penicillin resistance. Examination of 15,000 samples from 194 labs coast-to-coast found these singular variations of bacterial resistance to a conventional antibiotic:

- 41 percent of samples from the Southeast,
- 32.8 percent from the Midwest,
- 25.7 percent from the Northeast,
- 23.2 percent from the West (excluding California).

However, nothing was mentioned in relation to selenium.

I decided to do a little scientific sleuthing on my own and find out the possible reason why the degree of penicillin resistance in the West had been lower than elsewhere in the country. I made a number of phone calls to Utah State University in Logan, which is an agricultural school. I spoke with people in the Soil Testing Lab and the Animal, Dairy, and Veterinary Science (ADVS) department about this matter and whether it could tie in with selenium somehow.

The answers I got surprised me. Jan Kotuby-Amacher, the current director of the Soil Testing Lab, pointed out that farmers in Utah and many of the surrounding Western States tend to add *more* selenium to their soils and animal feeds than farmers elsewhere in the country were apt to do. Clell Bagley, a veterinarian connected with ADVS, reminded me that cattle, hogs, and sheep in ten Western States "are usually over- rather than undersupplemented in selenium." Thus, through forage crops like alfalfa grown in selenium-enriched soils and regular feed supplemented with extra selenium, such animals would acquire elevated levels of this trace element in their systems. The meat consumed from this slaughtered livestock would, therefore, transfer greater amounts of selenium into those who regularly dined on beef, pork, or lamb.

All of this explains in a logical fashion *how* those statistics for the prevalence of drug-resistant bacteria could be lower in the West than other parts of the country, where agricultural emphasis on selenium isn't so great. According to Frank A. Gilbert, the author of *Mineral Nutrition and the Balance of Life* (Norman: University of Oklahoma Press, 1969; p. 244): "Animal products, such as meat, eggs, and milk, seem to be the most important and *constant* source of selenium to which the inhabitants are exposed."

So, based on the evidence given, may I suggest regular supplementation with selenium *and* vitamin E? The two together are a formidable arsenal in checking the spread of dangerously mutating viruses.

A Quest for Better Selenium

According to *Free Radical Biology & Medicine* (20:139-43, 1996), when selenium is used in large dosages with other antioxidants such as vitamins C and E it can reduce by 50 percent hospital-induced sepsis (bacterial blood poisoning) and acute respiratory distress syndrome. Such mineral-vitamin antioxidant combinations can also shorten hospital stays for a variety of other conditions.

The distribution of selenium in the food chain can easily be summarized in the following simple table:

HIGH-SELENIUM FOODS	Fresh-water and salt-water fish (red snapper, salmon, swordfish, tuna), lobster, shrimp, oyster, organ meats (beef liver and kidney).
MEDIUM-SELENIUM FOODS	Nuts (especially Brazil), garlic, radish, horseradish, onion, chives, sunflower seeds, medicinal mushrooms (reishi, shiitake), raisins, brewer's yeast, cereal grains (sometimes).*
LOW-SELENIUM FOODS	Poultry, dairy products, eggs, fruits, vegetables, drinking water.

*Dependent on the selenium content of the soils they're grown in.

Some novel ideas are being batted around within the scientific community about how to get more drugs and a few nutrients like selenium into the food chain, which would pretty much eliminate the need for getting a booster shot every ten years. During the week of May 19-23, 1997, roughly 2,000 public health professionals were gathered in Detroit for the thirty-first annual Centers for Disease Control and Prevention (CDC) national immunization conference. They were hearing pretty incredible things about how some of tomorrow's immunizations might be given.

- Eat a tomato and never get rabies.
- Take a pill to prevent tetanus and tiny organisms will be released in your body for the rest of your life, eliminating the need for a booster shot every decade.
- Give your child a peanut butter and jelly sandwich made from genetically-altered peanuts that are chock full of selenium and vitamins C and E, precluding the need for regular immunizations against common childhood infections.

Sounds like science fiction, doesn't it? But according to astounding information coming out of some sessions, researchers are looking for every way imaginable to deliver serums and some nutrients other than by hypodermic injections. No one likes shots when it comes down to the nitty-gritty of things—toddlers to grandparents hate them with a passion. Scientists, knowing this fact all too well, have been studying the matter for some time now and figuring out new strategies of immunization that have reasonable potential for succeeding.

Beside boosting immune system functions (especially that of cellular immunity), selenium also: encourages sperm production; assists in prostate gland functions; helps in thyroid hormone activity; modifies blood coagulation to minimize clots; normalizes cardiac arrhythmias; prevents cardiovascular disease; improves psychiatric and mood disorders (especially in schizophrenics and hypoglycemics); protects against circulatory diseases; and reduces some inflammation attendant to autoimmune diseases such as rheumatoid arthritis and lupus erythematosus.

But getting an organic selenium compound that will perform these and other tasks efficiently without creating toxic situations in the body can be a rather tricky affair for the uninitiated. Fortunately, information is available that enables consumers to know in which direction to proceed safely. "Selenium: A Quest for Better Understanding," by Vladimir Badmaev, M.D., Ph.D., Muhammed Majeed, Ph.D., et al., appeared in the July 1996 issue of *Alternative Therapies* (2(4):59-67).

The authors stress that the form of selenium-containing amino acids that the body can best use are the "L-" forms, *especially* L(+)Selenomethionine. It has a much slower turnover rate within the system than other forms of selenium do. It is also virtually nontoxic thanks, in large part, to being coupled with the sulphur amino acid, methionine (from which it derives the last part of its name).

"The bioavailability of selenium was evaluated in a double-blind study with 10 volunteers, 5 of whom received 50 mg. elemental selenium in the form of L(+)selenomethionine alone," and the remainder getting the same amount of similar selenium form but with one little difference: their 50 mg. of L(+)selenomethionine was "supplemented with a small amount of naturally derived pure alkaloid piperine" (derived from black pepper) "in the form of a preparation known as Bioperine."

Over the next 6 weeks, "serum selenium levels were evaluated before the study and at 2-, 3-, and 6-week intervals. The serum selenium levels were approximately 30 percent higher in the group receiving selenium with Bioperine . . . None of the volunteers in the experimental groups reported any adverse effects from the supplementation."

Not long ago, Dr. Francis Crick, codiscoverer of DNA's double helical structure and winner of the Nobel Prize in Chemistry in 1962, was asked by a reporter how he managed to stay so healthy and active as he approached his eighties. His terse reply was, "I take a broad spectrum supplement, good antioxidants, . . . *yes, and also selemethionine.*"

Silicon
TONIC MINERAL FOR BONES, MUSCLES, AND ORGANS

Relief for Mitral Valve Prolapse and Angina

Cheryl Jarman runs a teaching center for folk medicine in the Piney Woods country of East Texas. Located in the small town of Hudson (just outside of Lufkin), her Remedies of the People Institute has taught hundreds of eager students in the last five years the finer points embracing good folk medicine: correct plant identification with walks in the nearby woods; right methods for their preparation; and proper procedures for the administering of medicinal herbs.

She called my research center on a recent morning and spoke with me on botanical-related matters. At that time I was working on this particular mineral entry and inquired of her what success she had had with the plant commonly known as horsetail or shavegrass, which happens to be incredibly rich in silicon. She proceeded to tell me the following true story.

"About five months ago I had a woman in her mid-thirties come into our classroom for a session I was then teaching. Afterward, she told me about an apparent genetic disorder she had which greatly affected her cardiovascular system. She suffered recurrent chest pains, shortness of breath, and a loud, crisp systolic clicking in the area of her heart.

"She had been to see her doctor, who ran a number of tests on her and eventually diagnosed it as mitral valve prolapse. Since it wasn't too serious, he told her she would 'just have to live with it' and sent her home. Understandably, she was quite upset with his poor manners and decided to come here to one of my classes for further instructions.

"I made it clear to her that in Texas, an herbalist like myself cannot prescribe or diagnose. But since I taught classes in the botanical arts, I could share with her what others have used. I told her that some who've experienced angina pains, which are somewhat similar to her own pains, had been using horsetail and alfalfa with great success. She asked how much of each to take. And again I reminded her, for my own protection, of state laws which prohibit herbalists like me from prescribing.

"But I told her about an older Hispanic fellow in Nacogdoches, up the road apiece, by the name of Juan Lopez who had been using both herbs quite successfully for his own angina problems. She contacted him and he told her he had been taking two capsules of horsetail herb in the morning and two again in the evening, and taking one capsule of alfalfa three times a day, with each meal. Well, she started doing this and within just four days her chest pains ceased and she experienced more energy than she did before.

"In two weeks she returned to her physician, who noticed an absence of the clicking sound in her chest. 'Whatever you're doing, keep it up,' he told her and dismissed her from his clinic. Both herbs have helped others in similar situations."

For those wishing to contact Cheryl with specific herb questions, they may call or write her teaching center for further instructions: Remedies of the People, Rt. 4, Box 2695, Lufkin, TX 75904, (409)-875-4335. She also conducts classes in herb wildcrafting during the spring, summer, and fall months. "We have just about every kind of herb you'd want," this 37-year-old herbalist told me over the phone. "We call this part of East Texas 'God's Country,' and rightly so with the rich variety of vegetation that grows here."

Keeping the Musculoskeletal System in Great Shape

I've known Daniel B. Mowrey, Ph.D. since 1979 when he and I were regular contributors to *The Herbalist* magazine. I'll never forget one cold winter day when he and I and a couple of other writers had to pose for some pictures in a farmer's pasture near Utah Lake. We were stomping our feet and rubbing our hands together in order to keep the circulation going, while the professional photographer doing the shooting tried to decide which pose we should assume next. I remember grumbling to Dan under my frosty breath. Under such intensely cold circumstances, we found it difficult to "look happy and radiate personal warmth!"

Dan received his doctorate degree in psychology and psychopharmacology from Brigham Young University in Provo, with related studies in biochemistry and biology. For a time he was con-nected with the faculty of that school. Since then he has served in an advisory technical capacity with many different herb companies, assisting them in toxicology testing and herbal formulating.

Dan thinks the world of horsetail because of its high silicon content. He believes there is nothing better to tone the muscu-loskeletal system (includes all muscles, bones, and cartilages of the body). Dan wrote the following about this herb's wonderful miner-al properties in the September 1996 issue of *Delicious!* (vol:62) mag-azine.

"This plant is the source of one of the most important trace ele-ments in human nutrition—silicon—which is involved in the processes that form bone, cartilage, connective tissue and skin. Connective tissues in structures such as the aorta, trachea, tendons, bones and skin are unusually rich in silicon. The growth and repair of tissue requires a matrix to which minerals adhere and upon which new tissue builds. Silicon is heavily involved in the metabolic processes of the matrix and is also an integral part of the matrix itself."

Officer Injured in High-Speed Chase Helped with Silicon

One of the more unusual cases in which silicon has proved its repairing abilities on injured muscles and tendons came to me by way of the wife of a Salt Lake City police officer. I met her at a book signing I was doing in downtown Salt Lake City. As I did the auto-graphing, she asked what my next book would be about. Upon hearing that it was on vitamins and minerals, she volunteered the following story.

Her husband and some other local law enforcement officers were involved in a high-speed chase along a 20–square mile area of Salt Lake County. They were in hot pursuit of a parole violator, who vowed he wouldn't be taken alive. Her husband is part of the Violent Crime Task Force called out in such emergency situations.

The 45-minute highway chase at speeds clocked in excess of 100 mph ended when the suspect ran over a spike mat that had been spread across the road. Although the stolen car's tires were gone, the man threw the stickshift into reverse and attempted to back off the mat on nothing but the wheel hubs. Her husband, along with some other officers in full flak jackets, had come up from behind with their guns drawn and ready. As the vehicle surged backward, the left side struck her husband's hip and he fell onto the spikes, injuring himself quite badly. Other officers approaching around the front left side yelled for the parolee to surrender. When he didn't, they opened fire, striking him in the left thigh. He was hospitalized under heavy guard and then promptly taken into custody.

Doctors told the injured officer's wife that his wounds were quite serious, but not life-threatening. They said it would take "many months for him to heal." Being a believer in natural remedies, she went to a local health food store and spoke with an in-house herbalist who recommended a homeopathic product called silica terra, which is an absorbable form of silicon derived from ground quartz or powdered rock crystal. The herbalist, who was apparently well versed in homeopathy, mentioned that silica combined with calcium and other minerals to help harden bones, and that it increased the production of collagen, the tough connective tissue that holds everything together and gives bones greater flexibility. The herbalist said that silica would help to repair the muscle and tendon tears that the woman's husband suffered as a result of his fall.

The woman was also advised to place her husband on an *alkaline* diet, which would enable the silicon to work better in his system. The suggested foods she could pick from included fish, goat's milk, legumes, oats, brown rice, whole wheat pasta, granola, root and leafy vegetables, nuts (especially almond, cashew, hazel, and walnut), tomato juice, and carob. The injured police officer liked his red meat, potatoes and gravy, plenty of desserts, and lots of coffee.

"Getting him to change even just a teensy-weensy bit," his wife sighed, "was like pulling teeth. He threw a fuss and I told him I'd never seen such a big baby in my life! That quieted him down. We compromised: *no* goat's milk, *no* brown rice, and *no* veggies; in return he agreed to eat everything else the consultant in the health food store had suggested."

The woman had her husband start taking a silica supplement every day. In addition, the alkaline diet put a great deal of other minerals (besides silicon) into his body, which gave him roughly a 20 percent acid to 80 percent alkaline blood balance. This really helped accelerate his recovery more rapidly, since the mineral salts detoxified all of the heavy acids out of his system that had built up over a long period of time due to his eating habits.

To make a long story short, this police officer recovered from all of his muscle and tendon wounds due to the spike mat fall in *just two months,* much to the amazement of everyone, including his doctors and fellow officers. The doctors had predicted a minimum of four months and a maximum of six months, but he was "up and ready for action," his wife said, in a matter of eight weeks.

Other Herbs with Silicon in Them

Besides horsetail (which is obviously the richest source of silicon), borage (1.5 percent-2.2 percent) and stinging nettle (up to 3 percent) also contain generous amounts of silicon (in the form of silicic acid).

I have had my own success stories with silicon. A man in the Bronx, New York wrote to me some time ago asking what I would recommend for his Cushing Syndrome. I suggested the above three herbs, one capsule each three times daily with meals for six weeks. He followed my advice and reported his "moon-shaped" facial appearance disappeared, as well as the purple stretch marks on his thighs and upper torso.

Silver

A PRETTY PRECIOUS METAL WITH SOME HEALTH SURPRISES

Silvery Sayings

Silver has been a favorite metal of many cultures through the ages, and as such has engendered some favorite sayings along the way.

- The ancient Egyptians preferred calling the metal "white gold."

- Judas' act of betraying Jesus into the hands of his Jewish enemies for "30 pieces of silver" has led to the frequent expression within the business world to describe someone's treachery, "he (or she) would sell him (or her) for 30 pieces of silver."

- Wishful optimism: "Every cloud has its silver lining."

- Glibness of speech: "Silver-tongued orators."

- Wealth and success: "Golden apples framed in silver."

- Graceful aging: "He/She looks so distinguished with his/her silver hair."

- "All is not gold that glitters"—an implied reference to silver by the Spanish novelist Miguel de Cervantes Saavedra (1547-1616) in his farce *Don Quixote*.

- "They . . . love silver better than their own lives"—used by French humorist and satirist François Rabelais (1494-1553) in his novels *Pantagruel* and *Gargantua*.

A King's Ransom

Spanish conquistadores scoured the viceroyalty of Peru for silver and extorted truckloads from the hostage Inca king Atahualpa

(1500?-1533). Author John Hemming explained it better in his book, *The Conquest of the Incas* (New York: Harcourt Brace Jovanovich, Inc., 1970):

> *The Incas now offered his famous ransom. 'The Governor [Francisco Pizarro] asked him how much he would give and how soon. Atahualpa said that he would give a room full of gold . . . He would also give the entire hut filled twice over with silver. And he would complete this within two months.' The Spaniards were staggered by the unexpected proposal. 'Certainly an offer of vast proportions!'*
>
> *The [Spanish] envoys were not allowed to visit the entire city [of Cuzco], but what they did see intoxicated them. 'They said there was so much gold and silver in all the temples of the city that it was marvelous. . . .'*
>
> *Over eleven tons of gold objects were fed into the furnaces at Cajamarca [by the Spaniards and their Inca slaves], to produce 13,420 pounds of 22-carat 'good gold'; the silver objects yielded some 26,000 pounds of good silver. Much of this consisted of vases, figures, jewelry and some furnishing ornaments, the masterpieces of Inca goldsmiths and silversmiths. Its destruction was an irreparable artistic loss.*
>
> *It is impossible to give the value of the ransom in modern terms. The purchasing power of gold and silver have altered since the sixteenth century, and so have the relative values and desirability of goods and services. The treasure was worth far less in Peru than it would have been in Europe.*
>
> *Nevertheless, it is interesting to know what Atahualpa's ransom would fetch on the present [1970] bullion market. The gold would be worth £2,570,500 ($6,169,200) and the silver £283,850 ($681,240), a total of £2,854,350 ($6,850,440).*

So where did all of this Inca silver finally end up? According to Allen A. Boraiko in his article, "Silver: A Mineral of Excellent Nature," which appeared in the *National Geographic* (vol:303) for September 1981, it went to the following places:

Most of the Inca silver was melted for King, Spain, and God. God's share of New World silver reappeared in Spanish colonial churches as crucifixes, chalices, and sumptuous silver altars. The king's portion, or "royal fifth," helped finance ruinous wars and inflate and wreck Spain's economy in a flood of silver reals.

Silver Surprises in Taxco

During March 1977 I was in different parts of Mexico doing field work in medical anthropology. With me at the time were several other anthropologists and, of course, an interpreter for those of us who couldn't speak Spanish fluently. One of our stopovers was in the famed "silver city" of Taxco, built by Hernando Cortez, the Aztec conqueror, in the mountains southwest of Mexico City. A local official informed us that, at last count, there were approximately 10,000 *tasqueños* hammering and casting silver. It revealed to our small group that their attachment to the metal ran so deep it almost bordered on obsession.

While the others explored the craftsmanship aspects connected with silver, I investigated solely the medicinal uses for this very precious metal. Here's what my scientific sleuthing turned up after several days of visits and numerous inquiries among city doctors and *curanderas* (female folk healers):

- Dr. Jesus Alvarez, a pediatrician in the city's only hospital, made his morning rounds in the pediatric ward accompanied by a nurse. I watched as they carefully introduced silver nitrate ointment into the eyes of several-hours-old newborns. "We do this," he explained through my interpreter, "to protect them against neonatal gonococcal conjunctivitis and infections generated by the herpes virus, which is quite prevalent here. Problems of this sort can happen as an infant passes through a mother's infected birth canal and comes out covered with herpes viruses." He reminded me, though, that such a practice is "fairly common where you come from" (meaning the United States).

- In the hospital's critical care unit, Dr. Frederico Sanchez and staff were busily engaged in treating a 27-year-old factory worker suffering severe third-degree burns on his back due to a gasoline tank explosion. The team gave calcium fluid resuscitation before applying about a 1/16th-inch layer of silver sulfadiazine over the injured areas. This sulfa medicine is standard therapy for burns and works by killing any fungus or bacteria that may occur in burns. But then Dr. Sanchez would do something later on that is seldom practiced elsewhere in conventional burn therapy: "We will give him some intravenous solutions of colloidal silver 12 to 24 hours from now." The good doctor then added this brief explanation: "We give our burn patients this colloidal silver—a little at a time and highly diluted—to help boost weakened immune functions and prevent the inward risks of staph infection."

- Silvia Maria Guzman y Fuentes, one of several widely respected curanderas in the area, demonstrated to my interpreter and I how she made her own colloidal silver. She took an old metal sewing thimble and dipped it into some powdered silver. She emptied the excess back into the container until only about 1/8th or "a pinch" remained. This she added to a quart of boiled water that had already cooled, corked the top, and vigorously shook the contents for a couple of minutes. This silver solution, she told us, would be applied directly to eczema, psoriasis, or rashes to help reduce the itching or inflammation. The afflicted parts would be bathed with some of this colloidal silver or else it would be squirted on from a clean spray bottle.

- Adriana Gomez, a much younger and lesser-known curandera, used her own colloidal silver to successfully treat bed bug bites (which this community seemed to suffer a great deal from). She would soak pieces of wadded cotton with a little bit of this liquid silver and then tape it directly over the bite itself. She mentioned it worked just as effectively for *all* insect bites and stings. Remembering this some years later, I experimented with it myself and sprayed some colloidal silver on mosquito bites and even on severe sunburns. I was truly amazed at just how well it worked: The inflammation and itching of both disappeared in minutes!

- Adriana also encouraged some of her teenage patients suffering from acne to rub their faces daily with cotton balls soaked in colloidal silver. She claimed it improved their complexions in a hurry.

- A number of the residents in Taxco routinely purify their drinking water with colloidal silver. The general method for doing this is to add one tablespoon of the colloidal solution to every gallon of tap water, shake the glass or plastic jug thoroughly, and wait 30 minutes before using. Mixed this way, I discovered, it is completely tasteless and with hot Mexican food works as a wonderful digestive aid to prevent heartburn, flatulence, and diarrhea. (By way of interest, Russian cosmonauts have been using silver ions aboard their aging Mir space station to sterilize all of their recycled water.)

- Many of the doctors and folk healers whom I interviewed in Taxco regularly put silver wires *into* or silver foil dressing *on top of* wounds with one great advantage: There was never any bacterial infection since silver kills or deactivates *every* type of known bacteria without the slightest side effects.

- Keeping the skin healthy, at least on the face, neck, throat, forearms, and hands, by sponging or washing them every morning with diluted colloidal silver (1 teaspoon colloidal silver to 1 quart boiled and cooled tap water, then mixed well) is a common practice for a number of Tasqueña women.

Getting the Silver Your Body Needs

In order for silver to be of value within the body, it must first be chelated into a form that the system can easily assimilate. Some types of elemental silver that have been introduced into the human body without first being converted into a more usable form have eventually proven to be quite toxic. Just look at all the trouble dental amalgam has caused for many people. But what folks seem to have forgotten in their mad rush to replace all of their fillings with something safer is that the elemental silver has only been a *small part* of the problem. Other trace elements such as mercury, tin, copper, and zinc were the rest of it.

Both colloidal silver, which I'm not a big fan of, and ionic silver, which I eagerly support, may be purchased from health supplement producers (see Product Appendix for further information on both on pages 382 and 383 from two different suppliers).

Sodium

STONE AGE SURVIVAL GENE NOW HEALTH HINDRANCE FOR MILLIONS

Life Was Rough in One Million B.C.

My colleague and friend of many years, Vaughn M. Bryant, Ph.D., has been a professor of anthropology at Texas A & M University since 1971. His work with prehistoric human feces (called coprolites) to reconstruct ancient paleolithic diets has made him world-renowned. In 1979 he gave a lecture entitled "Prehistoric Diets" before the faculty and student body. His presentation was the twelfth in the University Lecture Series, a distinguished information program that presents annual lectures deemed to be of exceptionally scholarly merit. A portion of his remarks has been reproduced here with his kind permission.

Archaeological evidence reveals that life on the plains of east Africa was difficult for our earliest ancestors. Tools made from chipped pieces of volcanic rock, quartz, and flint, along with animal bones shaped into daggers and clubs, were unsophisticated in style, yet adequate for cutting meat, shaping wooden spears, and skinning dead animals.

"Using the recovered records of these ancient east Africans, we can reconstruct a hypothetical scene from their daily lives. Ambling slowly across the tall grass plain is a group of twenty to thirty individuals. Out in front are the adult males, lean and trim even though they average just under five feet in height. Behind them the slightly smaller females and their children beat the grass searching for insects, small animals, bird nests, seeds, roots, or other items they can eat. As they feed on the tough grass seeds, roots, tubers, and nuts, we can see why they need their large molar teeth and powerful jaws to pulverize their food. Occasionally someone catches a small rodent lizard or insect and eats it raw as the search for food continues. The group wanders on until near dusk when one of the men finds the remains of a half-eaten zebra killed earlier in the day by a lion. After chasing away a group of buzzards and hyenas, the group feeds on the fresh meat and cuts it from the bones with flakes of chipped flint made from

*river cobbles. As darkness falls, the group moves on to an area of high
ground where they pile rocks and brush in a semicircle to protect them
from the many predators and the chill of night. Perhaps in the dim-
ming light of early evening they may have huddled together against
the evening chill and munched on whatever leftover seeds, nuts, and
dried pieces of meat they had carried back to camp at the end of each
day.*

Stone Age Gene Responsible for Hypertension

When these early sub-humans or hominids roamed the grassy
African savannahs, they carried a gene that helped them retain salt
and water so they could survive their low-sodium diet and the
intensely hot climate. But today that old gene makes millions of people prone to high blood pressure if they consume too much salt. A
newer mutant version of the same gene, though, protects other people from the potentially deadly condition of hypertension.

Scientists from Utah, Europe, and Asia reached that conclusion
in a study that appeared in the April 2, 1997 issue of *Journal of
Clinical Investigation.* Their research focused on the angiotensino-
gen (AGT) gene which millions of people still carry, but especially
African Americans. This research is very important for several different reasons. For one thing, it could eventually lead to a simple test
to identify hypertensive patients who can benefit from a low-salt diet
and from medicines that reduce salt retention. For another, it may
account for why African Americans are more susceptible to hypertension than whites, Hispanics, and Asians. Also, it supports the 30-
year-old theory that modern heart disease, hypertension, obesity,
and diabetes could very well stem from genes that once enabled
hominids to survive dietary shortages but now contribute to disease
in societies whose nutrients are relatively abundant.

In affluent societies, hypertension is a common disease. But it
is not so in poor third-world nations where sodium intake is minimal at best. Other genes could play a role in other forms of high
blood pressure, but salt-sensitive hypertension is due to the lingering presence of this original form of the Stone Age AGT gene. The
irony is, though, that it is no longer needed.

The study shows that evolution of human genes lags far behind evolution of human culture—in this case, the change from scarce to abundant dietary salt. In truth, we still have one-million-year-old genes inside of us, but our nutritional patterns have drastically changed.

A geneticist, Dr. James Neel of the University of Michigan in Ann Arbor, put it this way: "For years now I've been propounding the 'thrifty-gene theory' which says that some diseases of civilization—coronary heart disease, diabetes, obesity, and hypertension—are nothing more than our old prehistoric genes responding to an entirely new environment. This study is really the first evidence at a molecular level that my theory holds water."

Tracking a Gene

The AGT gene was first implicated in hypertension in the early 1990s in a study involving 300 pairs of siblings in Utah and France. Investigators discovered differences in the gene in people with and without hypertension. One of those differences was found to be crucial. A segment of the old gene makes human cells produce larger amounts of a hormone that elevates blood pressure. In the mutant gene, the segment is different, so cells produce less of the hormone, named angiotension II.

The hormone raises blood pressure by constricting blood vessels and stimulating the kidneys to retain sodium from salt, which in turn makes the body retain water. The old gene would have assisted early humans in Africa in maintaining normal blood pressure and volume as they sweated in a hot climate with inadequate dietary salt. Once humans began migrating to cold climates, though, and used salt to preserve food during the wintertime, the old gene combined with dietary salt intake led to excessive salt retention and high blood pressure.

People with the mutant gene produce less of the hormone, are less efficient at retaining sodium, and can eat more salt without suffering high blood pressure. The scientists cooperating in this significant study were able to demonstrate that the hypertension-susceptibility form of the gene is really the Stone Age gene by analyzing blood from chimpanzees, gorillas, and baboons. All three classes of primates had the old form of the gene in their blood, but not the mutant gene.

Another Utah study reported in the scientific literature in 1993 found pregnant women with the Stone Age gene had higher rates of preeclampsia, a form of high blood pressure that can kill the mother and fetus.

Over many generations, slightly higher death rates among women and fetuses with the million-year-old gene would slowly favor the spread of the mutant gene through the human population. This would eventually result in a dramatic reduction in salt-sensitive high blood pressure, observed Jean-Marc Lalouel, a physician-geneticist and principal author of the study that also included 11 other coauthors.

Turning Back the Clock on Your Own Prehistoric Gene

Having now clearly defined the ancient genetic link to hypertension, it remains to be seen what can be done with this old AGT gene that has never been able to "catch up" with our constantly changing environment. Following the common medical recommendations of going on a low-sodium diet and restricting one's salt intake certainly make good sense. Taking natural antihypertensive herbs such as barberry, black cohosh, boneset, cleavers, garlic, hawthorn, onion, parsley, skullcap, and wild black cherry in place of synthetic drugs especially designed for such a problem is a healthier and better approach.

But there are some other dietary alternatives that can allow someone suffering from hypertension the best of both worlds: enjoying a prudent salt intake while at the same time keeping the blood pressure level fairly stable. One of these was outlined in the January 1985 *American Journal of Clinical Nutrition* (41:52-60). Twelve normotensive men eating a controlled diet providing about 3 grams of sodium each day were given a salt supplement containing an additional 3.6 grams of sodium daily for 14 days. During the high-salt period, urinary excretion of calcium and potassium was much higher than during the low-salt period. Consistent with the theory that calcium plays a critical role in the regulation of blood pressure, men given a higher calcium intake (689 mg. per 1,000 kilocalorie) had much lower systolic blood pressure than those consuming less calcium (538 mg. per 1,000 kilocalories). The study suggested that a definite increase of calcium and a probable intake of more potassium would easily offset the negative influence that extra sodium might have on blood pressure. (Consult the food and herb lists under Calcium and Potassium for what to eat in this regard.) Average daily intakes of supplemental calcium (600 mg.), magnesium (1200 mg.), and potassium (800 mg.) should keep blood pressure within a safe range in spite of prudent salt intake.

Another solution to this problem is to use substances in which the predominant compound sodium chloride is surrounded by an array of other minerals. These many other trace elements act as buffering agents to pure sodium chloride, so it doesn't adversely affect the kidneys and blood pressure. Three common and affordable items that easily meet this criteria are ocean kelp, ionic mineral liquid concentrate from the Great Salt Lake in Utah, and Celtic Sea Salt from France. The health merits of each are discussed separately.

For many centuries most coastal Asian countries have taken advantage of the marine vegetation that grows abundantly in their coastal waterways. Marine algaes and ocean seaweeds have become important food staples in most Oriental cultures. It has only been in the last few decades that people in North America and Europe have become more fully aware of these mineral-rich food alternatives.

Kelp is probably the most recognized of the edible seaweeds. According to a definitive work on the subject, *The Seavegetable Book* (New York: Clarkson N. Potter, 1977) by Judith Cooper Madlener, the kelp species is very high in vitamins A, B-complex (especially B-6 and B-12), D, E, and K, and has a balanced complement of trace elements that include (but are not limited to): boron, bromine (very high), calcium, cobalt, iodine (very high), iron, magnesium, nickel, nitrogen, phosphorus, potassium, silicon, sulphur and tin. While they obviously have many individual effects within the body, they are united in one very specific function, which is to help check the biochemical influences of two other major mineral ingredients, namely chlorine and sodium, that combine to form sodium chloride.

Kelp is relatively inexpensive and can be obtained from most super-markets and health food stores in tablets, granules, or powder. The latter two forms make it easy to season a variety of foods that would ordinarily call for table salt. Psychologically, it takes a little getting used to. I mean, how often have you had *green* eggs and ham for breakfast? One may call to mind an adorable children's book of the same name by the very popular writer, Dr. Seuss, when first faced with such a meal situation involving the generous use of granulated kelp from what had formerly been the salt shaker.

The next of these three salt alternatives is an ionic liquid min-eral product (see Product Appendix pages 382–83). Beside the prin-cipal ingredients of chlorine and sodium, this liquid salt seasoning contains barium, bromine, boron, calcium, cesium, chromium, dys-prosium, fluorine, gold, lithium, magnesium, molybdenum, phos-phorus, potassium, selenium, silver, strontium, tin, and vanadium, among others. Their chief purpose is to balance out the sodium chloride, although they may only appear in extremely minute amounts that are usually measured in pp*m* (parts per million). This product can be sprayed on snack foods like homemade popcorn or potato chips, shelled nuts and seeds, celery sticks or radishes, fresh tomato, or peeled and depitted avocado to give them a really great flavor and taste.

The final item, Celtic Salt, comes from the Brittany region of northwestern France. This is a peninsula situated between the English Channel on the north and the Bay of Biscay on the south and comprises five areas: Ille-et-Vilaine, Côtes-du-Nord, Finistère, Morbihan, and Loire-Maritime. The economy of this picturesque and historic region is based on agriculture, fishing, salt production, and tourism. Another little industry is the making of the distinctive Breton cider from special apples grown extensively inland.

The coast, especially at the western tip, is irregular and rocky, with natural harbors at Brest, Lorient, and Saint-Malo, and, of course, numerous islands scattered about. Celtic Salt (so named after the Celts who settled this region many centuries ago) is obtained from ocean water which is taken through a mile-long decanting lake. This precipitates the particles at the bottom. The water then becomes a lovely sky blue and is guided in spirals along a series of concen-trating ponds for up to two miles. When the salt eventually reaches a certain concentration level, the excess magnesium salts known as bitters are removed. The remaining salt is wind- and sun-dried. What remains is a salt that is biologically active, pure, and moist. Nothing else is added to it.

Besides its obvious seasoning purposes, a number of medicinal claims have been made for it as well. One that recently came to my attention was contained in a letter postmarked April 30, 1997 from Geoff Sandford of Artarmon, New South Wales, Australia. I reproduce parts of it herewith that are pertinent to Celtic Salt, with the fellow's kind permission.

Dear Mr. Heinerman,

I appreciate the informative discussion of Saturday morning last [April 26, 1997 by telephone], especially your reference to the inadvisability of removing the fibre from the juice during juice preparation.

For your info[rmation], I have suffered C[hronic] F[atigue] S[yndrome] . . . for 20-30 years. The problem steadily worsen[ed]. It has only been in the last <u>six months</u> (!) that I have been able to get to the most powerful root causes.

<u>*And what an education that has been!!!*</u>

For approximately a decade I have been working at getting to the bottom of it, but, even using the best naturopathic advice, I was only nibbling around the edges.

The biggest single leap forward was in 1994 when I had the mercury fillings in my teeth (all 14) replaced with composites. Thanks to liberal consumption of Calli tea and Fortune Delight [Sunrider products], only using filtered water (and additionally consuming Celtic Salt which aids detox) I was able to progressively detoxify my body. Although three years later, I feel that I am only about halfway.

But the major root causes proved to be real shockers! I live 350 m[eters] from a T.V. transmission tower (and have been there for 20 years) and this has been debilitating me for years. Actually, it has been getting progressively worse [when] they attach[ed] two more microwave transmitters to it. We are living in electromagnetic <u>soup</u> . . . and guess who are the <u>croutons</u>! Well, I swapped my steel frame bed with I/S [inner spring] mattress for timber and foam [in] early Nov[ember 1996] with a marked effect.

Then on 12 Feb[ruary 1997] a <u>bioelectric</u> expert installed a device to eliminate the <u>neg.</u> radiations—a further marked change took *place.* (*I have had an Elanra negative ion generator unit for 2 1/2 years.)*

Then two weeks ago, I had a top piece of U. S. technology demonstrated to me—a Vitavac cleaner from Vitamix Corp.!!! It extracted all of the old [dust] mite feces from the mattress and carpet and eliminated a 45-year-old source of assault on my immune system!

So, finally, I have eliminated the <u>saboteurs</u> of my immune system.

Sincerely Yours,

/s/ Geoff Sandford

[NOTE: For information about the aforementioned products, please consult the appendix.]

Those who've used Celtic Salt regularly attest to its benefit minus any disturbances in their blood pressure. This buffering action to the salt's sodium chloride content may be attributed to some of its many mineral compounds that include: beryllium, bismuth, cadmium, copper, curium, europium, fermium, francium, gallium, holmium, indium, iridium, lead, mercury, neodymium, rubidium, scandium, thallium, and titanium, among others.

Salt Substitutes Used by Some North American Indian Tribes

Certain nineteenth-century Native American tribes residing in the American West relied upon several different types of plants for their salt needs. The unique manner in which they utilized each one to season their foods makes interesting reading and a fitting conclusion to this section on sodium.

Atriplex canescens. Nevada Indians called the saltbush by the name of *noo-roon-up*. The Cahuilla Indians of Southern California would take the sweet and salty berries, sun-dry them, and then grind them into powder to sprinkle over food. They would utilize the slightly salty seeds for the same thing. The seeds would be parched, ground into flour, and mixed with hot water to make mush or small cakes that would accompany every meal in lieu of salt itself. Indian "popcorn," Yuki style, was made of gathered beetle larvae and cicadas from the saltbush, which were roasted over an open fire and then liberally seasoned with some of the berry or seed powders to give them a delicious, salty flavor.

Heracleum lanatum. The Yuki Indians of Mendocino County, California called the cow parsnip by the name of *mun-shŏk.* The hollow basal portion of the plant was dried in short cylinders and eaten with other food in the dry state or else placed in the frying pan and cooked into the substance to be eaten.

Petasites palmata. The Wailaki Indians of Mendocino County, California called the Yuki salt plant by the name of tel-dink'-o. The plant ash was used in place of salt to season cooked food. To obtain the ash the stem and leaves were first rolled up into balls while still green. After being carefully dried for awhile they were placed on top of a very small fire on a flat rock and slowly burned. The resulting ash proved to be an acceptable ingredient in their pinole (finely ground flour made from parched corn), acorn bread, and acorn soup, not to mention being sprinkled over roast venison, broiled fish, or fried rabbit.

A number of different natural herb blends are currently available which make ideal salt substitutes and have virtually no sodium in them. They contain many different herbs, spices, and other seasoning materials including: onion, peppers, parsley, celery seed, basil, bay, marjoram, oregano, savory, thyme, cayenne pepper, coriander, cumin, mustard, rosemary, garlic, carrots, orange peel, tomato granules, lemon juice powder, citric acid, and oil of lemon. While certainly much fancier than anything early Native Americans used, they serve the same purpose of flavoring foods much as salt would do, but without harming the body as salt does.

Sulphur
THE MINERAL OF MANY UTILITIES

Stop Toothache in a Hurry

In May 1997, while working on the Selenium entry for this book in my research center, there came an overseas call from Sao Paulo, Brazil. An engineer named Paulo Rogerio had bought my book, *The Healing Benefits of Garlic* (New Canaan, CT: Keats Publishing, Inc., 1994) from a bookstore when he was visiting New York City the year before.

He read my recommendation to crush a peeled garlic clove and then put it next to a tooth that really hurt. "I tried your remedy, Dr. Heinerman,." he said in slow, deliberate English. "And your idea worked! My toothache stopped and I felt better. Now I believe in you."

I explained to Paulo that some of the many organic sulphur components contained in this spice acted on the nerves to stop the production of substance P, a potent pain transmitter. I wished him well in his endeavors to learn massage techniques and then turned him over to my capable secretary Susie White, who graduated from the Salt Lake School of Massage in June of that year and could give him more information on enrollment procedures.

Keep Cancer Out of Your Life . . . Forever

It is said that only two things are absolutely certain: death and taxes. Everything else is pretty much left to chance. But I would like to add a third certainty to the former pair: You need *never* get cancer if you consume sulphur-rich foods throughout your life on a fairly regular basis. Of the *top ten* nutraceuticals—*nutri*tive substances with phar-ma*ceutical* properties—currently being investigated with federal funds, garlic is *numero uno* (the others, in descending order, are: vitamins A and E, carnitine, magnesium, cranberry, probiotics such as lactobacillus acidophilus, evening primrose oil, ginkgo biloba, and calcium).

Thank Stephen L. DeFelice, M.D., chairman of the Foundation for Innovation in Medicine and the man who founded the term "neutraceuticals" in the first place. He picked garlic right off the bat because of its enormous sulphur content. He believes that if anything can stop cancer, this particular neutraceutical will. The evidence bears him out on this matter. *Science News* (151:239) reported in its April 19, 1997 issue that oncology researchers from Memorial Sloan-Kettering Cancer Center in New York exposed fresh human prostate cancer cells to S-allylmercaptocysteine (SAMC), a sulphur compound that forms as garlic ages, and watched in amazement as cancer cell growth diminished "two to four times more quickly than normal!"

The only aged garlic extract in the world with ample SAMC to get the job done of keeping cancer out of the system permanently is Kyolic Garlic. Not only is it the favorite garlic product that scientists like to work with, but it's also the best-selling garlic on the planet, *bar none*! I like Kyolic EPA myself—it blends together aged garlic extract with fish oil. I've been taking 2 to 3 capsules of this every day for a few years now. I believe that if I stay the course with this herbal supplement for the rest of my life, I won't ever get cancer! (See Product Appendix for more information on pages 383–84.)

Some of the more important sulphur compounds to look for that really do a masterful job in keeping cancer out of the body for good are as follows:

Indoles and Isothiocyanates (Sulphoraphanes). These are formed when plant sugars break down during processing, cooking, or chewing. Indoles act as blocking agents; isothiocy anates apparently pull double duty by both blocking and suppressing cancerous changes. These two chemicals are particularly important because they stimulate production of potent phase-2-enzymes, which help clear toxins. In one study, an increase in phase-2-enzymes alone successfully reduced the binding of a carcinogen to DNA by nearly 90 percent. *Food Sources:* Cabbage, kale, kohlrabi, Brussels sprouts, bok choy, cauliflower, garlic, onion, mustard greens, horseradish, broccoli, and watercress.

Thiols. These are a group of sulphur-containing nutrients with fantastic free radical scavenging capabilities. "Thiol" (as in the bactericide mer*thiol*ate) suggests that the compound has a sulphur atom bound to one of hydrogen. Thiols include sulphur antioxidants such as cysteine and glutathione. Cysteine is a sulphur amino acid that is a real biochemical workhorse. It neutralizes poisonous chemicals and carcinogens within the body through an enzymatic reaction process that occurs mostly within the liver. In the event of heavy metal toxicity, cysteine is good for removing such elements as aluminum cadmium, and lead from the body.

Glutathione, the other sulphur antioxidant, is regarded as the most important member of the body's "toxic waste disposal team." Glutathione protects us not only from the bad health effects of auto emissions and secondhand smoke, but also from electromagnetic radiation, chemicals, and excess sugar buildup that could lead to cancer, some forms of mental illness (manic depression and schizophrenia in particular), and cataracts. Glutathione is very dependent on the sulphur amino acids cysteine and methionine for its existence; as long as the diet contains enough foods rich in both of these amino acids, glutathione levels are likely to remain adequate. As we become older our levels of glutathione in the liver, spleen, kidneys, pancreas, and eyes (lens and cornea) eventually decrease.

Dietary intake of thiols comes from a daily consumption of those foods (and some herbs) containing the sulphur amino acids cysteine and methionine.

Food Sources

Eggs. By far the very best source of element sulphur; an average egg yolk yields 0.165 percent of this mineral, which is the equivalent of 165 milligrams of sulphur per 100 grams of yolk. Furthermore, the sulphur amino acids cysteine and methionine account for 91 percent of the sulphur in the yolk (each one contributing about 45.5 percent of it). Since the human body requires a minimum of 800 mg. of sulphur daily, just one egg a day can supply 10 percent of this need.

Meat. Certain types of meat are excellent sources for cysteine (and its oxidized form, cystine) and methionine. Salt-water fish (more than the fresh-water variety), duck, turkey, pork (ham and sausage more than bacon), and some wild game (antelope, deer, elk) have high amounts of each. Also, less conventional meat sources rank high in both sulphur amino acids: buffalo, emu, and ostrich!

Grains. Just a few grains and cereals have relatively moderate amounts of thiols: wheat germ, granola, and oatmeal (in that order).

Vegetables. Alfalfa, asparagus, broccoli, Brussels sprouts, cabbage, cauliflower, horseradish, mustard greens, red clover, and stinging nettle have respectable amounts of thiols.

Fruits. Some fruits rank high in sulphur content: figs, dried apricots, plantain (cooking banana), and ripe papaya and pineapple. In fact, three of this number contain high sulphur enzymes called sulhydryl proteases: ficin (figs), papain (papaya), and bromelain (pineapple). When consumed with other foods containing more cysteine they become very activated in the system and perform valuable pharmacological activities: reduce joint and muscle inflammation; decrease back pain due to deteriorated discs; and destroy intestinal worms. Because of their strong potency, it is best to take them *in the foods* in which they're found instead of through individual supplementation. By way of interest, meat tenderizers usually are high in papain content. Moistening a mosquito or other insect bite or sting and then rubbing a little meat tenderizer over it will quickly stop the itching and reduce the inflammation.

Dairy. Goat 's milk and ricotta and cheddar cheese are the only dairy sources with some thiol content to them.

Nuts and Seeds. Almonds, cashews, pecans, and pistachios are wonderful sources of thiols.

Legumes. Most legumes such as soybeans are extremely limited in sulphur amino acids; the sole exceptions are Bengal gram chickpea and lentils.

Foods likes these are relatively rich in sulphur compounds. The nonanimal sources (except for fish) will definitely reduce your cancer risks by a wide margin.

Other Sulphur Benefits and Sources

Since sulphur is found in every cell of the human body in some form or another, it obviously stands to help us in other ways than those already mentioned. Because so much of it is concentrated in the skin, hair, and nails, sulphur is necessary for their health integrity. Many of the problems associated with these three areas of the body—eczema, psoriasis, wrinkles, and dryness (on the skin); unmanageable hair, evolving hair loss, and baldness (on the scalp); and fungal infection, brittleness, and breaking (of the nails)—can easily be remedied most of the time with adequate intakes of sulphur.

One of the most frequently used homeopathic medicines is flowers of sulphur, derived chiefly from volcanic craters and hot springs in the U.S., Sicily, and other parts of Italy. This may prove to be a useful source of immediate sulphur for those who think they're deficient in it.

More sulphur in the system also prevents the caramelization or glycation of the blood which all of us experience to some degree or another as we grow older. According to a report featured on the ABC television network news program, "World News Tonight," which aired February 4, 1997, the blood in each of us very slowly becomes caramelized over an extended period of time. This "browning" effect of the blood is believed to be due to the intermingling of consumed fats and sugars that are "cooked" within the body by its own internal heat sources. When our blood eventually acquires a darker than usual color and becomes somewhat of a "syrupy" consistency (both indicative of glycation), literally everything inside us (from cells to organs and muscles) becomes "gummed up" or biochemically ruined to some extent.

In order to reverse this evolving process of aging within, it is essential that we always have enough sulphur and silicon within our circulating plasmas. The very best sources for these on a regular basis are garlic and onion (for their sulphur content) and stinging nettle for the silicon (which I prefer over horsetail for daily consumption). There are commercially available garlic products that combine sulphur compounds with the omega-3 fatty acids from marine lipids. I advise taking 3 tablets every morning with food. Stinging nettle may be taken in capsule form (2 per day) if you wish. Also, liquid mineral drops and seawater products are additional sources of sulphur and silicon. (see Product Appendix on pages 383–84 and 382–83 for specific information.)

Finally, a few things need to be said with regard to methylsulfonylmethane (MSM). The public knows very little about it, but chemists know a great deal. This protein-modifying sulphur compound with the hard-to-pronounce name is a naturally-occurring substance in minute quantities in most plants, but: is especially concentrated in pine tree bark, needles, and seeds (pine nuts). Early Native American tribes residing in mountainous areas heavily forested with pine trees understood the great nutritional value of pine nuts, though they didn't know *why* pine nuts kept the skin supple, the joints flexible, and muscle tissue pliant. But during the fall they would gather and store away large amounts of pine nuts for winter use for these very reasons.

In a printed document available from the United States Patent Office in Washington, D.C. (secure a copy by referring to U.S. Patent Number 5,071,878), specific reference is made to MSM as being capable of softening, smoothing, lubricating, and preserving the pliancy of human tissues and of reducing the brittleness of finger and toe nails. But you'd have to eat a lot of pine nuts fairly regularly in order to bring this about. However, it is simple and easy to get adequate MSM into your system to reverse caramelization of your blood from commercially available supplements. (See Product Appendix for more information.)

The patent office document also mentions that methylsulfonylmethane has proven helpful in treating the following array of disorders in humans and animals alike: gum disease, canker sores, acne, pruritis, eye inflammation (due to allergic reactions to dust or plant pollen), rheumatoid arthritis, lupus erythematosus, depression, wounds, intestinal parasites, arteriosclerosis, poor circulation, diabetes, acute pain, sun and wind burn, pleuritis, fatigue, leg cramps, "traveler's diarrhea" (due to giardiasis), emphysema, excruciating pain due to arthritis, bursitis, low back stress, and tendonitis, and multiple sclerosis and lymphoma.

As may be seen from the evidence given, sulphur is, indeed, "the mineral of many utilities."

Tin

Discovering the New World of Tin

"Like Old World explorers setting off for uncharted lands brimming with material riches," began the colorful article in *Science News* (136:23; July 8, 1989), "organic chemists have been probing carbon's *look-alike atoms*—largely silicon, but most recently tin. As a starring element in everything from protein and diamonds to pencils and ice cream, carbon has earned celebrity status among atoms. But silicon has gained in prestige, and new research is raising the status of tin considerably."

All three elements share the same column in the Periodic Table of the Elements and exhibit many similar chemical behaviors. Though scientists are still unraveling the fundamentals of silicon and tin chemistry, they have already learned how to couple silicon and tin atoms to carbon, *and to each other,* to form some very interesting polymers that have vast potential for making fibers, hard surface coatings and other materials. "It's as though we've discovered a new continent," one organic chemist at the University of Wisconsin at Madison told a reporter.

Tin Does the Body Good

The following information on the nutritional significance of tin was compiled from an article on the same that appeared in the *Journal of Nutrition, Growth and Cancer* (1(4):183-196; 1983). The highest concentrations of tin in the body appear to be in the thymus gland, followed by the spleen and bone marrow. The appearance of tin in the lymphatic system is believed to protect the body against cancer (including lymphomas).

Just as iodine has an affinity for the thyroid, so does tin have a real love affair with the thymus gland. But too much tin, as well as too little of it, can depress the competence of immune functions.

Other areas of concentration for extremely minute amounts of this trace element are the intestinal tract, brain, kidneys, testicles, and ovaries.

Tin (as well as silver and zinc) interacts favorably with the sulphur amino acid cysteine in preventing tooth decay, diabetes, psychosis, and seizures. In conjunction with a number of other sulphur compounds, tin plays a small but vital role in heavy metal detoxification through the microsomal enzyme system located in the liver.

Ideal sources of tin include virtually all plant seeds (sunflower and crushed cherry pits are the best) and nuts (almonds and Brazils are the best here). Anything with trace amounts of tin in it (reckoned in so many parts per *billion*) will yield a bitter flavor, which goes for those medicinal herbs that have strong anticancer properties (think of chaparral or wormwood).

Vanadium
AN ELEMENT FOR BLOOD-SUGAR-ASSOCIATED MENTAL
AND EMOTIONAL PROBLEMS

Debated Nutritional Value

According to a report published in *Federation Proceedings* (45:123-32, Feb. 1986), the total body pool of vanadium in humans is no more than 100 mg. at most; Within the body, vanadate and vanadyl ions form complexes that inhibit or stimulate the activity of many enzymes. Vanadium is known to affect liver, kidney, and cardiac functions, elevate blood pressure, and control elevated blood glucose levels in animal models. Elevated vanadium levels, on the other hand, have been found in manic depressives, suggesting a lack of other trace elements such as chromium, manganese, and zinc.

In his *Doctors' Vitamin and Mineral Encyclopedia* (New York: Simon & Schuster, 1990), Dr. Sheldon Saul Hendler wondered whether or not vanadium has any *legitimate* nutritional value: "Whether [this is so] is a question that has been extremely difficult to answer; at present the only thing we can say is, *maybe*. We certainly have a lot to learn about [it] . . . more study is badly needed."

Intake and Sources

The daily intake of this trace element appears to be quite low, about 20 micrograms (1 microgram is 1/1,000th of a milligram). Vanadium works best in harmony with chromium, manganese, and zinc for most blood-sugar problems, especially hypoglycemia, which often causes symptoms of mental and emotional disturbance.

The vanadium content of most foods is nothing to brag about. Black pepper, dill seed, aniseed, celery seed, and fenugreek seed have the highest content. Grains, seafoods and seaweeds (like dulse, bladderwrack, Irish moss, and kelp), meats, and dairy products are somewhere in the middle. On the low end of the nutritional totem regarding this element are fresh fruits and vegetables (with the sole exception of parsnips) and beverages.

Zinc
THE INTRIGUING WORLD OF A VERY FUNCTIONAL MINERAL

Killer Nutrient in Rattlesnake Venom

During the epoch-making journey of the pioneers from Illinois to the Salt Lake Valley during the spring and summer of 1847, a number of very large rattlers were encountered as the pioneers crossed the Plains. Several diaries and journals record that on May 23rd of that year, a large snake measuring almost an inch in width and nearly 3.7 feet in length bit one Nathaniel Fairbanks on the upper calf of his left leg, while he and two friends were carelessly jumping from one ledge to another on some nearby bluffs.

"In two minutes he felt his tongue prickle and begin to numb. By the time he reached camp, his face and hands felt like a foot that had fallen asleep." According to *Science Digest* (vol:20) for May 1984, this would have been due to the zinc content in rattlesnake venom. "An enzyme is formed from the interaction of the metal and a protein molecule in the snake's venom. It's the enzyme that then chews the blood vessels . . . and in turn causes destruction of muscle tissue in victims." But when the zinc is removed, these powerful numbing effects are no longer observed.

"The pioneers immediately applied tobacco juice and leaves and turpentine to the wound; they also bound tobacco leaves over the fang marks and down his leg which was quite swollen." It just so happens that tobacco juice and turpentine are both rich in the sulphur compound methylsulfonylmethane. Within hours the terrific pain had subsided and by the next morning pioneer Fairbanks felt a lot better.

The Many Health Benefits of Zinc

That was one of the bad sides to zinc. Fortunately, there is an array of good benefits to greatly offset the few negative ones. For brevity's sake, I've arranged a list of some of the more important uses with the appropriate suggested daily intakes for each and a reference source for further information.

Acne. Zinc cream helps clear up teenage acne. *Let's Live* (Mar. 1997, p.82).

AIDS. Zinc supplementation reduces many symptoms of AIDS. *Journal of Nutritional Medicine* (231:463-469, 1992). 50-75 mg. daily.

Blindness. Macular degeneration is a common vision problem in older people. Of 151 patients taking 100 mg. tablets twice daily with meals, all had "significantly less visual loss" than others getting only placebos. Sheldon Saul Hendler, M.D., Ph.D., *The Doctors' Vitamin and Mineral Encyclopedia* (New York: Simon & Schuster, 1990, p.199).

Body Growth. Growing children need ample dietary zinc to reach full physical maturity. *Los Angeles Times* (February 1, 1973, Part VI, p. 26). 10 mg. daily for ages 1 to 10.

Bone Fractures/Bone Loss. Zinc, in conjunction with calcium, boron, vitamin D, nitrogen (through protein), magnesium, fluoride, and several other trace elements, is important in developing peak bone mass. Skeletal muscle and bone (calcified bone and marrow) together account for 90 percent of total body zinc. *American Journal of Clinical Nutrition* (64:375-76, 1996) and Myrtle L. Brown (Ed.), *Present Knowledge in Nutrition,* 6th ed. (Washington, D.C.: International Life Sciences Institute/Nutrition Foundation, 1990, p. 251). 50 mg. daily zinc gluconate.

Cancer. Cancers of the esophagus, lungs, prostate, and throat have all been significantly reduced with daily intake of 50-75 mg. of zinc gluconate. (Provo, Utah) *Daily Herald* (December 11, 1977), p. A-4; and Hendler, op. cit., p. 198.

Common Cold. A randomized double-blind placebo test conducted by Dartmouth College Health Services concluded that treatment with Cold-Eze Zinc Gluconate Lozenge within 48 hours of the onset of a cold, delivered 93 percent of the zinc ions to mucosal surfaces resulting in a 42 percent reduction in the duration of the infection. *Journal of International Medical Research* (20:3, Jun. 1992). In

April 1996 a patent was issued for a specific type of zinc lozenge as a "Cure for Common Cold" (U.S. Patent Number 5,409,905) to patent holder George Eby, who published research to this effect 14 years before. *Natural Foods Merchandiser* (October 1996, p. 119); and *Antimicrobial Agents & Chemotherapy* [25:20-24, 1984). A definitive paper on "Zinc for Treating the Common Cold" reviewed all clinical trials since 1984 and was published in *Alternative Therapies* (2(6):63-72., Nov. 1996), but completely missed an important clinical study conducted earlier that summer. A team of medical researchers headed by Michael Macknin, M.D. of the Cleveland Clinic tested a homeopathic zinc lozenge (13.3 mg. zinc) on 50 clinic employees who developed symptoms of the common cold within 24 hours of enrolling in the experiment. Another 50 employees in the trial served as the placebo group, receiving similarly administered lozenges that contained 5 percent calcium lactate pentahydrate instead of the homeopathic zinc gluconate. The zinc group had significantly fewer days with manifested symptoms than did the placebo group: coughing (2 days compared with 4.5 days); headache (2 days and 3 days); hoarseness (2 days and 3 days); nasal drainage (4 days and 7 days), and sore throat (1 day and 3 days). The study, which was eventually published in *Annals of Internal Medicine* (125:81-88, Jul. 1996), proves that zinc gluconate definitely shortens many of the symptoms of the common cold, except for fever, muscle ache, scratchy throat, or sneezing. A couple of months before his favorable research appeared in print, Dr. Macknin purchased 9,000 shares of common stock in the lozenge manufacturer, the Quigley Corp. of Doylestown, Pennsylvania and then sold them after his paper was published, thereby reaping a quick $145,000 in profits. He still holds additional Quigley stock worth about $185,000 (*Newsday* Jan. 30, 1997). The New York media heavily publicized this research, resulting in a total sellout of the product in all New York City health food stores. (I am indebted to Lori Stewart, my publicist, of Jane Wesman Public Relations, Inc. in Manhattan for the *Newsday* clipping and for calling this to my attention.) Dr. Macknin was subsequently ostracized (but not by name) for this investment by Sheldon Krimsky, Ph.D., a science policy expert at Tufts University. *Tufts University Health & Nutrition Letter* (May 1997, pp. 4-5). The moral of this story is *zinc works* for the common cold.

Crippled Sexuality. (*Prevention* magazine, Apr. 1978, pp. 73-77). 50-150·mg. daily for four months for rekindling dampened sexual desire and drive.

Crohn's Disease. (*Let's Live Nutrition Insights,* 1996, p. 14). 30 mg. daily zinc picolinate plus other nutrients: vitamin A, 50,000 I.U.; omega-3 fatty acids, 2-3 grams; vitamin E, 800 I.U.; vitamin B-12, 1,000 mcg.; and vitamin C, 1 gram 4 times daily.

Cuts. Daily application of Polysporin First Aid Antibiotic from Warner-Wellcome Consumer Health Products. Each gram contains polymyxin B sulfate, 10,000 units and Dacitracin Zinc, 500 units in a lactose base. Also very useful for minor burns and scrapes. (Personal communication from Arnold Smith in Trenton, NJ, dated Feb. 11, 1996.)

Drug-Resistant Bacteria. (*Science News* 150: 335, Nov. 23, 1996). This is probably the only instance wherein zinc supplementation would *not*—repeat *not*—prove advisable. New microbes and drug-resistant versions of old ones have the ability to produce an outer coating known as lipid A, which depends on a zinc enzyme for its synthesis. Biological systems overwhelmed with such drug-resistant bacteria do better with chromium, molybdenum, selenium, and sulphur and vitamin A, C, and E supplementation than they would with zinc.

Free Radical Cell Destruction. (*Let's Live,* Jan. 1994, pp. 32-36). Recommended daily intake of 75 mg.

Eating Disorders. (*Let's Live,* Aug. 1996, p. 22 and Oct. 1996, p. 10). Jonathan Wright, M.D. and Alex Schauss, Ph.D. both recommend 30 mg. twice daily of zinc sulfate septahydrate in *liquid* solution.

Enlarged Prostate. (Hendler, op. cit., p. 203). 75 mg. daily.

Fatigue. (*Let's Live,* Dec. 1996, p.68). 75 mg. daily.

Genetic Defects. (*Scientific American,* Feb. 1993, pp. 56-65). Maintenance doses of 75 mg. daily of zinc gluconate during periods of sexual activity for both male and female, and continued supplement therapy in same dose for the female during entire nine-month gestation interval.

Influenza. (University of California at Berkeley Wellness Letter, Nov. 1996, pp. 1-2). Four to eight zinc gluconate lozenges sucked on daily for a total of 52 to 104 mg. for flu and cold.

Infertility. (Hendler, op. cit., p. 202). 50 mg. of zinc gluconate daily should increase sperm count and motility of sperm cells "within a few months."

Immune Dysfunctions. (Delicious!, Nov. 1996, pp. 58-59). During long-term zinc therapy, make sure that for every 10 mg. of zinc you get 1 mg. of copper as well. Zinc absorption is greatly enhanced by soy protein, glucose, lactose and red wine. Poorly absorbed forms of zinc are zinc sulfate and zinc oxide. Better absorbed are the chelated forms: zinc citrate, zinc gluconate, zinc monomethionate, and zinc picolinate.

Low Infant Birth Weights. (Journal of the American Medical Association 274:466, Aug. 9, 1995). "[Medical doctors] demonstrated that supplementing pregnant women with a daily oral dose of 25 mg. of zinc throughout their pregnancies beginning at an average of 19 weeks' gestation resulted in a significantly larger birth weight." Also helpful in preventing premature births and fetal miscarriages.

Mental Retardation. (Journal of the American Dietetic Association 84:457, Apr. 1984). Daily supplementation of 3 mg. for infants and 10 mg. for children one through five years of age will help to prevent mental retardation. Consultation with a doctor is always recommended when consistent zinc therapy at such an early age in life takes place.

Respiratory Infection. (European Journal of Clinical Nutrition 50:42-46, 1996). Daily supplementation of 10 mg. zinc sulfate in children ages one through five resulted in a reduced incidence of fever and upper respiratory tract infections. (See under *Immune Dysfunctions* for better absorbed forms of zinc.)

Sensory Dysfunctions. (Let's Live, Feb. 1997). Adult men need 15 mg. daily and adult women 12 mg. per day to improve their tastes, smells, and moods.

Spotted Nails/Stretch Marks. (Let's Live, Sep. 1977, p. 36). 25-50 mg. daily of zinc gluconate for up to three months should alleviate these physical signs of mineral deficiency.

Sunburn. (*Let's Live,* Apr. 1997, p. 84). Zinc oxide in cream or lotion form has been approved by the Food and Drug Administration as a very effective sunscreen for fair skin. Joan Lunden, the news anchor for 15 years on ABC Television's "Good Morning, America," is one of those utilizing this for better sun protection.

Uncontrollable Crying. (46th annual meeting of the American Fertility Society in Washington, D.C., Oct. 1990; as reported on CNN). Up to 25 mg. daily of absorbable zinc will help women suffering from premenstrual syndrome relieve some of their symptoms such as crying jags, eating binges, anxiety, and bloating.

Zinc Insufficiency. (*Prevention,* Nov. 1977, p. 49; *American Journal of Clinical Nutrition* 30:1721, Oct. 1977; *Healthwise* II (6):2, Jun. 1988; and *Journal of Animal Science* 70:178–87, 1992). Chemotherapy causes tremendous zinc deficiency. The frequent consumption of whole grain products and use of bran to lower cholesterol and regulate stool result in zinc loss due to phytic acid. But consumption of zinc-rich foods—oysters, 143 mg.; clams, 21 mg.; cooked oatmeal, 14 mg., other seafoods, organ meats, nuts, and legumes—and 25 mg. daily of zinc monomethionine clears up such insufficiencies very quickly. (See Product Appendix, p. 382.)

Zinc Oversufficiency. (*Newsweek,* Jan. 20, 1997, p. 48). "A zinc overload, however, can interfere with the body's ability to absorb copper, which can lead to a weakened immune system, among other woes. The medical consensus for now is that a handful of lozenges a day for a few days is probably safe but that prolonged use could throw your body out of whack. Eager gobblers should also bear in mind that some subjects of the Cleveland Clinic study reported experiencing nausea while taking zinc."

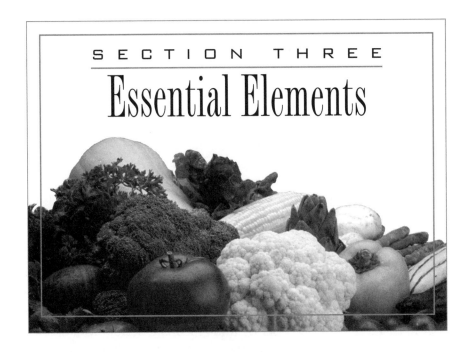

Essential Elements

Hydrogen

THE MOST ABUNDANT ELEMENT IN THE KNOWN UNIVERSE

Getting More Hydrogen into Your Body

Those who've written books on vitamins and minerals have never thought of including hydrogen, deeming it unnecessary and not very feasible to do. But hydrogen *is* an important element all the same: Without it there would be no light or warmth from the sun, nor any water either for that matter. Depending on what hydrogen is coupled with largely determines whether it is good or bad for you.

When this usually colorless, odorless, tasteless gas is linked up with oxygen, as the simple chemical formula H_2O suggests, water is formed. Most of the living tissue of man is made up of water; it constitutes about 92 percent of blood plasma, about 80 percent of muscle tissue, about 60 percent of red blood cells, and over half of most other tissues.

Therefore, getting more hydrogen inside of you in *this* form is good for your health. Everyone should be drinking more water every day, at least 6 to 8 full glasses as has been suggested by some doctors. But very few of us are doing this. When ample water is taken into the system, then the kidneys and liver can do their jobs of filtering out and eliminating poisons that regularly accumulate therein. *Water is a great detoxifier,* but we don't get enough of it. By drinking more water than we presently do and laying aside coffee, tea, colas, and soft drinks, we can put more hydrogen into our bodies where it will do us a world of good!

Getting Excess Hydrogen Out of Your Body

The above subtitle may seem contradictory at first glance and could lead to confusion in the minds of some readers. After all, I just got through lauding the benefits of drinking more water, which obviously contributes extra hydrogen to the system. But then I turn right around and appear to be advocating just the opposite. What's going on here, anyway?

As stated before, the *type of material* to which hydrogen is bonded can make it safe or harmful to human health. For instance, when hydrogen is combined with oxygen and sulphur, sulphuric acid is formed. This very definitely isn't good for our bodies at all. But within the body it reacts with nitrogen to form ammonia, which is an essential part of waste elimination, therefore making it quite helpful.

Hydrogen, in fact, has become a constituent of a great many organic compounds, some of which nature is responsible for and others which our own technological ingenuity has come up with. Take ethylene, for instance, which is composed largely of hydrogen and some carbon. This naturally-occurring plant growth hormone promotes aging, ripening, and wilting. It's produced as plants ripen and rot. That's why avocados, bananas, and peaches ripen faster in brown paper bags than sitting on a kitchen table or countertop.

But through technology, ethylene has been manipulated just enough to form the potent fumigant ethylene oxide, which is used for foodstuffs, imported medicinal herbs and spices, and textiles, as well as for sterilizing surgical instruments. But now the hydrogen has been so rearranged into an entirely new form that it can be highly irritating to the eyes and mucous membranes, not to mention inducing pulmonary edema in higher concentrations.

Another chemical alteration is the process known as hydrogenation. Your brain may not be all that familiar with it, but the rest of your body certainly is, from all the times you eat French fries, doughnuts, fried shrimp or chicken, chicken-fried steak, sweet and sour pork, or a host of other items routinely dropped into restaurant deep-fat fryers for a couple of minutes. The oils used to cook such things in were previously subjected to a fairly high temperature in the presence of hydrogen gas together with finely divided nickel, which acts as a catalyst. By means of this hydrogenation process, oils are able to reach a much higher point of heat (194° F.) without smoking and breaking down. Also, with it liquid oils can be rapidly converted to solid fats, which happens all the time in the manufacture of shortenings and margarine.

Foods that are cooked in or made from such hydrogenated oils and fats aren't good for your health. But don't take my word for it. No less of an authority than the Harvard Medical School *Harvard Heart Letter* for July 1994 proclaimed the same thing in a leading article, "Trans-fatty Acids: The New Enemy."

This respected monthly medical newsletter warned its readers that "trans-fatty acids are found in many foods . . . and new data indicate they increase a person's risk of a heart attack and [are] dangerous." The report went on to explain that when fat molecules are partially loaded with hydrogen, their configuration is substantially altered "from a form called *cis* to a form called *trans* by chemists."

The report went on to mention that "the amount of trans-fatty acids in typical margarines ranges from 10 percent to 30 percent of total fat and often exceeds 25 percent in cookies, crackers, pastries, and deep-fried foods such as French fries and doughnuts." And although such products are usually marketed as containing "No Cholesterol" or as being made with "100% Pure Vegetable Oil," which claims are generally accurate, yet "the implication that these oils are healthy choices is *not*."

Considerable research has shown, according to the article, that such "trans-fatty acids *raise* the 'bad' low-density-lipoprotein (LDL) cholesterol and *lower* the 'good' high-density-lipoprotein (HDL) cholesterol in a person's blood—alterations that increase the risk of a heart attack." In addition to this, "trans-fatty acids may also interfere with the production of prostaglandins, which are essential for the regulation of clotting and other bodily functions."

The report spoke about two major epidemiological studies conducted at Harvard Medical School in relation to the inherent dangers connected with trans-fatty acids. In the ongoing Nurses' Health Study, which consisted of some 85,000 participants, "women who ate large amounts of margarine and shortening used in cookies, white bread, and other baked goods had a 70 percent higher risk of heart disease than women who consumed little or none of them." Even "modest" consumption of trans-fatty acids has a detrimental impact on human health. In the same Nurses' study, women who ate four or more teaspoons of margarine a day (1-4 grams of trans-fatty acids) had a 66 percent higher risk of heart disease than those who ate margarine less than once a month.

Also, a separate study published in *Perspectives in Applied Nutrition* (2(4):36-37, 1995) found that foods fried in hydrogenated oils took much longer to digest and be evacuated from the stomach than did non-fried meals. Trans-fatty acids are a *major* contributing factor to so much acid indigestion and heartburn evident throughout the world today.

Having now described why too much hydrogen (in the form of hydrogenated oils) is bad for you, let me share some ways that you can get rid of it. First and foremost, *do not eat foods* with trans-fatty acid content in them. French fries, Danish pastry, doughnuts, corn and potato chips, cake and pie, berry muffins, margarine, and pizza (in that order) are very high in trans-fatty acids, according to information appearing in *The New England Journal of Medicine* (329:1969-70, 1993).

Secondly, embrace a lifestyle that includes regular aerobic exercise (such as brisk walking, biking, or swimming); a diet rich in fruits, vegetables, legumes, and whole wheat; the restriction of saturated fat and salt in the diet; and the reduction of risk factors for heart disease, such as high blood pressure, smoking, and obesity. I would also include some deep-breathing exercises in a place where the air is pure and invigorating. It's amazing how something so simple can do the body so much good in terms of actually cleaning it out. Drinking some warm peppermint or spearmint tea before and after deep breathing exercises will bring more oxygen into the system; both herbs are great oxygenators. This additional oxygen in the circulating plasma will help to flush hydrogen-nickel compounds hiding deep in muscle and tissue fat out of the body. It may sound preposterous on the surface, but *it really does work* to remove the harmful effects of previously ingested hydrogenated foods.

Another thing I would encourage the reader to do is incorporate certain spices into the diet that are more capable of reducing the cholesterol brought on by this bad form of hydrogen. Such herbs might include basil, cayenne, garlic, marjoram, onion, oregano, parsley, rosemary, sage, thyme, and turmeric. You can cook with them as well as take a couple of others in supplement form.

Oxygen and Nitrogen
THE GASEOUS ELEMENTS OF LIFE

Nutrients Taken for Granted

Oxygen is a colorless, odorless, tasteless gas. It makes up about 90 percent of water, *almost 67 percent of the human body,* and one fifth by volume of air. It is found in the sun, too. Nitrogen is also a colorless, odorless, tasteless gas. Although earth's atmosphere is 78 percent nitrogen, free gaseous nitrogen cannot be utilized by animals or by higher plants. To enter such living systems, nitrogen must be "fixed" (combined with oxygen or hydrogen) into compounds that plants can utilize, such as nitrates or ammonia. The basic living material of the human body, a semigelatinous, grayish to colorless fluid called protoplasm, contains nearly 4 percent nitrogen.

We inhale oxygen and exhale carbon dioxide, whereas nitrogen enters our bodies in the form of protein and exits as urea. But as vital as these elements are, you won't ever find them mentioned in any published reference works on vitamins or minerals. The reason they're not, I assume, is because they're taken so much for granted that no nutritional writer considers them necessary to include in books and articles on supplements.

After all, you can look until you're blue in the face (due to a lack of oxygen, no doubt) and never find any bottles labeled Oxygen or Nitrogen in the supplement section of your local health food store or nutrition center. You have to go to the mountains for *fresh* supplies of the former and to your local supermarket meat section for choice cuts containing the latter.

A Golden Window to Earth's Oxygen Past

About 80 million years ago the dinosaurs so realistically depicted in the movies *Jurassic Park* (1993) and its sequel *The Lost World* (1997) probably kicked up their heels instead of plodding about. Michael Crichton, the doctor-turned-writer, and Steven Spielberg, the film maker, both paid very close attention to getting the dinosaurs figured in their books and films anatomically correct by consulting with paleontologists (scientists who know a lot about dinosaurs from the bones they study). But one little matter escaped their otherwise sharp eyes for detail: they didn't give any consideration to the *air quality* these big behemoths breathed every day.

In fact, based on recent analysis of very ancient air from that distant period of time, those genetically recreated Crichton-Spielberg dinosaurs wouldn't stand a lick of a chance of surviving today, if such things were scientifically possible to reengineer. Here's why: dinosaur air *then* contained roughly *35 percent oxygen,* whereas our air at present squeaks by with only 21 percent oxygen.

The "proof in the pudding" as they say lies in that wonderful substance known as *amber.* Secreted long, long ago from coniferous trees, this soft, gluey resin captured enough air molecules as it hardened, dropped to the ground and eventually became buried. Gemlike in its rich shades of yellow, orange, brown, and even blue, and found all across the globe, amber has been used for decoration since the Stone Age, when Caveman 0g probably fashioned one into a crude ring and presented it to Cavelady Ogina.

Early humans regarded amber as something extraordinary. So, too, have modern geologists and geophysicists, like Gary P. Landis of the U.S. Geological Survey in Denver and Robert A. Berner of the Department of Geology and Geophysics at Yale University in New Haven, who have lavished a great deal of praise and attention on this warm-feeling, transparent, and piney-scented material. At an annual meeting of the Geological Society of America held in October 1987 in Phoenix, these two men presented very compelling evidence to show that the Cretaceous period had an exceptionally *high oxygen* content. They arrived at this evidence by crushing some ancient amber in a vacuum system in order to release the gases trapped in bubbles as small as 10 micrometers. They then analyzed the gases by quadrupole mass spectrometry to find out how much oxygen dinosaurs really breathed into their massive bodies.

Then in October 1993, both men presented additional amber data of a slightly later period, to show why all of the dinosaurs suddenly died. Instead of going out with the traditionally accepted, giant asteroid slamming into the earth theory, Landis and Berner suggested something even more logical: How about these huge monsters going out with *a gasp?*

Dinosaurs evolved breathing oxygen-enriched air. But later-dated amber showed only a 28 percent oxygen capacity. The dinosaurs, which were lacking the lung capacity to make the necessary adjustment, suffocated when atmospheric oxygen plummeted following an episode of intense volcanic activity.

Oxygen, the Life Within

Oxygen is, indeed, the very breath of life which keeps every one of us functioning for his or her allotted space of time upon this planet. Genesis 2:18 informs us that God made man out of the dust of the earth and then "breathed into his nostrils *the breath of life,*" after which "man [then] became a living soul."

It is interesting to note that oxygen requires iron in order to be effectively transported throughout the body. Here's how it's done. Red blood cells constitute slightly less than 50 percent of the body's blood volume. These tiny cells act as cellular lungs, intended only to ferry oxygen to every tissue and remove carbon dioxide. Shaped like plump, round cushions dimpled in the center, red blood cells consist mainly of water and a red protein called hemoglobin. It is the power of this protein that gives the red blood cell its vast oxygen-carrying capacity.

Constructed from more than 10,000 atoms, a hemoglobin molecule consists of four elaborately entwined strands of amino acids called globin. In the middle of each strand is the heme, a disk of carbon, hydrogen, and nitrogen atoms with a single iron atom wedged in the center. The iron atom in heme acts like a magnet, snapping up oxygen, then clinging tightly to it.

But the real wonder to hemoglobin doesn't lie in its power to seize oxygen, but rather in its ability to release it. Were iron atoms to float freely in the bloodstream, they would bind irrevocably to oxygen, keeping it from the body's other tissues. But embedded in the heme disk and surrounded by the tangled folds of globin, iron forms only a temporary bond with oxygen. The hemoglobin molecule can thus tighten or loosen iron's grip according to the pressures of surrounding gases.

Where oxygen is plentiful—as in the lungs—iron exercises its full powers, vacuuming up oxygen molecules. But by the same token, where the oxygen reserve is minimal—as in muscles after exercise—the hemoglobin molecule eases iron's hold, forcing it to surrender the gas to other tissues. Thus deprived of oxygen, hemoglobin immediately draws in carbon dioxide, turning a breathless blue as it transports the waste back to the heart and lungs.

The oxygen-carrying capacity of our blood is tremendous. Although one hemoglobin molecule can haul only four oxygen molecules at a time—one clamped to each heme disk every red blood cell contains about 270 million of these complex proteins. And, in turn, so many red cells crowd the bloodstream of the average individual that stacked end on end, such cells would soar for 31,000 miles into space.

The heart is the instrument by which the body circulates oxygen to the brain, first of all, and then everywhere else on a continuous basis. This terrific pump expels with every beat 2 ounces of oxygen-rich blood, 5 quarts a minute, and an estimated 220 million quarts over a 70-year lifespan.

Dealing with "Dirty" Oxygen

Just as the food we eat and the water we drink, so is the air (oxygen) we breathe contaminated with a whole host of chemical poisons too numerous to mention. I've been to many of the great capitals of the world and have been forced, while there, to inhale their polluted stench:

- The smog in Mexico City was so bad it stung my eyes.
- The air in Manila almost strangled me with an invisible pair of gigantic hands thoroughly contaminated with chemical particulates.
- Shanghai's pollution made my throat burn.
- The atmosphere hovering over Calcutta reminded me of pig sties.
- The night air in Cairo stunk fiercely of urine, camel dung, and burning garbage—a cross between a landfill and a urinal.

But I dealt with each situation in rather ingenious ways to modify the air enough so that my lungs could at least get a good share of the oxygen they were used to receiving.

Mexico City: I ate food laced with chiles and cayenne and sipped tequila periodically, having discovered that fiery spices and burning Mexican whiskey drives out heavy metal air pollutants faster than you can say Montezuma!

Manila: I feasted on ripe mangos, papayas, guavas, and avocados and drank a lot of coconut milk while I was there. These things soothed my inflamed sinuses and lungs, releasing them from their tight grip of pain.

Shanghai: Two things worked like a charm here: drinking lots of green tea and rice water. The fluoride in the tea washed away all of the sulphur dioxide my body had accumulated while there and the rice water acted as a liquid lozenge to cool my poor throat.

Calcutta: I made a strong tea from peppermint leaves every other day and not only drank it *warm* but also practiced a bit of aromatherapy and *inhaled* its fumes with my head above the teapot and a towel over it. Peppermint is one of the best oxygenators for putting more oxygen into the body that I know of.

Cairo: Figs, dates, and grapes helped me to rally there. I not only ate them with considerable relish, but would suck on them like lollipops in the mouth, so I could tolerate the stench better.

I might also add here that citrus juices and vitamin C are equally helpful in coping with the deleterious effects of metropolitan smog: The ascorbic acid tends to flush many of the heavy metal contaminants from body tissue before they have a chance to build up.

Solution for Indoor Pollution

Want to have more oxygen in your home and get rid of the harmful formaldehyde, xylene, benzene, and other polluted gases that synthetic carpeting, particleboard, foam insulation, upholstery, curtains, wall paint, and even so-called air fresheners can contribute? Well then, plan on filling your den with common house plants such as the Boston fern, English ivy, and spider plant. Not only are they inexpensive, ecologically sound, and aesthetically pleasing, but they do a mighty fine job of filtering toxins from your home, especially in the winter months when you're likely to be cooped up inside a lot. Did you know, for instance, that a single Boston fern can remove 1,800 micrograms of formaldehyde from the air (nearly the total amount found in a recent EPA study) in about an hour? An 8-inch hanging Boston fern costs an average of $15; a five-inch potted English ivy runs around $15; a ten-inch potted Areca palm costs about $35; a ten-inch hanging spider plant costs around $12 and removes 97 percent of room carbon monoxide *in less than 32 hours;* and an 8-inch Janet Craig/striped dracaena costs about $35. They all look nicer, are more affordable, and actually are livelier than dull, expensive, and inanimate self-contained air purification systems for homes and offices.

The Healing Benefits of Oxygen

Oxygen has great therapeutic value. If you don't believe this then the next time you accidentally burn yourself (but not seriously), conduct a little experiment (if you dare) to prove I'm right. Cover one part of the burn with your usual slathering of creams and ointments. But leave the other part exposed, spray ice water on it periodically to reduce the pain, and run alternating currents of hot and cold air across the afflicted surface.

You won't need long to discover that the warm, moist environment created by all those creams and liniments is like a living nursery for opportunistic bacteria to enter your system. But that portion of skin that has been lovingly caressed with cold water mist and hot-cold air currents is going to feel better and heal more rapidly.

At the annual meeting of the Acoustical Society of America held in Honolulu in November 1988, scientists from Johns Hopkins University in Baltimore presented findings to the effect that loud noise and 1,200 parts per million (ppm) of carbon monoxide *together* pose a far greater hearing loss risk than either of them do alone. Their findings also suggested that carbon monoxide and other chemicals cause hearing damage by restricting the flow of oxygen to nerve cells in the cochlea of the inner ear. These "hair cells" demand more oxygen as sound levels increase.

So, patrons of smoky honky-tonks and mechanics who inhale exhaust while working around noisy engines, take heed and be sure you get adequate oxygen into your system. What's that . . . you want me to talk louder because you can't hear me?

Are you or someone you know prone to blood clots due to sluggish circulation? Well, we already know that a little jogging, a dip in the pool, or a leisurely bike ride will help to lower this risk. But, according to the *Medical Tribune* (Jan. 25, 1978) deep breathing exercises, such as are practiced in yoga or many stretching routines, can offer the same prevention against blood clot formation. A doctor in a certain hospital instructed 600 patients who were recovering from surgery to practice deep breathing techniques for 15 minutes every day. The blood flow in their legs increased by as much as 33 percent during these inhalation-exhalation sessions. The extra oxygen taken was just enough to prevent clots from happening.

Speaking of blood clots, those that reach the area of the brain and burst open can cause immediate strokes. The best therapy for rehabilitating those who've suffered loss of speech, memory, or use of one side of their bodies is hyperbaric oxygen. Be advised, however, that this *isn't* a type of therapy that can be practiced at home. It requires considerable medical skill, special equipment, and highly trained personnel to run. But for strokes, diabetic gangrene, serious skin burns, and other difficult problems conventional medicine can't easily treat, hyperbaric oxygen therapy may just be the remedial answer some people have been looking for. (See Product Appendix, p. 384.)

Putting Yourself in a Good Mood with Negatively Charged Oxygen

Over the years much has been said in newspapers, magazines, and science journals about the separate impacts that negative and positive air ions have upon the human body. A great deal of favorable publicity extolling the wonderful health virtues of the former and denouncing the terrible effects of the latter has been circulated by neg ion proponents.

Air ion formation commences when sufficient energy acts on a gaseous molecule to eject an electron. Most of this energy usually originates from radioactive substances within our planet's crust. The remainder comes from the shearing forces of water droplets in water-falls or the friction that develops when great volumes of air move rapidly over a land mass (the foehn, sharav, and Santa Ana winds are representative of this action), or from cosmic rays. The displaced electron quickly joins an adjacent molecule, which becomes a nega-tive ion. This leaves the original molecule a positive ion. Molecular collisions transfer the charge, so that the positive charges come to reside on molecules with the lowest ionization potential, while elec-trons are attracted to the species of greatest stability.

Next, small numbers of molecules of water vapor, hydrogen, and oxygen cluster about the ions to form small air ions. In normal pollutant-free air over land, there are 1,500 to 4,000 ions per cen-timeter. But negative ions are more mobile and Earth's surface has a negative charge, so neg ions are repelled from the planet's surface.

Polluted air creates not only a choking atmosphere but also one filled with garbage ions carrying a positive charge. These exert a real "ball-and-chain" effect on brain and nerve behavior, resulting in per-sonality disorders. In fact, the *Journal of Personality and Social Psychology* (49:1207-20, 1985) reported "students in polluted settings describ[ing] their moods and emotions in more negative terms, express[ing] less liking for individuals not sharing their fate, giv[ing] lower evaluations of their surroundings, form[ing] more negative atti-tudes about social stimuli, and spend[ing] less time in the setting."

The solution, of course, is to get such individuals exposed to neg ions as quickly as possible. Thunderstorms, waterfalls, ocean waves, and even *cool* running showers all generate an abundance of neg ions that exhilarate the body, lift the spirit, change the mood, and brighten the mind. Despicable attitudes disappear and violent behav-ior ceases after that. There are also a variety of machines on the mar-ket that claim to produce friendly neg ions. But nothing comes close to what nature itself puts out for giving oxygen molecules that nega-tive charge that has become synonymous with *good* air.

Oxygen Burns Stored Fat

Want help in losing weight? Then stoke your biological furnace with more pure air derived from unpolluted settings: mountains, hills, deserts, and seashores. The rich oxygen you inhale is carried direct-ly to cell mitochondrion where energy is created and preserved. Your body's internal combustion gets accelerated to the point that more stored fat is chemically burned off.

Nitrogen Functions through Intermediates

Nitrogen is critical for the health and well-being of the body. But because it is a gas, it cannot operate alone but must always be con-nected with other things in order to be useful. Amino acids are the building blocks of proteins, and are comprised of nitrogen, hydro-gen, oxygen, carbon, and sometimes sulphur. Amino acids are the building blocks of proteins; twenty different amino acids have been isolated and identified in body and food proteins thus far.

Amino acids are required for the synthesis of all enzymes, including digestive enzymes and those that are required for oxida-tion, reduction, and all chemical processes within cells. Enzymes are catalysts for chemical reactions in living cells. Ribonuclease, the enzyme that breaks down ribonucleic acid (RNA), is made up of a chain of *only* 124 amino acids, one of the shortest enzyme chains around. Nitrogen figures prominently in every amino acid link form-ing this particular chain.

Amino acids are needed for the production of certain hor-mones, including insulin, thyroxine, epinephrine, parathyroid hor-mone, calcitonin, and some of the secretions of the pituitary gland. Hormones are regulatory substances secreted principally by endocrine glands. They are transported in the blood to the specific organ or tissue where the special effect of the hormone is produced. While the majority of hormones are either proteins, polypeptides, or derived straight from amino acids, they all share a small amount of nitrogen in their sequential makeups.

Finally, all antibodies contained within our circulating plasmas depend very much on nitrogen for their formation and immune-strengthening activities. Blood antibodies belong to a class of pro-teins known as immunoglobulins. Antibodies show up in the blood in response to the introduction of a foreign protein (called an anti-gen). The antibodies produced combine with the antigen, which stimulates their creation, thereby forming what's recognized as an antigen-antibody complex. This reaction is termed the immune response. A great incidence of bacteria or viruses in the body fluids leads to a higher level of immunoglobulins in the blood and a greater capacity to protect the body against the invading agents.

There are ten *essential* amino acids which the body is unable to synthesize and which must come from various food sources. The remaining ten *nonessential* amino acids don't need to be provided ready-made in the diet, since the body can make them on an "as needed" basis using whatever nitrogen may already be available within the system.

A hen's egg is used as the nutritional standard by which to gauge the ideal or nonideal amino acid composition of many different foods. An egg provides all of the essential amino acids in adequate amounts for protein synthesis and without excess. Another way of looking at it is that an egg presents an almost perfect balance of nitrogen in relation to other minerals.

Without amino acids there would be no proteins. Protein is one of the most abundant components of the body, being exceeded only by water. One-half of the dry weight of the body is protein, and is distributed in the following manner: 34 percent in the muscles, 20 percent in the bones and cartilage, 10 percent in the skin, and the remaining 36 percent in other tissues and body fluids. Urine and bile are the only two body fluids that normally don't contain protein. Protein is made up of the same four basic elements that comprise amino acids—nitrogen, hydrogen, oxygen, and carbon—of which nitrogen is the most significant since it's always present in protein but doesn't show up in fat or carbohydrate.

To number *all* of the proteins there are would be to count each grain of sand on the beach or the stars in the nighttime firmament overhead. Scientists theorize that there could be anywhere from ten *billion* to one *trillion* proteins. The combinations of different numbers and kinds of amino acids (20 so far that we know of) and different sequential arrangements of the amino acids in the molecule make possible the astronomical number of different proteins in existence.

Dietary proteins provide amino acids to build and maintain tissues. This need continues throughout life. Although new tissues are largely formed in childhood, the process proceeds into adulthood; hair and nails continue to grow, and the outer layer of skin is periodically replaced. The total quantity of protein needed for maintenance *increases with age* until a fairly constant level is reached at around 18 years. This level pretty much continues throughout adulthood until about age 65, at which time there is a gradual to severe diminishing of protein being manifested in the form of "wasting" so typical in the elderly. It is at this later period of their lives that folks need to start thinking about *adding* more protein to their diets, but preferably from food sources such as avocados, nuts, and legumes instead of animal flesh all the time.

Proteins also provide the nitrogen and other nutrients that are necessary for the synthesis of all enzymes, certain hormones, all antibodies, and as precursors to some vitamins. Protein is also essential in the diet in order to help a person maintain equilibrium due to losses that routinely occur through the urine, feces, and skin. Even on a protein-free diet (with an adequate energy intake), nitrogen losses still occur through the urine, feces, and skin (by way of perspiration). Finally, protein contributes somewhere between 10 and 15 percent of the body's total energy output, the rest coming from dietary carbohydrates and fats.

Nitrogen Losses to Be Careful Of

The nitrogen in amino acids and their proteins is carried by the blood into the liver, where it is either separated from them and reutilized another way or else left intact with some of them and used in that manner. Keep in mind, though, that nitrogen is being recycled through our bodies all the time: It enters in the protein we eat and exits as the waste by-product urea. But the liver is the major clearinghouse through which all nitrogen entering or leaving must pass; therefore, it behooves us to keep our livers in great shape with the appropriate herbs, nutrients, and foods.

A factor by which clinical nutritionists, hospital dietitians, and medical doctors can determine the amino acid and protein requirements of an individual human being is known as the *nitrogen bal-*

ance. Describing the manner in which such is calculated takes too long and is a bit complex. Suffice it to say, the nitrogen balance is based on the principle that the amount of nitrogen consumed minus the amount excreted in different ways indicates the amount of protein needed by the body under particular conditions.

However, there are some situations which a person needs to be on guard for so far as the loss of too much nitrogen goes. Under these given conditions, protein intake *must be increased* or else the body's delicate nitrogen balance will swing too far into the negative, having a very bad impact on overall health. Situations in which nitrogen losses can be excessive and must be quickly reversed include, but are not limited to, the following:

- fasting (for religious or purification reasons)
- fever (due to illness)
- malnutrition (due to poverty, mental illness, or age)
- physical exercise (that is excessive and overdone)
- sickness (such as cancer, a wasting disease)
- surgery (in which drug therapy can promote *greater* nitrogen loss)
- wounds (like those experienced in major burns in which unbelievable amounts of nitrogen are lost within a very short time)

When substantial nitrogen is lost through any of these or other circumstances, it is absolutely imperative to get more nitrogen back into the system as quickly as possible from those sources known to be high in this trace element.

Nitrogen Sources to Depend on in Medical Emergencies

Certain foods and medicinal herbs are known to supply the body with good amounts of nitrogen for tissue mending, muscle rebuilding, weight, gain, and physical recuperation in general I've listed them below in terms of percentages of the total nitrogen supplied by the essential amino acids contained in each item.

Total Nitrogen from Essential Amino Acids	*Foods and Medicinal Herbs*
37% or better	Eggs, human milk, cow's milk, goat's milk, lactalbumin, casein, alfalfa powder, red clover powder
33 to 30%	Red (beef) and white (pork and chicken) meat, fish, beans, peas, soy beans, sorghum, sweet potato, yam, spinach, watercress, mustard greens, stinging nettle
29 to 25%	Lentils, oats, millet, cornmeal, sesame seed meal, cashew, white potato, rice and wild rice, wheat grass
24 to 20%	Barley and barley grass, whole wheat flour, almond, Brazil nut, peanut, cashew, pecan, pistachio
19% or less	Carrot, cassava, gelatin, blue-green algae, kelp, dulse, bladderwrack, slippery elm, marshmallow root, fenugreek seed, comfrey root or leaf

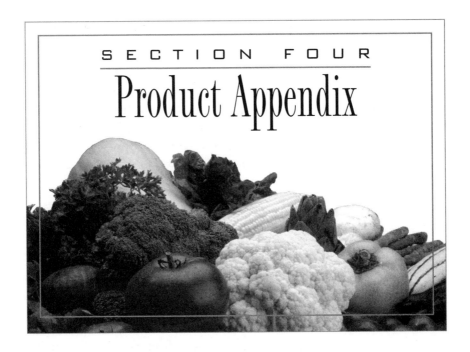

SECTION FOUR
Product Appendix

Anthropological Research Center
P. O. Box 11471
Salt Lake City, UT 84147
1-801-521-8824

Double the Power of Your Immune System (Video I) $30.00

Strengthening Your Immune System through Proper Diet (Video II) $30.00

Boosting Body Immunity through Weight Management (Video III) $30.00

Self-Treatment for Immune Disorders (Book I) $20.00

Living to Be 120 and Enjoying It More (Video IV) $30.00

The immune system videos are a series of filmed lectures that Dr. John Heinerman gave at Westminster College in Salt Lake City, UT and at two locations in Southeastern Idaho (Idaho Falls and Pocatello) between October 1996 and June 1997 to huge crowds in capacity-filled auditoriums. It is the most complete instructional video series ever done on the immune system anywhere. The immune system videos may be purchased separately or as *a unit of three for only $75.00* (a savings of $15.00).

Video IV was a public lecture give on longevity to a good-sized crowd at a bookstore in downtown Salt Lake City during a highly-publicized and very successful book signing of his book, *Heinerman's Encyclopedia of Anti-Aging Remedies* ($20.00) in February 1997.

We also carry the REX'S WHEAT GERM OIL ($65.00). It is the most potent vitamin E oil you can buy without a prescription. It is available in one quart metal cans. Suggested intake is one table-spoon daily with a meal.

Celtic Salt
Ye Are the Salt of the Earth
P. O. Box 6547
Tweed Head South
New South Wales 2486
Australia
011-61-755-242287

The world's finest and purest salt harvested from the Brittany region of northwestern France comes from a peninsula lying between the English Channel on the north and the Bay of Biscay on the south.

Flora Beverage Co., Ltd.
Bay 'F,' 2828 - 54th Avenue S.E.
Calgary, Alberta, Canada
T2C 0A7
1-403-236-0155 business/fax

In business since 1921. Manufacturers of Essex Botanical Herbal Drink (developed by the late Rene Caisse) and Hoxsiac Herbal Drink (formulated by Harry Hoxsey's great-grandfather). Both herbal for-mulations have been successfully used for many years in the alter-native treatment of cancer. Flora also sells Mojave Nectar (an herbal drink made from *Yucca schidegera*) which is a tonic beverage for recuperation from serious illness.

Lonza Inc.
17-17 Route 208
Fair Lawn, NJ 07410
1-201-794-2400 business / 1-201-794-2695 fax

Manufacturer of the world's finest dietary supplement, L-Carnitine L-tartrate, which is the stable form of L-Carnitine. L-Carnitine itself is very moisture-retaining and liquid-forming, especially when exposed to air. On the other hand, L-Carnitine L-tartrate is extremely stable under any type of environmental conditions.

Naturally Vitamins
14851 North Scottsdale Rd.
Scottsdale, AZ 85254
1-800-899-4499 business
1-602-991-0551 fax

The company's motto. is: "Our mission is to defend public health in a responsible and timely manner." They have succeeded in doing so with these top-quality products: A-Mulsin, Wobenzym, 25,000 IU Vitamin A softgel, Mind Actives, Inositol Powder, B-1, All-B, Supreme B, Super Stress, Pantothenic Acid, B-6, Foli Complete with B-12, B-12, Big Shot B-12, Vitamin C Chewable Juicees, Vitamin C 1500 Mg., Stomach Friendly C, Flavo Ester C 250 mg, Winterized C, Grape Ceed, A&D, Cod Liver Oil, Lipomega 3, Lipomega 6, Omega Marine Lipids, Primrose Gold, Lecithin 19 Granules, Lipo-Tone, Super Flavonoid Boost, Rutin 500 Mg., Cal Mag with Zinc and Bore Cal Forte, Chromium Picolinate, Manganese, and Green Tea capsules.

Pines International
P. O. Box 1107
Lawrence, KS 66044
1-800-MY-PINES / 1-913-841-6016 business
1-913-841-1252 fax

Owned and operated by American farmers in the "Heartland of America," this company produces very excellent wheat grass, barley grass, and beet root powder that is all-organic and all-nutritional. The fine products represented in this book include Mighty Greens (a superior chlorophyll blend derived from numerous green plants), Barley Grass Juice Powder and tablets, Wheat Grass Juice Power and tablets, and Organic Beet Root Juice Powder. Don't trust any other cereal grass or beet products but those bearing the Pines label.

Sabinsa Corporation
121 Ethel Road West, Unit 6
Piscataway, NJ 08854
1-908-777-1111 business
1-908-777-1443 fax

Manufacturers of Bioperine (an extract from black pepper), L-Selenomethionine and Zinc Monomethionine, and numerous other fine phytochemicals, herbal extracts, and Ayurvedic pharmaceuticals.

Total Life International, Inc.
P. O. Box 990
Monument, CO 80132
1-719-481-6080 business
1-719-481-6077 fax

The true worth of any company must never be measured by its sales success alone, but also by the principles of rightness and fairness exemplified by its leaders. Cofounders Roy R. Davis and Alexandra R. Lord worked against seemingly impossible odds to form a company that put the welfare of customers first and their cash last. In summing up the many adversities through which they've had to go, both cofounders felt like salmon during the spawning season: "We've swum *up*stream for so long in the odds that were against us, we really don't know how to swim the normal and easy way." Their bionourished™ formulations include: MSM Complete Renewal, Cool Whey, Cran+MSM, Fresh Country Chocolate, Fervor!, Fire!, and Colloidal Silver. The naturally-occurring protein modifying agent from pine trees known as methylsulfonylmethane (MSM) is a nutritional enhancer in all of their many fine products.

Trace Minerals Research
1990 West 3300 South
Ogden, UT 84401
1-800-624-7145 business
1-801-731-6051 business
1-801-731-7985 fax

"'Never underestimate the power of nature" is the motto by which this company operates. The secret to their mineral success lies in the source for such nutrients: the Great Salt Lake (the world's largest inland sea). The ionic minerals manufactured by them consist of: Arth-X Plus, Complete Calcium Hydroxyapatite, Complete Calcium & Magnesium, Electro-Vita-Min, Complete Chromium, With-In, Complete Magnesium, Inland Sea Water, ConcenTrace, Electrolyte Stamina Tablets, Powerhouse Sports Recovery, and Ionic Silver. They have a full money-back or product replacement guarantee if consumers are not 100 percent satisfied.

Vita-Mix Corporation
8615 Usher Road
Cleveland, OH 44138
1-800-VITAMIX (1-800-848-2649) business
1-216-235-3726 fax

Like some of the imperial dynasties of old, this company has been in one family for over three-quarters of a century. Founder William Grover Barnard I started it up in 1921 and demonstrated his innovative juicer that retains the fiber at the Chicago World's Fair in 1933-34, where it became an immediate hit with the public. His son William Grover Barnard II took over years later and greatly expanded operations. Following his retirement, the founder' grandson, William Grover Barnard III, inherited the corporate mantle of leadership around his very capable shoulders and is carrying the company into the twenty-first century. In 1996 Vitamix celebrated 75 years of trend-setting sales and service with the world's only whole food machine that wastes nothing and conserves everything, The company also makes a wonderful cleaning unit called a Vita-Vac with a microguard, antiallergen filtering system built into it for those who are hypersensitive to dust and pollen.

Wakunaga of America Co. Ltd.
23501 Madero
Mission Viejo, CA 92691-2744
1-800-421-2998 business / 1-714-855-2776 business
1-714-458-2764 fax

The world's premier selling garlic product, Kyolic Garlic, is the only aged garlic extract preferred by doctors and scientists for treatment and research purposes. Consumers in every corner of the globe have come to trust the Kyolic name for effectiveness, quality, and safety in garlic products they can believe in. Kyolic Garlic, Kyolic EPA (garlic extract and marine lipids), Kyo-Ginseng (aged garlic extract and ginseng root extract), and Kyo-Chrome (aged garlic and chromium picolinate), and Ginkgo Biloba Plus (extract of ginkgo and aged garlic) are some of their many fine products.

Health Restoration Center
26381 Crown Valley Parkway #130
Mission Viejo, CA 92691
1-714-770-9616

Dr. David A. Steenblock is one of America's finest authorities and specialists in the administration of hyperbaric oxygen therapy. His clinic has assisted thousands of stroke patients return to useful (and productive) lives after taking numerous hyperbaric oxygen treatments.

Index